10-08

BREAKTHROUGH

SUZANNE SOMERS

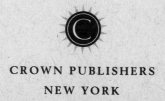

CROWN PUBLISHERS
NEW YORK

BREAKTHROUGH

LIFE-ALTERING SECRETS FROM TODAY'S CUTTING-EDGE DOCTORS

The information presented in this work is in no way intended as medical advice or as a substitute for medical counseling. The information should be used in conjunction with the guidance and care of your physician. Consult your physician before beginning this program. Your physician should be aware of all medical conditions that you may have, as well as the medications and supplements you are taking.

Published in the United States by Crown Publishers, an imprint of the Crown Publishing Group, a division of Random House, Inc., New York.
www.crownpublishing.com

CROWN and the Crown colophon are registered trademarks of Random House, Inc.

Grateful acknowledgment is made to Don Tolman for permission to reprint the excerpt of whole food signatures from his Web site, www.dontolmaninternational.com.

The illustrations on pages 76 and 77 (February 2007) and page 83 (May 2008) are reprinted by permission of *Life Extension* magazine.

Library of Congress Cataloging-in-Publication Data
Somers, Suzanne, 1946–
Breakthrough: eight steps to wellness / Suzanne Somers.
      p.   cm.
1. Self-care, Health.   2. Longevity.   3. Health.   I. Title.
RA776.95.S63 2008
613—dc22   2008027696

ISBN 978-1-4000-5327-8

Printed in the United States of America

DESIGN BY ELINA D. NUDELMAN

10 9 8 7 6 5 4 3 2 1

First Edition

TO ALAN:

TOGETHER WE WALK THIS PATH,

HEALTHY, VITAL, ENERGETIC, IN LOVE,

AND LAUGHING ALL THE WAY.

AND TO MY MOTHER:

IF I KNEW THEN WHAT I KNOW NOW,

YOU MIGHT STILL BE WITH US.

I GOT OLD BY MISTAKE.

—*Paul Colby, owner, The Bitter End, New York*

ACKNOWLEDGMENTS

A **PROJECT LIKE THIS** does not happen without help. The doctors interviewed in this book have been invaluable, always responsive to yet another e-mail or phone call, patiently answering all my questions. This has been quite an education. Thank you from the bottom of my heart to Dr. Jonathan Wright, Dr. Ron Rothenberg, Dr. Thierry Hertoghe, Dr. Jennifer Berman, Dr. Russell Blaylock, Dr. Eric Braverman, Dr. Steve Nelson, Dr. Howard Liebowitz, Dr. Prudence Hall, Dr. Khalid Mahmud, Dr. Michael Galitzer, Dr. Steven Hotze, Dr. Robin Smith, Dr. Candice Lane, Dr. Andy Jurow, Dr. Larry Webster, and Dr. Julie Taguchi. And to the professionals: Bill Faloon, cofounder of the Life Extension Foundation; David Schmidt, founder of LifeWave Nanotechnology; and Cristiana Paul, M.S.

Thank you to my darling daughter-in-law, Caroline Somers, who along with Danielle Shapero designed this beautiful book cover with their usual style and taste. Thank you to my editor Kristin Kiser, who has guided me with a gentle hand for the last fourteen books. She has been a great friend and ally, and I will miss her terribly. To Heather Jackson, my new editor, who has helped with the final editing of this manuscript and rolled with it so beautifully. I look forward to many books together.

Thank you to my publisher, Jenny Frost, and to her team: Tina Constable and Philip Patrick, who are not only talented but a lot of fun to hang out with; Heather Proulx, Lindsay Orman, Lucinda Bartley, and Julie

Miesionczek; Amy Boorstein, Linnea Knollmueller, Christine Tanigawa, and Elina Nudelman.

Thanks to Marsha Yanchuck, my trusted friend and assistant for thirty-five years, who compiled the back-of-the-book resource guide, a job that I am incapable of doing. Thanks to Julie Turkel, my friend and executive assistant, who set up all the interviews and keeps my schedule running smoothly; and to darling Jordyn Goodman, my other assistant.

Thanks to David Vigliano, my agent and friend, and thank you Marc Chamlin ("the Closer"), my lawyer for the last twelve books—it's working. And to Sandi Mendelson, my publicist forever, with gratitude and admiration.

Thank you to Cindy Gold for the fabulous jacket photograph, and to darling Mooney for keeping my golden locks hip and sexy.

Thanks to Dave Henson, my computer guy, and Sonia Greenbaum, my copy editor.

Thanks to Dr. Philip Miller for the Schopenhauer quote. It was exactly what I was looking for.

And lastly, thanks to Alan. He has been there for me daily—helping, encouraging, listening to me read to him, and suggesting.

CONTENTS

PART III
The Future of Medicine

INTRODUCTION

> All truth passes through three stages. First, it is ridiculed. Second,
> it is violently opposed. Third, it is accepted as self-evident.
>
> –Arthur Schopenhauer

IT IS THE YEAR 2041. This is me, Suzanne Somers, at ninety-four years old.
I am healthy, my bones are strong, my brain is working better than
ever. Sleep is sound and deep, usually eight or nine hours nightly. I don't
need sleeping pills; they're not necessary. I wake up happy, excited, and
active. Most mornings start with wonderful sex with my 105-year-old
husband, Alan (who has also embraced the same health regimen). The
two of us are enjoying our lives because along with our healthy, strong
bodies, we both have great wisdom and perspective—and this gives us an
advantage over younger people.

Our children and their friends come to me for advice. That's satisfying.
I am not one of those "old people" put in the corner or, worse, put in a
nursing home. Nope, not me, I got it early on. I wanted to live, really live.
So I jumped on the fast-moving train of new medicine and never looked
back. My friends laughed at me . . . called me a "nutcase" and a "health
freak," but who's got the last laugh now? Huh?

I won . . . I am vital, I am active; I am a *productive* member of society.

Because of my great health, I am not a drain on the system; I don't
need pharmaceutical drugs. It would be nice if the government could
grasp the wisdom of the supplements, bioidentical hormones, and detoxification that I have embraced for the last forty years. It would be great
if they could understand and attribute this nondrug regimen to my fantastic health and sharp thinking and provide it free of charge to all our

citizens. It certainly would save the government a lot of money in the long run, and bankruptcy would not be looming; unfortunately, big business is still in the way.

But I feel lucky—I understood early on. I was not going to blindly accept outdated medicine. I knew if I were to survive in this toxic, stressful, polluted world I had to approach my health differently. I also understood that drugs were not going to be the answer for me unless absolutely necessary. I did have cancer once, but thank God I banked my stem cells in my early sixties, so I would be able to rebuild my immune system if the cancer ever came back. That was a relief for me. I could let go of the worry. I've been fine ever since.

And those nanotechnology (nondrug) patches I have been using for the last forty years have really helped. Any time I experienced pain or low energy or sleep problems or weight problems, or the need for detoxification (if I wanted to kill off the free radicals that are part of today's toxic world), I put on one of the patches and the problems went away, with no need to turn to drugs.

I saw what happened to so many of my contemporaries, most of whom died early on from diseases that could have been rectified with hormones and cutting-edge, nondrug technologies. Instead, they chose the pharmaceuticals given them by their trusted doctors until they were "out of gas" and "wacky." I loved these people, but my theories were so radically different from what their doctors were telling them that I had to back off.

I hung in there with my beliefs. I knew this was the better way. Those around me lovingly smirked and mocked my approach, and now it's too late for them. "I told you so" seems empty.

I'm a believer in pharmaceuticals: My friend's nephew is a schizophrenic and those drugs have allowed him to live a somewhat normal life. I always say, "That's what drugs are for"—pain, infection, and mental illness. Without those drugs he would be in a mental home, but instead he gets to live with his family. They are a godsend for him.

I have stayed healthy all these years by eating good and real food; I realized early on the value of nutrients. It was simple, I thought: Good food results in healthy cells. I grew my own food and ate organic as often as possible. I never knowingly consumed chemicals. I replaced my declining hormones, which kept me happy and energetic, and I tried to avoid toxins in the house and the environment. I always knew chemicals could no longer be avoided completely in anyone's life, so I did what I thought was the smart thing; I went to those antiaging doctors and they gave me intravenous drips of vitamin C and glutathione and other treatments to "build me up."

My friends really got a laugh off that one, but again, who's laughing now? Those treatments helped me stay limber and healthy and have kept my brain sharp. Maybe that's what I am enjoying the most. I can think . . . my brain is not foggy, I am not forgetful. I remember dates and the past, I keep a journal on my computer, and hasn't the Internet been a great connection to information and the rest of the world? I could spend all day doing that but I really don't have time. I have my business and then there is daily exercise and Alan and I go out dancing once or twice a week. We both really enjoy that.

The second half of my life is filled with satisfaction. It's better than it's ever been. Who knew ninety-four was going to be such fun and so productive? Who knew my 105-year-old husband would remain so sexy? The new career I embraced at sixty-five has brought me great contentment and financial rewards.

My friends retired and became bored, but not me. It's as though I have found the golden key. I feel I have it all: a *great* family, *great* children and grandchildren, *great* great-grandchildren, *great* health, *great* marriage, and *great* sex! And it's not over. . . . I am ready and eager for what life brings next. I know I'm going to get old one day, but at the moment it doesn't even appear to be on the radar. . . .

Also next month I am hosting the wedding of my great-great-granddaughter at our house. So I'm very busy dealing with caterers and rentals; I am going to do the flowers myself—I mean, who grows more gorgeous roses than mine?

THIS is, of course, a hypothetical situation, but with the way I am living now, *I firmly believe* it is entirely possible that I will be living the life I just described into my nineties and beyond. Sound too good to be true? It's not—with breakthrough medicine, the future is now. It is never too late to start, but it is also never too early. If you're thirty-five, get ready! It's coming, and sooner than you think. When you are young, you never think about your health—it's a given; but the earlier you understand the benefits of embracing what you are about to learn, the better the quality of life you can continue to enjoy without fear that you will end up sick and in a nursing home.

Your future is not so far away. It's important, crucial, to take the steps now—today—to reset the course of your health. It's not difficult; it just requires a few simple but crucial steps to change the outcome of your life. It *is* a choice; continue your present unhealthful lifestyle, poor diet, and overuse of pharmaceuticals and experience a slow but sure, painful, unhealthy, sick life with dementia, heart disease, and probably cancer. Or choose to make a few simple changes starting today and enjoy a long life of vibrant, joyous energy and magnificent health.

I practice BREAKTHROUGH MEDICINE and I have never felt better, been healthier, or had more energy in my life. I wake up excited for each day to begin; my brain is sharp, my libido is active, and my outlook is always upbeat. I am experiencing this quality of life through the knowledge I have obtained from the doctors in this book. I have embraced a new approach to my health that is about prevention and not waiting for a debilitating diagnosis.

We *can* grow old in great health. We *can* age with our brains intact and our energy at youthful levels. The model of the aging person of today will no longer have to be a part of our future. There is no reason to fall apart the way our older population is now. Our bones do not have to turn to powder. Our brains do not have to become demented. Cancer and heart disease do not have to be an inevitable part of our future. But we have to start *now*!

The cutting-edge, Western-trained doctors in this book are truly onto something and they are excited; they all realize that the way medicine has been practiced for the past fifty years is no longer relevant in today's world.

We are under the greatest environmental assault in the history of mankind; we live in a world of unbelievable stress and pollution. Our bodies are no longer able to tolerate this assault and as a result people are sick. It is inevitable that something has got to change, and that is what this book offers. We can change our fate, we can take charge of our health. We do not have to expect sickness as we age. We can replace our lost youthful hormones, we can reverse the dietary habits that are starting to wreak havoc on our bodies, and we can supplement what is missing from our food supplies and what has been depleted from our soil. But we have to start now.

At present most of us are existing to some degree at the whim of pharmaceuticals. We have a pill to make us sleep, a pill to normalize our moods. We live on antacids for our churning stomachs and take tranquilizers to calm down; we take pills to lose weight, pills to control our water retention, pills for bloating, pills for headaches, pills for aches, pills for pains, and pills for erections! Yet with all this medication, nobody feels . . .

good. Nobody is thriving. Pills are not the answer; pills are a Band-Aid. And, ultimately, they are one's demise. The toxic buildup of pharmaceutical chemicals in our bodies eventually backs up. You see it everywhere; it's all around us: aging people who can't think or walk or take care of themselves. The present pharmaceutical model most conventional doctors follow can lead directly to the nursing home. None of us ever believe that *we* would be one of the ones to suffer this horrible end, this terrible fate. Yet without changing the way you approach your health at present, the likelihood is that you will one day find yourself sitting in your wheelchair, drugged into a medical stupor, and left to die alone, lonely, and sick. It happens every day.

Senior people always say the same thing: "As long as you have your health." We laugh it off when we are young, but imagine living the life you are watching with your aging, senile, feeble parent or grandparent. What makes you think the same won't happen to you? In many cases our aging parents did not experience anywhere near the chemical assault that we are in this millennium. This is a big change. Stress is blunting our hormone production earlier and earlier, chemicals have slipped into our food, toxins are all around us in our homes, in the air we breathe, in the water we drink. In fact, in Los Angeles we recently were "treated" to fluoride in our water. Fluoride is a toxic-waste by-product of the aluminum manufacturers, which *doesn't* prevent tooth decay, yet now we in southern California are drinking it, bathing in it, cooking with it, watering our vegetable gardens with it—and we are actually paying for it. What are we thinking?

It's no accident the doctors in this book realize that the present Western "standard of care" model is not working. There is no drug at the moment that can mask the real problem—which is toxicity, stress, pollution, and their effects on the human body. The interviews with these courageous doctors will change your attitude, change your health, and set you on a path of feeling well and energetic. They all share their life-altering secrets to successful health and aging and how to achieve it.

The true breakthrough is understanding that *you* are in charge of your health. Only you can turn it around, and the good news is that it is easy to do. Technology and new medical approaches have made it possible for all of us to live years beyond any time frame the human species has ever before imagined—but *without* quality of life! Who wants to live a long life without good health and a working brain?

Living to ninety and one hundred years (some say it could be more like 120 years) will be normal for those of us alive today. Imagine living that long with your brain intact, your body in good health, disease-free and with strong bones and lots of energy.

No longer do we have to expect disease as we age (and we are aging younger and younger; in fact, thirty-year-olds are starting to have problems once associated with much older people). Alzheimer's now affects people in their forties, fifties, and sixties. This has never happened before. What has changed? What are we doing wrong? Why hasn't the conventional medical community anticipated this? The sad but true fact is that dementia in thirty-year-olds is predicted in the next twenty years in epidemic proportions, due to years of high intake of chemicals from seemingly benign everyday habits such as consuming diet soda and food additives. Dementia in young people! This is unprecedented.

By embracing this information, by reading each interview with these amazing doctors, you will find the well-researched, cutting-edge information to live a long, healthy, energetic life without drugs. *Breakthrough* is in part a collection of interviews with the preeminent antiaging doctors of the world. Each of these doctors has had the courage and integrity to stand back and realize that the way he or she was taught medicine in our most prestigious medical schools is no longer working in the world in which we all live today. Technology now allows us to live longer, but we are stressed beyond belief. We are consuming chemicals in amounts (knowingly or unknowingly) that are lethal; we are severely hormonally imbalanced, and we are uninformed about the incredible positive effects of good nutrition. We are getting cancers at younger and younger ages. Alzheimer's is sucking the minds from our elders and sneaking up on the unsuspecting young. We all hope and pray it won't be us, but at present most people are on a fast-moving train to disaster and they don't know how to jump off.

From each of these physicians I set out to discover how to avoid this fate. Each interview is a personal appointment for you; in fact, it's better than an appointment. Over a period of weeks I had the opportunity to spend hours and hours probing their fantastic brains to get a sense of their individual passions. We went back and forth, so many phone calls, always with yet another breakthrough to share.

There is very little ego among professionals in the antiaging field. Because there is so much new information, each doctor is eager to share with others. They are one another's teachers. The several conferences a year that these doctors attend are not pharmaceutically funded (meaning they have to pay their own way), so no agenda dictates their ideas. Each doctor is there to share something they have uncovered by utilizing what was once known as the "art of medicine," the kind of medicine we have always hoped we would have, where the doctor actually sits back and thinks about what makes sense.

In essence they connect the dots. You see, the dots don't connect when dealing with pharmaceuticals; they become crutches or Band-Aids, never really healing, just maintaining and usually causing problems from side effects that are sometimes worse than the condition for which the drug was originally prescribed.

When it comes to good heath and aging, we simply need to put back what we have lost. Maintain our hormones at optimal levels and reconsider food as fuel: Both build health and give energy.

Bioidentical hormones are at the base of this approach, because hormonal decline creates a decline in *you*. Without youthful hormones you are no longer you. Anyone who is in hormonal decline can attest to that fact, and younger and younger people are in hormonal decline due to enormous stress and toxic overload. Bioidentical hormone replacement is a must to remain youthful, healthy, and energetic, but this book takes it further. We start with bioidenticals, but then we go body part by body part, identifying the weakness in the body and then strengthening it. There will be no more sudden deaths when you embrace breakthrough information, because you will now have the knowledge to catch a problem before it manifests.

The news is good. We no longer have to *expect* the inevitability of cancer, Alzheimer's, heart disease, or life in a nursing home. We have become so used to disease in this country that we are no longer shocked when an older person (and nowadays even younger people) gets a serious illness. I've already had my brush with a serious disease and, because of that, I realize information is the key to understanding how to avoid the lifestyle and dietary habits that had allowed my body to become weakened, the way it once was when I played host to breast cancer. I want to be around for a long time, so I take all this new information seriously.

It's no joke, this is serious . . . deadly serious. Women in particular are unwell: out-of-control weight gain, inability to sleep, stomach problems, aches, pain, stiffness, bad knees, bad hips, no libido, and then the life-threatening conditions—heart disease, diabetes, cancer, osteoporosis, heart attack, stroke, lupus, fibromyalgia, dementia, Alzheimer's, brain tumors, mental problems. Where are these conditions and diseases coming from? It is not normal to be sick because we are aging, yet that is what we have come to expect.

HOW do you feel about getting those twenty or thirty extra years technology now provides if you are not in good health? How do you feel about the possibility of a life without a working body or brain? That's not such a good thing. Suddenly those "extra years" are a burden. Quality of life is what living is all about. Technology has found the key to longevity, yet quality of life has not been addressed by the scientific community in those extra years.

Here's where breakthrough, the changing face of medicine, comes in! To live a long life in vibrant health requires a shift in thinking. All behavior patterns are broken by "shifts in thinking." Between chemicals, pollution, stress, and overuse of pharmaceuticals, it's a battle to maintain good health. The way we have been taking care of ourselves is no longer working, evidenced by the sickness we see around us. A change is necessary.

At present in our country we do not practice "health care." We think we do, but in reality we practice "disease care," meaning, we go to the doctor when we are already in a diseased state. To take advantage of the breakthroughs we have achieved in new cutting-edge medicine, a shift in our thinking is required: a commitment to practicing true health care from here on in to enjoy a long, healthy life.

So what does that mean? True health care means we go to the doctor when we are well. Most of us wait until we have "conditions" or disease before we drag ourselves to the doctor's office. We are not encouraged to be proactive about our health. We are not encouraged to think about health care in terms of *prevention*. Most of us go to the doctor like children waiting to be told what to do. Generally, we don't think for ourselves as to what we feel would be best for us. We've been lulled into thinking that our doctors know best. But our doctors are restricted by their workload and time constraints. If you are part of an HMO, you already know that your doctor has only about eight minutes to spend with you. It's hit or miss, maybe he or she will get it and maybe not. Because we have chosen not to be "in tune" with the language of our body (aches, pains, burning, coughing, etc.), we wait too long, until we are already sick, and then there is no choice but to resort to pharmaceuticals, antibiotics, or surgery. Surgery is fantastic and there are those of us who have had no choice but to resort to cutting and repairing. We are fortunate because American surgeons are the best on the planet, but what if we could be so in tune with our health that we catch a problem before it has the chance to manifest as something requiring such a drastic approach?

Medicine is advancing by turning away from the crutch of pharmaceutical drugs. According to Dr. Jonathan Wright, "We can achieve perfect health using nature's tools": hearing can be restored, macular degeneration can be reversed or at least stopped, and in some cases infections can be treated more effectively with natural approaches. There are intravenous treatments to flush out the toxins that are debilitating precursors to disease. Dr. Michael Galitzer feels we can beat cancer: "We can learn to live with cancer by staying a step ahead of it, building up the body to keep the cancer at bay."

We can restore brain cells by taking a simple, natural supplement that is neuron protective. We can heal the gut damaged by years of over-the-counter drugs, antibiotics, and poor nutrition. Often these conditions can not only be healed but reversed as well.

The first and most important step to real health care is to understand how your body works. This book will teach you that in layman's terms. Knowledge is power. Most of us sit in our doctors' offices quietly expecting them to know how our body is feeling. No one can possibly know your body as well as you do. We need to learn to *listen* to our bodies. If you have constant burning, swelling, indigestion, coughing, choking, or constipation, that is your body talking (screaming), letting you know that all is not well. We hear the chatter for months and sometimes years before we decide to find out what is going on. By then, we are usually in a condition that requires surgery or major drugs, most of which are designed to keep us on them for life.

Breakthrough medicine is a fast-moving train. There are thousands of incredible doctors around the world who have come to realize that the way they have been taught to treat their patients no longer works. It's a collective consciousness that brings these doctors together from all points of the world. It is as though they all came to the same conclusions at the same time. In this book I will take you to the best of them. This is your opportunity to tap into the latest and best breakthroughs medicine has to offer. These are doctors who have "stepped out of the box" to find a better way—medicine that uses pharmaceuticals only as a last resort. This type of medicine has been practiced in Europe for decades. Europeans are healthier than we are. They eat better food, real food; they don't use chemicals as liberally as we do; and they treat their ailments homeopathically, resorting to Western medicine and antibiotics as a last resort.

European doctors have been savvy to bioidentical hormone replacement for the last fifty years. They have understood the need to replace the hormones we lose in the aging process, not only sex hormones but also the major hormones—thyroid, insulin, adrenals, and cortisol. Dr. Thierry Hertoghe of Belgium is known as "the father of bioidentical hormones."

He explains in this book the advantages of real hormone replacement. Europeans did not buy into synthetic hormones the way we did in this country and because of that they have less cancer.

Breakthrough is new medicine that, among other things, takes advantage of bioidentical hormone replacement for women *and* men, understanding that the decline of hormones in all of us is commensurate with the decline in our health. Individualized bioidentical replacement rectifies the decline. Breakthrough medicine is also having the ability to understand all the "pauses" in the human system and how we can stop these pauses and actually reverse them.

According to Dr. Eric Braverman the pauses are:

- thyroid pause—weakened thyroid
- electropause—diminished brain capacity
- cardiopause—increased heart rate, due to decrease of pumping efficiency
- immunopause—weakened immune system
- menopause—loss of hormones in women
- andropause—loss of hormones in men
- osteopause—loss of bone density
- somatopause—loss of human growth hormone; muscles lose strength and tone
- dermatopause—loss of collagen and elasticity in the skin

All of these pauses are reversible if treated with bioidentical hormones and advanced techniques to head off future diseases or health problems.

The current medicine we are practicing for the most part is out of touch. Many doctors don't have the knowledge or the tools to do the job. So, we bombard cancer, attempting to kill it with radiation and poisonous drugs, and antibiotics mount the assault on infections. We surgically carve out diseased tissue as a routine practice. What we call modern medicine is really quite primitive and can accomplish only so much until we invent new tools—which usually mean more drugs. This is where breakthrough medicine, or what I call "commonsense medicine," comes in. We now have the information to understand that with a few simple changes we can push back time without drugs.

Breakthrough medicine has 8 Steps to Wellness:

1. Get BHRT
2. Avoid Chemicals and Detoxify Your Body

3. Take Nutrition Seriously
4. Create a Healthy GI Tract
5. Avoid Pharmaceuticals Unless Absolutely Necessary
6. Supplement Your Diet
7. Exercise Regularly
8. Get Proper Sleep

These 8 Steps to Wellness are the cornerstone of breakthrough medicine. This new kind of medicine builds the body up and restores us to youthful hormonal balance, pinpointing the weakest oldest organ or gland, then building up the organ most in decline. By doing so, the body no longer has to compensate for the weak link and all becomes well.

You will also find out about the latest breakthrough advances in technology, including nanotechnology, banking stem cells, and genomics (the science of the human genome), which will make it possible to understand the genetic origin of disease and then take action to extend life by preventing illness. Genomics will radically change medicine and make it predictive. Cognitive brain-science breakthroughs will protect the aging mind, refresh vital memories, improve physical agility, and promote human performance enhancement.

Right now, we can work with doctors who specialize in utilizing exciting new treatments to *build up* the body: hyperbaric oxygen for cancer patients, infrared sauna to detoxify, intravenous treatments such as vitamin C in large doses, intravenous glutathione, intravenous chelation treatments to detoxify from the excessive pollution and heavy metals we unknowingly take into our bodies, intravenous hydrogen peroxide treatments, and much more.

Breakthrough medicine understands the terrible impact of chemicals on the human body. Dr. Russell Blaylock's interview on this topic is life-changing. You will never drink another diet soda again!

Breakthrough medicine stresses the importance of good nutrition, the necessity of avoiding chemicals and toxic sprays and using green household products instead. This new approach also understands stress and how to eliminate it, the importance of avoiding pharmaceutical drugs unless absolutely necessary, avoiding over-the-counter drugs, and most important, SLEEP. Yes, something as simple as a good night's sleep and all its healing benefits are escaping most of us. Going to bed early will prolong your life and keep you healthy. But as you will learn, hormonal imbalance makes sleep impossible. Once you have been restored hormonally, sleep will return, and it is a blessing.

Breakthrough introduces you to the doctors who have chosen to move forward with true "health care," rather than the present "disease care." This is proactive medicine. We all know it is easier to rectify any problem if it doesn't get too far advanced. Why wouldn't the same theory apply to the body? The doctors in this book will help you find natural and effective ways to get off pharmaceuticals unless there are no other options. When you can heal yourself *without* drugs, why wouldn't you want that? This book will teach you the way to a natural healthy life, and explain the downward spiral of becoming pharmaceuticalized.

Ask yourself this question: Are you getting better on the drugs you are taking or just maintaining the status quo? If you are not getting better, this book offers solutions. Whenever you can heal yourself without drugs you are prolonging your life. *Breakthrough* will teach you to understand that the toxic buildup in our bodies is killing us, and just what to do to stop that buildup in its tracks.

There is an exciting new approach to health and medicine. These simple changes in the way you live your life are not difficult, and the results are amazing. Breakthrough medicine makes vibrant health attainable. It will allow you to live a long life, maintain your brain, vitality, and energy, with your organs intact and in full working order. This is true health and it is attainable through the information you are about to read. Enjoy.

ABOUT THE DOCTORS

My hope for the future is that these new ideas about prevention will take hold and the younger docs will adopt this information and gradually medicine will change.

–Khalid Mahmud, M.D.

THE DOCTORS IN THIS BOOK are brave and courageous people who recognize that our dependency on pharmaceutical drugs as the only method of controlling health is not making people well. They all believe there is a better way, taking advantage of the healing tools provided by nature, resorting to pharmaceuticals only as a last resort. These doctors are committed to healing and *prevention*. It is better to prevent than to be scrambling for a cure.

Looking for a cure means you waited too long.

I have had the privilege of meeting with many cutting-edge doctors from around the world by attending medical conferences, listening to them speak, and observing them share information with one another. These doctors practice breakthrough medicine by approaching health care proactively. They work with you to prevent anything disastrous from happening in the first place by staying on top of your health. This way they can detect and catch problems long before they are able to manifest into something unmanageable.

It is exciting to be around these new thinkers. These are Western doctors, men and women at the top of their game. These are honorable people, highly educated and intelligent, who have chosen to step outside the accepted "standard of care" box, which carries with it the risk of being ostracized by their peers.

The enthusiasm of these professionals is intoxicating. They are happy, passionate, and eager to pass on the best and latest medical information. Over the years in writing these books, I have had the opportunity to get to know many of the best of them on a one-on-one basis. They help me with my own health; in turn, I am able to help you get through the confusion that accompanies bodily decline.

I am proud to present these fine people. Take the time to read each interview, which represents hours and hours of conversation condensed into twenty or so pages. All these doctors have something to teach. They all have common areas of expertise regarding the "art of medicine," and each one has his own unique take and approach. I have asked the questions I believe we all have, some from my own health situation and others from the e-mails you have sent to me. The information gathered for this book has propelled me forward with yet new understandings of what is possible.

There is a choice. You can continue to follow the same standard-of-care pharmaceutical approach as always, or perhaps, after reading what these professionals have to say, you might choose to go in a new direction, utilizing alternative natural methods.

Now that I have embraced natural medicine directed by Western doctors, my health has soared to new heights. I consider interaction with my doctors as fine-tuning, constantly tweaking my health program for optimal energy and vibrant health. The same can happen for you.

PART I

Breakthrough Medicine

Unless we put medical freedom into the Constitution, the time will come when medicine will organize into an undercover dictatorship. To restrict the art of healing to one class of men and deny equal privilege to others will constitute the Bastille of medical science. All such laws are un-American and despotic and have no place in a republic. The Constitution of this republic should make special privilege for medical freedom as well as religious freedom.

—Benjamin Rush, M.D., signer of the Declaration of Independence, and physician to George Washington

I

WHAT IS BREAKTHROUGH MEDICINE?

IN THE OLD DAYS, a doctor would be able to have lengthy office sessions with a patient when he or she came in for a checkup or to complain of pain or illness. The doctor could spend time with the patient and really listen to what he or she was saying. They could work together to make a determination on how to proceed. A prescription pad was reserved for extreme illness, with doctors trying to find other ways to make a patient feel better. Rest, proper nutrition, and fluids were frequently the best remedy.

That doesn't happen much anymore. Doctors have only a few minutes to spend with each patient, and it is easier and faster to write a prescription for something that will alleviate the complaints. Next patient, please!

As I said in the introduction, our prescription-mad medical culture actually contributes to our feeling unwell. We never really get better; we just mask our symptoms. We don't follow a commonsense approach to medicine, because taking a pill is easier. But we are not feeling better, and we are frustrated with the downward spiral of our health.

Recognizing that many of us feel we have hit the wall with conventional medicine, antiaging is the likely outcropping to move medicine forward. At present its numbers are small but growing steadily. Breakthrough medicine treats people and patients like individuals who have their own special needs. It brilliantly brings together the personal one-on-one commitment we got from the medical community decades ago *coupled* with the cutting-edge technology of today.

Technology, so far, has been a double-edged sword for us. We are an aging society because we now have access to technology so sophisticated that the normal life span has been extended. In other words, technology today will not allow us to die. This is great news except for the sad fact that the health of most people has deteriorated to the point that quality of life no longer exists. As a result, many people are passing their last years suffering with various forms and stages of disability, uncomfortably waiting it out until the final curtain; that is, if their brain is still firing well enough to realize that they *are* alive.

Antiaging medicine and the forward-thinking Western doctors who have embraced it are able to use technology to help us not only prolong our lives but also have good quality of life. They have rejected the idea of the inevitability of disability and debilitating disease and have decided to band together and take matters into their own hands using natural methods as well as cutting-edge science.

The goal of antiaging medicine is to increase the life span as well as improve overall health. It emphasizes early detection of illness, preventive strategies, and lifestyle changes. This requires improving the diet, reducing stress, detoxifying the body, boosting the immune system, healing the GI tract, correcting hormonal imbalances, improving cardiovascular function, and rebuilding brainpower.

Change is never easy; as with all passages, most of us enter it kicking and screaming. We are comfortable with our pharmaceutical drugs. We are used to taking a pill for every ailment. We are used to side effects; for instance, a woman takes an antibiotic for a yeast infection, which then requires another antibiotic for the new strain of infection that has compromised the gut flora, so she takes yet another medication to rectify this new problem, and so on.

In its way, antiaging medicine has put the brakes on this crazy hamster wheel and said, "Slow down, it's not working; let's find another way." Let's reintroduce common sense and the "art of medicine." Let's take advantage of intravenous treatments, chelation, detoxification, nanotechnology. In other words, let's first try to improve health without chemical interference. Let's reserve pharmaceuticals for their original intention, which would be extreme medical intervention as in acute illness, infection, mental illness, and pain; then pharmaceuticals are the miracles they are meant to be . . . the last card in the practitioner's back pocket.

The new breakthrough doctors have pooled together their great mindpower to use nature's tools to find creative ways to stay healthy without risking debilitating side effects.

What makes us age? What makes us sick? Aging brings about loss of function, loss of organ reserve. A number of factors contribute to the deterioration of the body—nutritional deficiencies are at the top of the list. We patients still have not connected the dots relative to good diet, that the food we eat is responsible for building us up or taking us down. It is truly that simple.

Imbalances of hormones accelerate aging; toxins and poor-quality food accelerate the aging process at a cellular level. Yet through this new approach to medicine we are able to reverse and correct these imbalances before having to resort to pharmaceuticals. These stressors combine to produce changes in the cell's membranes; simple measures such as changing from omega-6 oils (safflower, sunflower, corn, soybean, cottonseed, perilla, walnut, and others) to omega-3 oils (flax, fish oil supplementation, and others) can drastically improve the elasticity of each cell membrane to allow for hydration and oxygen to flow in and out freely. Cells that are hydrated and oxygenated work optimally and reverse the aging process to create a smooth-functioning, healthy body.

As human beings we are "cells reproducing." In order to live long and healthy, this process must continue. On the other hand, cell dysfunction eventually culminates in disease as the body deteriorates. A simple step, like changing the oils you consume, can positively impact the health of your cells; there is no drug that can do that.

Antiaging takes free radicals seriously, knowing that free radicals damage cells, which causes the body's organs and systems to lose function capacity. Excess acid in the system increases free radicals, and 80 percent of chronically ill adults in the U.S. have too much acid in their tissues, which makes them prone to chronic degenerative diseases such as heart disease, stroke, and arthritis. Free radicals are a major contributor to all cancers, and a major factor in loss of collagen resulting in tissues that are old and withered. Free radicals damage the cell membrane, which interferes with the ability of each cell to send and receive messages from other cells and to absorb the necessary nutrients while eliminating waste products. Free-radical damage is most pronounced in oxygen-rich organs (eyes, brain, liver, heart, lungs, kidneys, and blood) and has been implicated in the following diseases: kidney disease, diabetes, pancreatitis, liver damage, inflammation of the GI tract, lung disease, eye diseases (macular degeneration, cataracts), nervous system disorders (Parkinson's, Alzheimer's, MS), diseases affecting red blood cells (sickle-cell anemia, pernicious anemia), iron overload, autoimmune diseases (rheumatoid arthritis, lupus), and most infections (tuberculosis, malaria, AIDS).

Clearly the need to understand the creation of free radicals and then to take the necessary steps to eliminate them is essential for our systems to be healthy.

Chemicals and toxins, plus stress and poor diet continually help create more and more free radicals, which is why antiaging medicine understands and focuses on the absolute necessity of neutralizing free radicals by utilizing antioxidants through the food you consume, intravenous treatments, and supplementation.

It's a new world. If we continue doing things the same old way—eating chemical-laden foods, using chemical toxins in our homes and offices—it will seriously affect the quality and length of our lives, and most likely will be the trigger for one or more of the previously mentioned diseases.

The public is responding. Growing numbers of people are turning to alternative antiaging medicine to address their needs. This new breakthrough medicine recognizes the wisdom and effectiveness of this approach to health, which blends mind, science, and experience. In 1993, a study published in the *New England Journal of Medicine* found that over a third of those surveyed chose alternative medicine over traditional conventional medicine because people have grown weary of the medical establishment's continued emphasis on diagnostic testing and treatment with drugs without focusing on them as the patient.

Here's the good news: It's not an either/or scenario. It's important to recognize that practitioners of alternative medicine are not opposed to conventional medical practices and do not hesitate to resort to them when appropriate, especially when dealing with patients who have life-threatening, acute illnesses. Antiaging medicine aims to stay a step or two ahead of sickness and disease; it also works at toxic avoidance and detoxification, knowing that toxins create malfunctioning cells and cell death is the gradual end to us as a species. It's that serious. I am a great admirer of antiaging medicine . . . it appeals to my common sense. Drugs will never heal; they abate. Restorative treatment as practiced in antiaging medicine approaches the body with true healing in mind.

2

DR. JONATHAN WRIGHT

Nature does nothing uselessly.

–Aristotle

SOMETIMES RENEGADES APPEAR; they are pioneers, fearless and educated, who take on the issues and are passionate about their beliefs. Dr. Jonathan Wright is one of those renegades; highly educated, with degrees in cultural anthropology and medicine from Harvard and the University of Michigan, and, yes, fearless—he has been harassed, ridiculed, and persecuted because of his rejection of the modern "allopathic only" approach to medicine throughout the years. The first prescription for bioidentical hormones written in the United States over twenty years ago was by Dr. Wright. He has been ahead of the curve ever since as a crusader and champion of bioidenticals and natural medicines in the United States. He fights tirelessly for the right to choose whatever type of medicine we desire and is respected for his abilities to treat patients successfully using nature's tools to heal the body—as a result his patients flock to him in his Tahoma Clinic in Washington State. "In forty years I've never healed a patient," says Dr. Wright. "They heal themselves." His modesty notwithstanding, over 35,000 patients have come to see him. A sought-after speaker in Europe, he's considered a hero in Japan, and more than 3,000 professionals have put their careers on hold to attend his famous seminars. Instead of aiming a chemical howitzer at health problems, which is the approach of today's standard of care, Dr. Wright attacks the patient's health with the deft precision of a martial arts master. On the one hand, he utilizes treatments and breakthroughs so sophisticated that the medical

establishment would rather ridicule than embrace them for fear of looking ignorant or worse; on the other hand, so much of what he does is like
the old country doctor who tells you to go home and drink plenty of fluids and get lots of rest. I was enthralled speaking to him, and the information that follows in this interview is life changing.

SS: May I begin this interview saying how much I admire you. Your
approach to today's health is cutting-edge and wise. You are best known
as the doctor who brought bioidentical hormones to the United States,
yet when I read your 1994 book on nutritional therapy, I realized your
"specialty," for lack of a better word, is nutrition.

JW: I focus on nutrition because none of us can do everything. But actually my practice is "using nature's tools to promote health." So that involves nutrition and diet; it involves vitamins and minerals, botanicals,
essential fatty acids, natural energies, magnetic energy, homeopathy,
bioidentical hormones, anything that's a natural tool to promote health.

And, yes, I did write the first prescriptions for bioidentical estrogens
along with progesterone, DHEA, and testosterone, all cycled according to
nature's timing, in the early eighties. Nobody else was doing it, and it
turned into quite a thing.

SS: Let's go through your program. Most people reach for antibiotics
the moment they don't feel well. Yet you seem to be able to do better
work with herbs and supplements and nondrug treatments.

JW: Let me tell you about a really simple one: BLADDER INFECTIONS.
Ninety percent of the time we can get rid of them with no drugs at all.

SS: Are you talking about "the honeymoon disease"?

JW: Yes, and sometimes people get it when they're not even having a
honeymoon, darn it. You probably know that approximately 90 percent
of all bladder infections are caused by a little bacterium called *E. coli*. I'm
not speaking of the dangerous mutant *E. coli* that killed people in restaurants a few years ago, I'm talking about regular old *E. coli* that happens to
be in every living creature that has a colon. Actually, it's a normal bacterium that *should* be there. It helps to finish the process of digestion and
also helps with some nutrient absorption.

But when these bacteria get into the wrong place, meaning the bladder,
they cause an infection. *E. coli* has the unique capability of clinging to the
inner lining of the bladder—imagine Spider-Man. *E. coli* sticks to the
molecules of a simple sugar called D-mannose that is found here and
there in the cells that line the bladder; by sticking, the *E. coli* can crawl,
like Spider-Man, to the next D-mannose and the next and the next and

so on. Like any living thing, they love to reproduce, and they do, causing an
E. coli population explosion, which from our point of view is an infection.
The whole time, the *E. coli* cling like crazy to the D-mannose inside the
bladder so they won't get washed out or rinsed out with every urination.

But we can actually put *E. coli*'s love for D-mannose to good use!
When a patient (usually a woman because women get more bladder infections than men) is given 3 to 5 grams of sweet powdery D-mannose (a
safe, simple sugar that by now is found in virtually every health food
store), only a small amount is metabolized. Most is "kicked out" through
the kidneys into the ureters, then into the bladder, where the bacteria say
"Party time! Look at all that delicious D-mannose!" They detach themselves from that little bit of D-mannose that is naturally in the walls of
the bladder and they grab on to these great swirls of D-mannose coming
into the bladder from the ureters. They float around enjoying all that
D-mannose, and the next time the woman empties her bladder, the infection is literally rinsed away! She never had to go near an antibiotic,
she's better, and the *E. coli* are happy, too, wherever they go, surrounded
by all that D-mannose. What could be better?

But remember two things: First, she needs to take D-mannose every
three to four hours while awake until the symptoms are totally gone,
which can take a few hours or one or two days. Second, D-mannose eliminates bladder infections nine times out of ten, not ten of ten, so if there's
no improvement in symptoms in twenty-four hours, it's best to get "regular" antibiotic treatment.

SS: Do you think we take too many antibiotics in this country?

JW: Antibiotics kill bacteria. We need to kill them, otherwise they'll
kill us with certain infections. But what could be better than making
these little guys happy (*E. coli*, for instance), because when you kill living
things, they quite naturally resist. Any organism that's being shot at, figu-
ratively, is going to fight back. That's precisely why we get drug-resistant
bacteria. But in the case of *E. coli*, that bladder infection couldn't possibly
become resistant to D-mannose, because if it did, the *E. coli* couldn't
hang inside the bladder anymore. So they're stuck, but they don't care.
They are happy and they travel on down to the sewage treatment plant
and they tell all their buddies how nice you were to them. You gave them
this load of D-mannose that they just love. So they're happy; they don't
develop resistance. And we're happy because we get to flush them. And
we did not have to use a drug. We used one of nature's tools.

SS: Why doesn't everybody know this?

JW: You know the answer, Suzanne . . . D-mannose isn't patentable.

You can get it at a compounding pharmacy or natural food store without any prescription. The patent medicine companies just aren't interested. And antibiotics are such a great business. Just think of all the other drugs you need to take to combat the side effects and secondary infections created by the first antibiotic.

When we need them, we need them, but we only want to use them if we absolutely must. And in a case such as this, the alternative medicine (D-mannose) is a much better option.

Let me tell you about a little girl who came to Tahoma Clinic with her parents when she was four. Her mother was an obsessive record keeper and she was able to show me that they had been, so far, to seventy-four different doctors. She and her husband had been told by the local children's hospital that their four-year-old was going to need a kidney transplant in the next two or three years because her kidneys were starting to fail because of all her infections. She had been on so many antibiotics she had become allergic to most of them. Her father didn't say a word, just stood there with his arms crossed.

When I asked the mom what kind of infection her daughter had, she checked her records, and it turned out to be *E. coli* every time. I told them their daughter could be treated with D-mannose. They were worried it would hurt their daughter, so I told them it was safe and natural.

Well, Mom started giving it to the little girl every three to four hours while she was awake. Her last infection went away in less than two days. She took D-mannose from the time she was four until the time she was eight and didn't get another bladder infection until the family went on a vacation and forgot the D-mannose. After that, she stayed faithfully on the D-mannose for ten years, had only that one bladder infection repeat, and she saved her kidneys. And that's that.

SS: That's a spectacular story, especially when you realize what would have happened to her if she'd stayed on the standard-of-care treadmill.

It seems that as we reach middle age, we decline in hormones and everything starts falling apart, things that people never would associate with hormones. For instance, a lot of older people have MACULAR DEGEN-ERATION. Is that a lutein deficiency, or is it hormonal in origin?

JW: Well, for macular degeneration, lutein helps, and hormones help also. Testosterone and estrogen are anabolic steroids (by anabolic I mean the term "naturally anabolic"). All the word "anabolic" means is tissue building. And if we need to rebuild our maculi, what we need to do is rebuild tissue.

But most of the time, and hold on to your chair, Suzanne, macular de-generation starts in the stomach.

SS: What? Tell me more.

JW: Now I did say *most* of the time. A number of years back there was a study that compiled all the significant risk factors for age-related macular degeneration, and one risk factor that puzzled the researchers was antacid use.

SS: Connect those dots for me.

JW: Mayo Clinic researchers (I get a lot of my stuff from the Mayo Clinic) in the 1930s published an article that tabulated the statistics on stomach function in people of all ages. They found that 50 percent of all the people they tested over age sixty had less stomach acid produced in their stomachs than is necessary to completely digest their food. When we don't digest our food, we don't get the nutrition out of it.

For instance, we could be eating the best organic free-range chicken in the world, but if we don't completely digest it, we won't get the amino acids out of the protein, we won't get the minerals broken out of the organic matrix they're in, and the vitamin B_{12} won't come out. Now, we're not going to starve to death. But we are going to be malnourished to one degree or another, because we are sold this bill of goods that if we have digestive difficulties we need to take an acid-blocking medication and shut off our digestion.

SS: So what is missing? Hydrochloric acid?

JW: You betcha, ma'am! It's a failure—usually partial, occasionally complete—of hydrochloric acid in your stomach. Along with Lane Lenard, Ph.D., I wrote a book about this problem and all its implications called *Why Stomach Acid Is Good for You*.

At Tahoma Clinic we've been following this very important clue since the 1980s, especially with "dry" macular degeneration, which is roughly 97 percent of all macular degeneration. The other 3 percent is called "wet." Why anyone calls the two types "dry" and "wet" is a mystery to me because the back of the eye is always wet, anyway. Wet macular degeneration is where new blood vessels form and grow over the macula and you can't see through them. All that dry macular degeneration means is that the macula is deteriorating, falling apart like an old barn in need of repair. No new blood vessels like the wet type.

So, how come things are falling apart? Maybe we don't have enough materials to repair with? Most of the time, it's that simple. So, when people come to our clinic, they can go one of two routes, and for one there is a money-back guarantee.

SS: What is that?

JW: It costs $9,000, and our money-back guarantee is that either we're at least able to stop your macular degeneration from getting any worse, and in many cases help improve your vision, or you get your money back!

But first we insist you be seen by two independent ophthalmologists. We are not ophthalmologists; we're natural medicine therapists, nutritional therapists. I sometimes like to call it applied natural biochemistry. And you have to see at least two, and they measure your visual acuity and confirm that you have dry macular degeneration. Then if we give you our treatment, and your visual acuity keeps getting worse, you get all your money back.

SS: [laughs] You're my kind of doctor.

JW: If you're able to stop macular degeneration so it doesn't get worse, we consider that a success. We don't fool around with trying to improve the stomach first, although we do work with that, too . . . macular degeneration is serious stuff; you could go blind. To get the job done as rapidly as possible, we give people a series of IVs that contain the very same nutrients that are needed to repair macular degeneration.

SS: Hmm . . . just like you replace missing hormones to restore quality of life, so in this case you restore the nutrients whose absence has led to the macular degeneration. It makes perfect sense.

JW: Let me tell you where I got one of several important clues. Here in Washington State, in the Yakima Valley, local farmers know that the soil is very selenium deficient, and the cows were getting something called white muscle disease due to selenium deficiency. So the farmers gave their cows selenium supplements and they got better.

Years ago, one doctor who lived in the Yakima Valley, Dr. Joseph Bittner, thought, hey, I'm eating the local produce, I have macular degeneration, maybe if I took some selenium just like the cows, it would help my eyes. So he did, and his eyes got better. He published this in his weekly column in the Yakima newspaper, and, fortunately, I obtained a copy. After that, for patients who came to me at Tahoma Clinic with macular degeneration, I would measure and replace their hydrochloric acid if the test showed it necessary, and it usually did. I'd have them take selenium and a lot of them got better. After I saw that work, I thought, well, what else helps the eyeball? It turns out that zinc is more concentrated in the macula of the eye than anywhere else, except the hearing apparatus. That gave me another clue.

SS: So this is detective work . . . common sense . . .

JW: Well, that's part of it. That is the art of medicine, putting things together.

Anyway, when I added zinc to the regimen, more people got better. Then I started putting these things into IVs and the results were amazing.

So that's why I use and believe in intravenous treatments, and now we've got about sixteen different things in the treatments including zinc and selenium. We are getting amazing results.

One woman came to me at Tahoma Clinic with rapidly deteriorating vision. This was 1986; we gave her the IV treatment and her vision returned. She came back in the nineties and her eyes were going bad again, and I asked her, are you still taking your supplements and she said yes. We went over her list and guess what was missing? Hydrochloric acid. Even though she was eating well and taking her vitamins and minerals, after a gastric analysis and factoring in that she was now in her sixties (remember the 1930s Mayo Clinic research, where after age sixty, the odds are 50 percent you will be experiencing a decrease in hydrochloric acid), I realized that a missing component to saving eyesight is poor nutrient digestion and absorption, and a very common reason for this is a lack of sufficient hydrochloric acid.

By the way, she had another episode of vision loss in the early 2000s, and the IV treatment reversed it again.

SS: Let's talk about HEARING LOSS. That's just part of aging, right? I mean, do we have to lose our hearing as we get older?

JW: No we don't, ma'am. We can now prevent or correct many cases of age-related hearing loss. Some of this is based on the work of Dr. Dennis Trune. He's at Oregon Health Sciences University and he's worked strictly with animals; but that's okay, animals can lose their hearing, too. His research involved the information that animal hearing loss can be corrected by replacing a natural bioidentical hormone (there you are) . . . this one is made by the adrenal glands, not the ovaries, not the testes, but the adrenals in both sexes, and it's called ALDOSTERONE.

When I became aware of Dr. Trune's work, I had been working with a patient who had lost his hearing. He'd been treated with Prednisone and it helped, but he didn't want to stay on that formerly patent medication forever because of all the side effects: osteoporosis, stomach ulcers, diabetes, all that kind of stuff. His twenty-four-hour urine test for aldosterone (which is more comprehensive than any single blood test) was low. So he took aldosterone and his hearing came back. We then retested his aldosterone and it was smack-dab in the middle range of normal, which is where we want it. He was able to taper off the Prednisone and his hearing stayed normal with "just" the aldosterone.

After a while he stopped taking his aldosterone, and his hearing started to go away again, rapidly. He went back on the aldosterone, and his hearing came back once again.

He's an engineer—I really like working with engineers, they always test theories and want proof—so he actually quit the aldosterone again and started to lose his hearing again. He told me his wife put an end to that and told him to get back to his aldosterone and stay there!

Since that time Dr. Trune referred to me another individual with age-related hearing loss, and I have two other patients myself, and all of them when tested were found to have low twenty-four-hour urine aldosterone measurements.

One gentleman, eighty-four years old, had developed his hearing loss more than ten years before. We checked his urine and sure enough his aldosterone was low. We thought, well, he's eighty-four, what do we expect? So he took aldosterone and in six weeks, Suzanne, he had a 35-decibel recovery in his right ear. Plus the discrimination (the difference between one sound and another) rose from 23 percent to 91 percent. Now his left ear, which had been labeled nearly useless, improved 10 decibels, not 35, but his discrimination between one sound and another in that ear went from 3 percent to 81 percent in six weeks!

SS: Is this only about hearing loss related to aging, or could you restore hearing loss in a rock 'n' roller who has been around loudspeakers all his life?

JW: No, that kind of hearing loss can't be restored—as far as I know—with just aldosterone. But for those in the "older age range," at least they should get a test and find out their aldosterone levels.

SS: What test do we take?

JW: I definitely recommend the twenty-four-hour urine test and never, ever believe the doctor who says, well, the normal range on serum aldosterone is 5 to 30 and yours is 6, so you must be okay. No, no, no, no, it's just like with bioidentical hormones, we want to put you in optimal ranges, which would be closer to 30. I'm kind of enthusiastic about this one. I've treated just four patients, but every one of them has recovered a significant degree of hearing. At this time, the only other doctors I know who are using aldosterone treatment are those who have attended my seminars.

SS: This is incredibly exciting. I know people who have lost their hearing and they become removed from others socially. To think it's this simple. I can't wait to pass this one on.

Two things I'm noticing with our older friends—both men and women are getting bald, and they have memory problems. Got any remedies for either of these, doctor?

JW: Well, for BALDNESS, some people would want to take that stupid Propecia as a partial remedy, but we can do that with natural stuff. Propecia (finasteride) blocks the transformation of testosterone into DHT. We know that from the commercial, and if we do make less DHT in our scalp, we lose less hair. The problem is, making DHT is a natural process. If we block DHT too effectively, as they did in the Prostate Cancer Prevention Trial, it can have unintended consequences. The men who took finasteride had a prostate cancer rate of 18.4 percent, and the guys who didn't take finasteride had a cancer rate of 24.4 percent, which is statistically significant. So finasteride did reduce the incidence of prostate cancer, but here's the bad news. Of the guys in the finasteride group who got prostate cancer, in 37 percent of them it was a highly aggressive type of prostate cancer that is much more likely to kill you. The men who did not take finasteride, even though they got more cancer, only 22.3 percent of them got the more aggressive types of cancer. That's likely why we're not seeing aggressive commercials for growing hair with finasteride or other DHT blockers—it looks like they would give us a higher chance of a more aggressive type of cancer.

So at the moment, nobody knows how to safely grow a full head of hair for men. They can certainly try with zinc because it is also a 5-alpha-reductase inhibitor and a nutrient, but a much gentler one than finasteride. But never take more than 100 milligrams of zinc a day because present research shows when we go too high on zinc, we raise our risk of prostate cancer. Fatty acids also inhibit 5-alpha reductase to varying degrees, so when you are trying to grow hair, you have to work with your doctor about finding the fine line—not too much, not too little—with zinc and fatty acids, which we need in our diets.

SS: So what about BALDNESS IN WOMEN?

JW: If a woman is in her twenties and thirties and losing a lot of her hair, what's happening is often too little stomach acid and pepsin. Because of that, protein isn't digested, and—what is hair made of? You got it . . . protein!

Now with women in their forties who are losing their hair, most often it's a combination of low stomach acid, low thyroid, and, of course, sex hormone loss—mainly estrogen and progesterone. In this case, we replace missing hormones with bioidentical estrogen, progesterone, and thyroid. Then we also replace the missing or low hydrochloric acid. But there is one more element on the outside track—DHEA. Sometimes DHEA is the key missing element.

SS: That's great, like a cocktail for hair loss. I also love that your remedies are about what's missing naturally rather than finding a drug to put a Band-Aid on things. So, in balding ladies, you get a gastric analysis and it's probably low stomach acid, low thyroid, and/or a lack of DHEA and/or natural sex steroids. What about BALDNESS IN POSTMENOPAUSAL WOMEN?

JW: You often see postmenopausal women with all those little curls close to their skulls; because they are losing so much hair, if the curls are not close to the scalp, everyone will see their baldness. Well, these women have very low stomach acid. They don't have much DHEA and their thyroids are weak. Of course, their sex steroids are low, too. If we are able to catch a woman before she's gone almost completely bald, we can stop the process and slowly get it turned around. It's a combination of fixing the digestion assimilation and bringing in the requisite hormones. That usually takes care of the problem. It needs to be known that lack of DHEA and low thyroid are bigger and bigger factors past the age of thirty-five. Now what was that other thing you asked about?

SS: Memory [laughs].

JW: There you go [laughs], I'm sorry to do that to you. So let's do MEMORY before I forget. Regarding memory, you have been right on target all along. Bioidentical hormones, and in this case the sex steroids (estrogen, progesterone, testosterone), are right up there among the most powerful things we can do to hold on to our memories. There is actually epidemiological evidence in women that the lower the estrogens, the higher the risk the woman is going to end up with Alzheimer's or senile dementia. There's no question about that. Even the National Institute on Aging has that on their Web site. And for men, the lower the free testosterone, the greater the risk of Alzheimer's.

Nobody knows why, but there are proteins that float around the bloodstream that grab on to sex steroids . . . testosterone for men, estrogen for ladies. (Of course, both sexes have a little bit of opposite-sex hormones; if we didn't, we probably wouldn't get along.) These proteins bind to the sex hormones and the hormones can't act anymore. Imagine taking your house key and gluing it to a giant beach ball, and then trying to unlock your door with it. Uh-huh! The binding protein is that giant beach ball, proportionate to the size of the testosterone or estrogen molecule. The testosterone and estrogen molecules can no longer fit into the receptor sites because they're stuck on this giant beach ball.

SS: That's a great visual. I've always had a difficult time explaining receptor sites.

JW: But men and women go to the doctor to measure their sex hormones, and the doctor measures their total testosterone and/or total estrogen, which is basically measuring the total of bound *and* free testosterone or estrogen. But you see, in our bodies, almost all of these hormones are "bound," the more so the older we are. To a doctor who doesn't get it, the amount can look okay. But remember that our bodies can make more and more of these binding proteins (beach balls) as we get older and older—so the free count goes down—but if you were to measure the free testosterone or estrogen, it would be abysmally low. Now what do you do about that? You take testosterone or estrogen . . . whatever you are missing. Also, we can sometimes use botanicals that—in a manner of speaking—"bounce" the bound sex steroid off the beach ball (binding protein) and back into circulation as the active free hormone.

SS: So this is how you restore your memory . . . bioidentical hormones, right?

JW: Well, there's another thing to think about—and this is not going to be popular back at FDA headquarters—concerning memory loss. It turns out that it is a normal, natural trace element. It's in the same family as sodium and potassium and rubidium. It's called lithium.

SS: Lithium—that's for bipolar syndrome, or severe depression, manic depression, or mental illness!

JW: Those conditions require super-pharmacologic doses, hundreds and hundreds of milligrams. You would never find those doses in nature. What I'm talking about is 5 to 15 milligrams a day. Now, if you went to look that up, you'd find that in about a half-dozen tomatoes there would be about 3 milligrams. But who is going to eat a half dozen tomatoes a day—or 30 tomatoes a day to get 15 milligrams?

SS: Well, this is interesting to me because I've been complaining to my husband that recently I'm forgetting things. Maybe because my mind is crowded with information from this book, but I know I am on plenty of estrogen. It's frustrating, because usually I can remember everything.

JW: There is so much literature in regular and mainstream medical journals about lithium and protection of neurons.

SS: You mean lithium can actually *repair* neuron activity in the brain? That would be fantastic.

JW: Yes, in some of these medical journals they say lithium is a "robust" neuroprotective agent. Now when a scientist writes the word "robust," that is the equivalent of jumping up and down and saying "Wheeee!" When research scientists investigating lithium's effects have attempted to damage animals' brain cells by giving animals toxins, whether it's a toxin the body makes itself, such as a glutamate, or whether it's a toxin from outside the body, such as aluminum, or by deliberately inducing a stroke and causing lack of oxygen (hypoxia), the animals who get lithium pre-treatment always have less neuronal damage than the animals who don't. That's a fact, always, always, always.

SS: But I've always heard that as we grow older we're all going to lose neurons; our brains are going to shrink. There's nothing we can do about it, right?

JW: An article in *The Lancet* described a "before and after" MRI study of patients over fifty-five years of age done by researchers at Wayne State University. With an MRI you get a picture of the brain that's hard to argue with . . . and they had all these folks take lithium. What they found in the majority of these cases was that lithium induced the formation of approx-imately 3 percent brand-new brain cells, those in the "gray matter." [Re-member Hercule Poirot and his "little grey cells"?] Now 3 percent doesn't sound like much unless you understand that 3 percent involves several billion new brain cells. When I read that, I thought, oh my, if lithium can do this for people who are over fifty-five, I want some of this stuff.

SS: So did you start taking lithium and how much?

JW: I started with 5-milligram tablets and I took two a day. I hap-pened to know it was perfectly safe because I have a long history of work-ing with people who have inherited alcoholic genes, either people who are alcoholic themselves or come from families with alcoholism. There are studies that go way back to the seventies that clearly show that alco-holics who take lithium have reduced cravings.

SS: This is incredible. I mean, who wants to lose thoughts? And my family history is rife with alcoholism. I've written three books on the sub-ject. Where can you get this?

JW: The Tahoma Clinic, www.tahomaclinic.com. Click on "dispen-sary" and then enter "lithium." They come in 5-milligram size, and one or two a day is safe. The "prescription size" is 300 milligrams of lithium car-bonate daily, 55 milligrams of that is lithium, and the on-prescription quantity for bipolar disease is one or two capsules three times a day. That's 55 to 110 milligrams of lithium three times daily for a total of 165 to 330 milligrams of lithium itself, and clearly requires working with a physician. Five to 10 milligrams daily is obviously much, much less.

A woman came to me at Tahoma Clinic and said she wanted lithium. "Why?" I asked. "Only your father and brother are addicted to alcohol, but you've never touched a drop." She said, "I know, but I'm a worrier, and I don't feel right, I get depressed off and on for no reason. I don't sleep well. It helped my father and brother and we're the same genetics, aren't we?"

She was right. Two months later she came back and said, "Lithium turned my life around. I'm much more social, and I don't know why but I can talk to people more easily, I'm sleeping through the night with no problem, and my low-grade depression is gone. I never realized but I had this depression all the time but now I sure feel better."

I said, "Thank you for teaching me something." You know, we physicians learn only so much from medical school and the rest from the people we are working with. But that's life, isn't it? We all learn from each other. From this I started working with people who had genetic predispositions to alcoholism and began suggesting low doses of lithium for them.

SS: But what about lithium toxicity? Do you ever worry about that?

JW: Sometimes individuals with "bad" manic depression get lithium toxicity. These folks are on the maximum doses of lithium. Lithium toxicity can cause kidney damage, high blood pressure, and feeling like you've got a bad flu in your gut all the time. But I learned how to deal with lithium toxicity from one of Dr. David Horrobin's lectures. He casually mentioned that essential fatty acids stop lithium toxicity.

So I tried essential fatty acids with manic-depressive individuals in early lithium toxicity who couldn't stop or decrease it because their symptoms (of bipolar disease) were so bad, and it worked.

Now I tell my patients, "You're not going to get in trouble with 5 or 10 milligrams of lithium, but just in case, would you mind taking some walnut oil in your salad or eat flaxseed or cod liver oil for your heart? This way it will minimize any chance of toxicity."

SS: What else does lithium do?

JW: Remember, lithium protects neurons against glutamate toxicity. There is a new FDA-approved drug for Alzheimer's called Memantine, which was approved partly because it was found to block glutamate toxicity. But it does virtually nothing for Alzheimer's disease. Myself, I'd rather try lithium first.

There's also preliminary research from Italy that found higher-dose lithium can slow or stop the progression of ALS—amyotrophic lateral sclerosis, Lou Gehrig's disease. Research in animals shows that lithium treatment reduces beta-amyloid, tau protein, and neurofibrillary tangle in brain cells. All of these are factors in Alzheimer's disease.

Suzanne, people who want to keep their marbles for as long as possible should keep their eye on lithium research and work with a physician skilled and knowledgeable in bioidentical hormones as well as lithium use.

SS: Let's talk about CORTISOL. People are so stressed in today's world, me being one of them. (Being a professional woman takes its toll.) I take hydrocortisone (bioidentical cortisol), 5 milligrams, four times a day about every four hours to mimic the way it pours in nature. My oncologist, Dr. Julie Taguchi, wrote me the prescription and she believes in cortisol replacement.

JW: Ah, Julie Taguchi, now she's one of the few oncologists who gets it. Cortisol. Most doctors don't get this . . . cortisol and hydrocortisone are the same thing. Many doctors think you are taking "supersteroids" if you mention cortisol; but if you use nature's quantities, you're just doing another type of bioidentical hormone. Cortisol is a natural steroid molecule made by the adrenals. It's another type of steroid, like estrogen, testosterone, aldosterone, all of these.

Dr. William Jeffries wrote a book called *The Safe Uses of Cortisol* in 1981, which really helped me in my practice. Dr. Jeffries pointed out that if we copy what normal adrenal glands do, we would understand that when under stress, our adrenal glands make much more cortisol. When we're not under stress, they make roughly the equivalent of 5 milligrams, four times a day, which sounds like what Dr. Taguchi has you doing. But when we are under stress we make bunches more. When a person who's taking replacement cortisol is under extreme stress, she probably should take 30 to 40 milligrams a day. Then it is important to cut back by 5 milligrams a day, until you're back to a total of 20 milligrams daily. You never want to go from 20 to 40 and then back down to 20. The body doesn't like that . . . it likes to taper its cortisol.

SS: I believe I'm not a whole lot different from all the other working men and women out there. I have overworked and taxed my adrenals and cortisol levels so often in my career that I'm not sure if they will ever be right again. I have "burned out" four times in my career, flatlined my adrenals, got depressed, couldn't sleep, gained weight, and woke up unhappy one Christmas morning (and I love Christmas). And it wasn't until I replaced my missing and burned-out cortisol with hydrocortisone that I got my adrenals operating correctly again. Now I sleep, depression is a foggy memory, and my weight is perfect.

JW: Well, that is the remedy for all who have overdone it, but why not go one step further? Why not get your own adrenal glands better?

SS: Huh? Isn't that what I am doing?

JW: Let me tell you about a patient of mine, a woman whose twenty-four-hour urinary cortisol and cortisone were measuring 5 and 6 respectively (normal in that test was above 30 and up to 110 for each metabolite). And she's flat on her back and she's got low blood pressure and she can't handle any stress. All she can do is get up, cook dinner for her family, and go back to bed. She felt so worn out. Her doctor had her on the "antidepressant of the day" because they told her she was just depressed. We were able to bring in some "live-cell adrenal" from Europe, because after 1994—in this "free country"—it became legal to bring in anything that is natural for treatment: the "DHEA law." We gave her the adrenal cells and thyroid cells and other cells, and within six months her own cortisol and cortisone had risen from 5 and 6 to 40 and 50. Now, I've got to admit that's still low, normal in that test being 30 to 110, but we had absolute documentation that her own adrenals had recovered themselves. She was up and out of bed and feeling good. She was also thirty-five; of course, the younger we are the better we recover.

SS: I thought replacing cortisol with hydrocortisone was repairing. Now I realize it's replacement but not necessarily repairing. In cell therapy you're talking about repair. Reactivating the gland to start producing as though I were in optimal prime, right?

JW: Right. Now, you are replacing and your body is responding, but you also have to remember to take your Cortef four times a day. I'm sure that's not easy to do . . . for life. Not many people are going to do that, humans being human.

SS: That's true. It is very difficult to remember precisely on time.

JW: Let me explain what I am talking about regarding bringing in cells. But first please write that only some of this was original with me—the pioneer in what I am about to tell you was a Dr. Paul Niehans. Google him; he was "the father of cell therapy." His book translated in English is called *Cell Therapy* (usedbooksearch.co.uk). He lived in the mountains somewhere in Switzerland in a small village, and he was simultaneously the town's only general practitioner and the only veterinarian. You could do that in the 1920s.

SS: You could do that because people weren't as sick as they are now.

JW: You got that right. One day Dr. Niehans was in his office with a woman who had just had her giant goiter removed. (For years, people living in the mountains got goiters and had them removed all the time.) They had no iodine, right? If a surgeon wasn't particularly skilled they would also remove the parathyroid glands. They are called parathyroid glands because they are embedded in the thyroid and are critical to life. They regulate calcium, and if you don't have these glands, your calcium drops, drops, drops. When your blood calcium drops that far, you get incredible painful spasms. They are called "tetanic" spasms—like people with tetanus get—because they are so bad. After a couple of weeks of this people usually die.

SS: Goiters sound old-fashioned. You don't hear about people getting them anymore.

JW: No, you don't, because of the tiny amounts of iodine in salt. I am hoping you are taking IODINE.

SS: Yes, I take it twice a day, 5 milligrams each time.

JW: Good for you. It's one of the best things you can do to protect yourself against recurrent breast cancer. Yay, yay, yay, you're on the ball . . . but then again, you always were.

SS: Thank my oncologist, Dr. Taguchi. Now, are we still talking about CELL THERAPY?

JW: Yes. Dr. Niehans is visited by this woman with terrible spasms due to having had her goiter removed by someone who removed her parathyroids, too, and she asks can he please, please do something for her? She's going to die. So he rounds up a pregnant sheep and dissects the parathyroid glands from the sheep's fetus. (You probably know that transplanted fetal tissues are very rarely rejected, because they do not stimulate the recipient's immune system, just like they don't stimulate their mothers to reject them.) It doesn't matter if it's animal or human fetal tissue. . . . Dr. Niehans took the fetal parathyroids and squished them up so they would fit into a syringe and injected them into the pectoral muscle of the woman, and within two weeks the woman's blood calcium was back to normal, and her spasms had gone away. She was fifty-five at the time and lived well into her eighties.

SS: So, was this the first stem cell treatment?

JW: No, no, stem cells are totally undifferentiated cells that have the possibility of turning into any other kind of cell, if you can figure out how to get them to do that. Dr. Niehans took the next step. He took cells that had already turned into parathyroid cells, except they'd done that in the fetal sheep. He took the actual cells that the woman was missing from the fetal sheep and implanted them in her.

SS: Replacement again. It's all about replacing what is missing. That's the key . . . the ticket to today's aging. That's the advantage you are all talking about.

JW: Yes. This is cell therapy. When I give lectures on bioidentical hormones, I'll say, using the actual molecules is good, but it is even better to rejuvenate our own glands.

SS: You mean you see a day when, instead of taking bioidentical hormones or rubbing on the bioidentical cream, you would use cell therapy to restimulate your glands or organs to start producing these hormones or molecules on their own again? This is fantastic.

JW: Dr. Niehans started with replacing parathyroid; by the time he was finished with his career, he had given over fifty thousand injections of fetal animal cells to humans and in some cases it was disease specific. For example, he found that injecting fetal heart cells would improve the health of people who had congestive heart failure and they would come out of it.

Now to get specific to your circumstances, Suzanne, when I work with women with weak adrenal glands (and I run into this more often with women than men, it's just the way it is), I tell them, and I am telling you, if you can afford it, go to Dr. Niehans's clinic in Switzerland and get adrenal fetal cells. Of course, now we are doing it at my clinic in Tahoma so you could also come here. As Dr. Niehans said in his book, you never, ever treat an endocrine gland in isolation. That's how we administer hormones; you don't just use estrogen, you use estrogen, progesterone, and DHEA. Then you might need a little testosterone, thyroid, and melatonin. You do the whole network.

Dr. Niehans said relative to cell therapy, "You give them a preponderance of adrenal cells, a little bit of thyroid cells, a little bit of pituitary cell, and a little bit of hypothalamic cells [the preponderance of the cells that are the weakest]." When these women come back, they feel like a different person.

SS: Does this last? Are you now patched up for good and ready for another fifty years?

JW: It lasts anywhere from two to five years, then you go back and get a booster. It's really quite amazing; a person has a weak liver, they get a preponderance of liver cells. If they've got weak kidneys, they get kidney cells. The whole thing is called "cell therapy." What I'm saying is with cell therapy injections, you, Suzanne, literally have a shot at making your own adrenal cells better.

SS: So you don't have to go deaf, you don't have to be hormonally imbalanced, you don't have to go bald if you're a woman, you don't have to lose your eyesight from macular degeneration, you don't have to suffer from adrenal exhaustion, you can regenerate your organs. I mean, this is all very exciting stuff.

JW: Right now we're the only clinic in the country that's doing much of this.

SS: You mentioned IODINE. So many women (myself included) have painful cystic breasts. Is iodine the remedy and why?

JW: If you have enough iodine, it makes your estriol levels (estriol is a hormone) go up and that protects against breast cancer. The only other marker to follow relative to breast cancer protection is your 16-hydroxy estrogen marker. You can check this level with a twenty-four-hour urine test.

The urine test is the only way to really measure your estriol levels. Estriol is one of the most abundant estrogens produced by the body, but the body clears it very rapidly. You can always find considerable estriol in the urine but very little in the blood. That's why I do the urine tests rather than blood tests to measure these hormones. Unfortunately, most doctors don't understand this and they rely on blood tests.

SS: So are you saying that if you take iodine and estriol you won't have fibrocystic disease?

JW: Actually, if you take the right amount of iodine your fibrocystic disease will go away no matter how bad it is. I learned that from Dr. John Myers in the 1970s, and it works every time. (Very few things in medicine or anywhere else work every time, but this one does.) You don't need to take estriol; if you take enough iodine, your body will make enough estriol for you.

SS: How much iodine is that? I would love for this to go away in my body.

JW: First let me tell you about Dr. Myers. He originally worked in a dog lab with dogs (beagles) who had fibrocystic disease. (Beagles commonly get this disease.)

SS: Who knew?

JW: Myers was a surgeon. He performed an experiment with two groups of female dogs with fibrocystic disease. From one group he took the ovaries out and in the other he did "sham surgery," which left the ovaries in. In both groups he then swabbed the vagina area with iodine on repeated occasions. The beagles with ovaries had their fibrocystic breast disease go away completely; the beagles who'd had their ovaries removed had no improvement at all. He concluded that the ovaries use the iodine to make another molecule—he thought this molecule might be di-iodotyrosine but he had no proof—which in turn eliminated the fibrocystic breast disease.

SS: Why in the vagina?

JW: Myers pointed out that when we swallow iodine most of it goes to the thyroid gland. He found that when he took out the ovaries in these dogs he wanted to put the iodine as close to the ovaries as he could get, so that it wouldn't get to the thyroid first. No ovaries, no effect.

At a seminar in 1976 that I attended along with about thirty other doctors who had been invited, Dr. Myers introduced two women with the very worst cases of fibrocystic disease that the thirty doctors could find. These brave volunteers had such pain that if they hugged their husbands it would be excruciating. Dr. Myers asked them to lie down on the table, and all these doctors were asked to palpate, palpate, and these ladies were wincing and groaning, because it was like hard painful marbles in their breasts.

Then Dr. Myers, with a nurse, takes one woman at a time into the exam room and swabs their vaginas with iodine. Thirty minutes later the women come out and the doctors are asked once again to palpate their breasts (good grief).

SS: Somebody's got to do it!

JW: You're right, but at this point the women are smiling. I'm not kidding; only one half hour later, the breasts of these ladies were perceptibly softer. It's no longer like marbles in there. Dr. Myers said, "Gentlemen and ladies, you do that twice a week until the fibrocystic disease goes away."

SS: These women had their ovaries, right?

JW: Correct. I went back to my clinic and we did that for our patients. For about a year and a half we must have seen every woman for twenty miles with fibrocystic disease. It got to be so common that the nurses were doing the treatment (you can do it for yourself also; it doesn't really require a doctor), and all these women were cured of fibrocystic disease.

SS: So this is for short-term use?

JW: Until the fibrocystic breast disease goes away, however long that takes. Generally, it's six weeks to three months.

SS: If you stop using the iodine, does the pain come back?

JW: Only if you totally stop all iodine intake for quite a while.

SS: And how much iodine does a woman take?

JW: Remember, Dr. Myers recommended using a swab saturated with iodine (not iodide, there's a subtle but definite biochemical difference) and he didn't even measure the dose. However, once the fibrocystic disease is gone, a woman can—just like you—safely use a total of 10 to 12 milligrams of a combined iodine/iodide preparation daily. The liquid form of this iodine/iodide preparation is called Lugol's Iodine, the tablet form is called Iodoral.

SS: Why iodide, too?

JW: Although breast tissue is more iodine dependent, thyroid tissue is more iodide dependent. Over our lifetimes, we need both; for the short-term elimination of fibrocystic disease, iodine is "the one."

SS: What about the bioidentical estriol you mentioned? How does that connect here?

JW: At that time women were being told that if they had fibrocystic disease, their chances of cancer were higher. Many of the women starting fibrocystic breast disease treatment asked if they could measure their cancer risk. Since we knew from the research of Dr. Henry M. Lemon done in the 1960s while at the University of Nebraska that if a woman's estriol was low, her chances of cancer were higher, we measured the estriol in twenty-four-hour urine specimens. We found that an unusually high percentage of women with fibrocystic breast disease had low estriol.

Much to my surprise, when we rechecked these same women after the iodine treatment had eliminated their fibrocystic disease, we found all the estriol measurements were now much higher! That's how I "accidentally" found that iodine stimulates more estriol production. Now, I'm guessing that the estriol also has something to do with normalizing the breast tissue, not just the iodine; of course, I don't know for sure. However, even if estriol doesn't do that, it is definitely cancer protective.

Bottom line: fibrocystic breast disease goes away, every time, with application of iodine. Thank you, Dr. Myers!

SS: All without a single drug. That is the amazing part. Now, let me ask you, when I was a child and I skinned my knee, my mother would put iodine on it. Is that what we are talking about?

JW: No, that's got alcohol in it, and that would hurt. You go online and look for Iodoral (an iodine supplement). If people are taking Iodoral, I ask them, please, please work with a physician skilled and knowledgeable in nutritional medicine and bioidentical hormones, because if you take too *much* iodine from any source, you can suppress your thyroid gland.

Or there is an over-the-counter form made by a small Seattle company (I'm not involved with them) called Tri-Quench. One drop of that a day is safe. Or you can get your doctor to prescribe Lugol's Iodine. One drop of that a day is safe. Iodoral is the same as two drops of Lugol's.

SS: [Reader: I have been taking Lugol's at this point for six months and my fibrocystic disease is gone, gone, gone.] Okay, I've got one for you. . . . I'll bet I know forty women with IRRITABLE BOWEL SYNDROME—IBS. Is it about bad food, bad diet, eating on the run, not chewing your food? What is it, and what can you do about it?

JW: You've got part of the answer. Doctors often refer to IBS as a wastebasket diagnosis, meaning we don't know what the hell is the matter so we call it irritable bowel syndrome. In a way it is; the bowel is sitting there being irritable.

SS: Well, is it the food we are eating?

JW: Yes, it's all about the refined foods, all the foods with chemicals in them, such as this sucralose stuff, which of all things is chlorinated sugar. Nature never chlorinates sugar molecules! That stuff is toxic. By the way, a way to really cut down on the sugar cravings is with the supplement chromium. It's a supplement, but you've got to use enough of it.

SS: How much do you take?

JW: First, let me give you a safety parameter. According to Dr. Robert

Anderson, one of the key chromium "gurus," you do not want to go above 70,000 micrograms of chromium a day, which is a ridiculously high amount that no one would do anyway.

SS: Seventy thousand micrograms. That sounds like a lot.

JW: It is. And that's the funny part. Who is going to take that much? At the Tahoma Clinic we recommend between 5,000 and 6,000 micrograms daily until the sugar craving goes away, and then cut back to about 1,000 micrograms daily.

SS: So IBS . . .

JW: Yes, symptoms: either too many bowel movements in a day, eight to ten movements, or constipation, sometimes with cramps and a lot of gas. That pretty much describes IBS. Really, get all the junk out of your diet and everything will go back to normal. Eat whole nourishing types of food, no chemicals. But really the big deal is FOOD ALLERGIES.

SS: My daughter was having trouble with her weight until she discovered her food intolerance. She gave up eggs and lost twenty-five pounds.

JW: Yes, you have to find out your allergies and intolerances and be really strict about avoiding them. When you put them back in, you must pay strict attention to your reaction. If it is not good . . . stay away from them. But now we're into an area that is so essential to understand. The food we eat has a lot to do with determining our health.

At present, food allergies and food intolerances are only totally "curable" by giving up the offending foods. Dr. James Breneman (who at the time was chair of the food allergy committee of the ACAAI) wrote the book *Basics of Food Allergy.* Essentially he said, remove your allergies, meaning, get the offending foods out of your diet and the problems they cause will go away. He wrote that 50 percent of all undiagnosed symptoms—that's not 50 percent of all symptoms, but 50 percent of those that no one can diagnose—are due to food allergies and food intolerances.

You see, you can't get a patent for this kind of treatment, but it works; it relieves a substantial proportion of IBS symptoms, and it's a lot better than all the drugs most patients are given for this condition.

Speaking of food allergies, intolerances and weight loss—like your daughter's circumstance—Dr. Theron Randolph first wrote about that in the 1940s. I had one woman patient who was miserable. She had cut her caloric intake down to 300 calories a day, otherwise she would gain weight. That's hardly any food. It turned out that she was intolerant to everything but onions and milk. No kidding! So for one month the only thing she ate was 1,000 calories of cream of onion soup every day. Obviously she couldn't stay on that for life, so we had to desensitize her to a whole bunch of other foods.

SS: How do you desensitize a person to food intolerances?

JW: Actually, in much the same way that "mainstream" allergists desensitize people to ragweed or whatever, with very tiny doses of ragweed antigen over a period of time.

SS: Very tiny doses of ragweed? Or pollen? Or whatever they're allergic to? Sounds suspiciously like homeopathy. . . .

JW: Shh! Don't tell anyone, but the original version of the American College of Allergy and Immunology—the name has changed several times since its inception—was started by a group that included two homeopathic doctors. Of course, no one will officially admit that today.

SS: What do you think is responsible for the epidemic of obesity in this country?

JW: Well, if you really take a look at the big upswing that started in the 1980s, it was at the same time that high fructose corn syrup came into the food supply big time. Linus Pauling said, fructose is infinitely worse for the metabolism than sucrose. There are many biochemical reasons, but fructose is much more fattening than sucrose.

SS: And it's in everything.

JW: Everything. Sure, there was obesity before then, but this was the major stimulant for the epidemic proportions. And this was also the major kickoff for diabetes. My undergraduate degree at Harvard was a twin major—premed and cultural anthropology. Medical anthropologists tell us that one-third of the population has the genetic predisposition toward diabetes, but it doesn't necessarily activate unless there are "precipitating environmental factors."

SS: So in that same vein, do you mean we could be genetically predisposed to, say, breast cancer, but it wouldn't activate unless we were exposed to or, worse, ingested chemicals?

JW: Yes. Preagricultural man who was hunting and gathering did not have many carbs because he wasn't exposed to them. We've all heard of the lean times and the fat times; those who could fatten up easily had a competitive advantage over those who could not fatten up easily. That's why there are so many of us with those genes. But now we are hit with an onslaught of carbs, carbs, carbs. In fact, it became nutritional dogma that we should all be eating diets high in complex carbohydrates. And while that may be good (if the carbs aren't refined) for two-thirds of the population who don't have that genetic predisposition, it's a disaster for the third who do have that genetic predisposition. And, of course, unnatural chemicals are toxic to man and will give your body the opportunity to activate your genetics.

I have another little tidbit you might find interesting: What is the common skin condition that is 80 percent likely to predict the presence of type 2 (adult onset) diabetes?

SS: I have no idea.

JW: It's real easy; it's those little guys called "skin tags." They usually occur on the neck, armpits, and in the groin. Some people will just have one or two, some people will have a whole crop. They're caused by a virus, but this particular virus loves the genetics that lead to blood-sugar metabolism problems. If you have skin tags your odds of getting type 2 diabetes are much higher when you're older.

SS: What is your opinion of statins?

JW: Patent-medicine statins (which are incredibly higher doses than found in nature) are awful. The worst thing patent-medicine statins do is shut down production of cholesterol, not only to the liver but to the brain. All cell membranes contain cholesterol; when brain cells are damaged, they literally try to make a little more cholesterol to repair themselves. But if that's shut down by statins they can't do so well.

You've probably heard of Dr. Duane Graveline, an astronaut and a flight surgeon. He suffered the worst example of statin toxicity. He lost his whole memory for a week and had to be hospitalized, just from one dose of statin. He has subsequently written a book called *Lipitor, Thief of Memory*.

SS: Yes, I've read that book. If 50 percent of all adults are on statins, what is going to happen to their brains in twenty years?

JW: It's going to erode their memories. Ironically, Merck & Company holds the patent on combining the natural substance coenzyme Q_{10} with statin to prevent a lot of the statin side effects, but none of their patent-medicine statins have coenzyme Q_{10}. But they do hold the patent. I've got their patent number copied into my computer. I've downloaded it from the U.S. Patent Office.

This patent prevents some of the side effects from their patent statin, so it's possible they are not using the combination of coenzyme Q_{10} and their statin because doing so might admit liability. If they release this information, everyone will know, and they may have to admit that their drug was harmful.

SS: How long has Merck held the patent combining Co-Q_{10} with statin?

JW: In 1990, two patents were issued covering the use of Co-Q_{10} in combination with statin drugs to prevent, treat, or ameliorate the complications brought on by the drugs. The first patent (U.S. Patent #4,929,437), issued by Jonathan A. Tobert and assigned to Merck & Co., clearly states that by lowering Co-Q_{10}, the statin drugs can cause predictable elevations of liver enzymes with liver damage. It also states that by giving $Co-Q_{10}$ along with the drugs, this complication can be prevented or treated if it already exists.

A month later, a second patent (#4,933,165) was issued to Nobel laureate Michael S. Brown, M.D., who is well known in scientific circles for his work in fat and cholesterol metabolism. This patent, which was also assigned to Merck, states that statin drugs, by causing a reduction in $Co-Q_{10}$, can produce complications of muscle pain, weakness, and myopathy. The patent covers a combination product of $Co-Q_{10}$ added to a statin to prevent these complications, plus the use of $Co-Q_{10}$ for the treatment of those complications.

Incredibly and inexplicably, Merck never exercised these patents, never made combination statin–$Co-Q_{10}$ products, and, even more ominous, never attempted to educate physicians or patients about the very dangerous statin–$Co-Q_{10}$ connection. Even though patients are informed of potential side effects of muscle weakness and soreness and liver-enzyme elevation, they are not told that this is likely due to the drug's reduction of $Co-Q_{10}$. Nor are they told that by supplementing with $Co-Q_{10}$ they could prevent or eliminate these problems. And there have been consequences.

SS: Tell me about the importance of cobalt.

JW: Well, and thanks for getting all this information out for your readers, every once in a while a woman takes bioidentical hormones and they don't work. It's only a small percentage of women who try bioidentical hormones, 3 percent to 4 percent. These women can take more and more and more, and it still doesn't work, or maybe it works a little bit. Here is the problem.

When these ladies do a twenty-four-hour urine test, we find that all the estrogen is in the urine. It's not staying in their bodies; it's not being retained long enough. Of course, it can't help them that way.

SS: One of the doctors I interviewed told me he had one patient for whom bioidenticals were not working. He had to give her 14 milligrams of estrogen four times a day and finally she absorbed it. So was it all going out in her pee?

JW: Yes, but he was assuming it was an absorption problem. Usually these women were Premarin (patented horse hormones) takers, which had screwed up their livers. So their livers had developed extra "muscles" to deal with it; actually it's not really muscles, it's enzymes. With all those extra enzymes, the liver just processed the weaker human estrogen (weaker than Premarin) at "superspeed," and got rid of it. These women would have 600, 800, even 1,000 or 3,000 micrograms per twenty-four hours of total estrogen (premenopausal normals are 200 to 250 micrograms per twenty-four hours) in their urine. The blood levels showed that their estrogen was low, but that was because it was all in the urine, where it is useless. So, in fact, they were absorbing it, but kicking it out.

SS: So what do these women do? They've got to have hormones.

JW: Aha. We give these women physiological doses of COBALT! Another trace element. ["Physiological" here means amounts normally found in the daily diets of some areas of the world.] This activity of cobalt was figured out by a couple of researchers named Mahin Maines and Attallah Kappas. They told us that when certain enzymes in the liver get overactive, there are several trace elements that will settle them down, and at the top of the list was cobalt.

SS: So where do we get cobalt?

JW: Unfortunately, it's not concentrated in one food, darn it. So we put women on a quantity of cobalt that's in the upper end of the physiologic range: 500 to 600 micrograms a day. Cobalt is a fairly safe trace element, so we're copying nature. We put them on cobalt and tell these women to keep taking their estrogen. The cobalt slows down the liver from kicking all the estrogen out of their bodies. When we finally get the estrogen in the urine and blood levels to optimal levels, we have them stop taking cobalt. The liver has readjusted and the cobalt is no longer necessary.

SS: And the woman did not have to take a drug. Is cobalt a prescription?

JW: Yes, back in the early fifties doctors got way too enthusiastic about cobalt. They were using it for anemia that wouldn't get better any other way. But they were giving doses of 10,000 and 30,000 micrograms a day. That level will give you heart failure, but at 600 micrograms a day it won't.

SS: Well, you are a font of information. I'm proud to know you and I admire the work you are doing. It is truly cutting-edge and progressive. It's been fascinating having this conversation with you, and I know it will be for my readers as well. How wonderful to know that we don't have to live a life of taking prescription drugs that don't heal us and that will eventually make us wacky. Of course, as I always say, there are important uses for prescription drugs, but when you can fix your body naturally without a drug, why wouldn't you want to? It is inspiring to learn that we can find safe ways to correct and replace what's wrong or missing by gathering information and then being lucky enough to find doctors such as yourself who understand that nature has provided the tools to correct the problems in our bodies.

JW: I thank you so much for getting all this information out not only to women but also to their husbands. Your work has been dramatic. The increased numbers of women who are interested in nature's approach to getting and staying well has changed drastically since your books have come out.

SS: Thank you very much, it's been a privilege. One last question . . . What in your opinion is the best thing we can teach our children?

JW: Hmm . . . The best thing we can teach our children is to take personal responsibility for their own health when they are old enough to understand how to do so and investigate, investigate, investigate. And number two, copy nature. If we copy nature, we won't go wrong!

SS: Thank you for being a great teacher.

DR. JONATHAN WRIGHT'S BREAKTHROUGH BREAKOUTS

- Instead of antibiotics, D-mannose, found in health food stores, can be effective in curing bladder infections.
- Macular degeneration often originates in the stomach due to poor nutrient digestion from lack of sufficient hydrochloric acid—IV treatments of zinc, selenium, and other minerals can *also* reverse eyesight loss.
- Hearing loss determined by lab work in older patients can be restored through replacement of the bioidentical hormone aldosterone.
- Very small doses of lithium can stave off memory loss as we age and are neuroprotective and neuroreparative.
- Iodine can cure painfully cystic breasts.
- Cell therapy can rejuvenate glands and organs that are no longer working properly.
- A way to cut down on sugar cravings is with the supplement chromium—dosages are between 5,000 and 6,000 micrograms daily until the sugar cravings stop, then they're reduced to 1,000 micrograms daily.
- Women who have been on synthetic hormones such as Premarin will often have trouble processing bioidentical estrogen. One possible solution is to try 600 micrograms of the trace element cobalt until estrogen reaches optimal levels.

3

DR. RON ROTHENBERG

Old age, like everything else, to make a success of it, you've got to start young.

    —Theodore Roosevelt

I HAVE KNOWN Dr. Rothenberg for several years. He is the Doctor Dolittle of antiaging medicine—excited, enthusiastic, knowledgeable, and the person the other doctors come to for clarification. He is a highly sought after speaker and teacher who understands thoroughly the need to approach aging not as a disease but as a condition that can be greatly slowed or reversed. Dr. Ron Rothenberg's specialty is preventive and regenerative medicine. He is also the founder of California HealthSpan Institute in Encinitas, California. His past careers include everything from pediatrics to emergency medicine, and he is a graduate of the Columbia University College of Physicians and Surgeons. He is a full clinical professor of family and preventive medicine at the University of California, San Diego (UCSD), School of Medicine.

Dr. Rothenberg is one of the first physicians to develop antiaging/preventive/regenerative programs for patients and has been doing so for the past ten years. He describes himself as an "old-timer" in this rapidly evolving field. He lectures regularly at national and international medical conferences where he shares the possibilities for this new approach to health and aging, and has educated over 25,000 physicians this way.

Dr. Rothenberg's patients are both men and women, with about one-third of them being physicians themselves. That should tell you something. From hormone replacement to nutrition, exercise, and lifestyle changes, Dr. Rothenberg's approach is cutting-edge, enabling thousands to reverse poor health, resetting them on a path where quality of life is the standard.

SS: Hello, Dr. Rothenberg, thank you once again for your time. Describe preventive and regenerative medicine.

RR: Well, it's about keeping people as happy and healthy as possible for as long as possible. The new model of medicine is about not accepting losses, but instead asking, can we actually change the process?

Up until now conventional gerontology was a matter of telling the patient, "Let's do the best we can, but you are developing osteoporosis, so just try to not fall and break a hip." Of course, we are all going to die sooner or later, but what I am doing in my practice is to maintain optimal function so the patient can stay happy and healthy until the very end. Instead of a gradual decline we want "rectangularization" of the function curve. Stay as strong, healthy, and smart as possible till the end, then fall off the curve and die fast.

SS: So, you are saying we don't have to degrade as we age. That's exciting. I don't think any of us care if we are old, we just don't want to be frail and sick. What is the difference between geriatrics and antiaging medicine?

RR: In a way, they are opposites. Geriatrics is the specialty of taking care of medical problems with elderly people. It's a disease model. Geriatrics acknowledges that the person is going to become sick and frail, and this model of medicine does its best to keep the person alive with whatever function.

Preventive/regenerative/antiaging medicine believes disease and falling apart is not the inevitability, especially if you start young enough. The sooner you start to plan against aging, the more you are able to avoid the conditions of frailty. There are only a few things that happen to people: cardiovascular disease, cancer, autoimmune disease, infectious disease, trauma, injuries, and frailty. All of these things overlap, so you've got to plan to prevent them. That is preventive medicine. Some people don't like the word "antiaging," but the concept is maintaining mental and physical function and not accepting losses without a fight.

I see in your books, Suzanne, that you connect the dots, and I try to as well. That's how this works, thinking it through. Connecting inflammation with cardiovascular disease, cancer, frailty, failure of the immune system, and preventing all of the above with a combined plan.

SS: We have to because we are living longer.

RR: Yes. Today's technology and medicine are going to keep the baby boomers alive until we are at least one hundred, like it or not. So what is the journey going to be like? We know the conventional medical model is to stay alive with disability. But who wants to stay alive with the last years in a nursing home and the last months in an intensive care unit? No one in the world. So, how does that happen? It's because today's medicine is great at keeping us alive, but the quality of life hasn't kept up. That's the gap.

SS: How much of a part do pharmaceutical drugs play in your program?

RR: Rarely, that's the beauty of this. I am not opposed to pharmaceutical drugs; they certainly can be lifesaving, but I always try natural approaches first. For example, if the patient has high blood pressure, I would try lifestyle, nutrition, exercise, amino acids, and nutraceuticals. If that approach was not effective, I would pull out the prescription drugs. I would carefully consider which one had the least side effects. I would continue preventive/regenerative programs and maybe the patient could discontinue the drugs at a later date.

Let me explain how I develop preventive/regenerative programs for patients. When a patient comes to me, I have lab test results drawn previously so I can see their hormone levels, cardiac risk factors, inflammation, and vitamin levels immediately. I get imaging studies when needed. Then an extensive medical history and physical exam, tests of biological age, nutrition, and fitness evaluation. Then we come up with a plan together.

SS: When you say patient, do you mean women's hormones or men's hormones?

RR: Yes, hormones are the backbone of my program and, yes, I do treat both men and women. My practice is evenly divided, but lately there has been a lot of fascinating new information that has come out relative to men. Both men and women need testosterone, but there have been myths about testosterone, and the old dogma goes like this: "Men have more testosterone than women, and men have more heart attacks than women, so it must be the testosterone—there must be something dangerous about it." But it's just not true. Here's the truth—it's just the opposite. In fact, andropause (failure to produce enough testosterone in men) is a dangerous disease, a critical disease, a lethal disease. First of all, did you know that testosterone is getting lower every year?

SS: What do you mean? In the general population?

RR: Yes, in the 1980s the average testosterone level in men was in the 600s or so, but when you look at men of different ages today, it's somewhere around the 400s. That is a dramatic difference.

SS: Caused by what?

RR: There are various theories. It may be caused by xenoestrogens from insecticides, plastic milk cartons, and toxins, increased stress, increased obesity. The sperm count is also going down, and hopefully we will figure out how to combat this so that there will still be a human race, but at this rate . . .

SS: How frightening.

RR: Right. The next problem is that low testosterone levels are associated with everything negative from cardiovascular disease to diabetes to cancer. Very powerful studies have come out recently concluding that high testosterone equals low mortality, meaning that the men who have the highest testosterone levels live significantly longer. An important study by K.-T. Khaw et al. was published in *Circulation*, the journal of the American Heart Association. This isn't a "fringe type" alternative study, this is mainstream medical literature sent to cardiologists. Unfortunately, many cardiologists don't read their own journals. I'm not trying to criticize, just trying to make a point. This was a ten-year study of eleven thousand men from ages forty to eighty. The results conclusively showed that the higher the testosterone levels, the lower the mortality from heart disease to cancer. The article even points out that, paradoxically, the fear of cancer has kept men away from testosterone treatment. Yet it has been proven that men with the highest testosterone have less of all types of cancer. If you do the arithmetic, at any given moment, the group with the lowest testosterone has twice the chance of dying. This is dramatic.

SS: It's dramatic, all right, but then there's the confusion. Men tell me all the time, "I have so much testosterone, and my doctor tells me I don't need any of it." Usually these are men who don't look well—I always presume that they have a high total of testosterone, but in most cases it is bound up, useless testosterone. Why are conventional doctors so ignorant of this fact?

RR: There are three possible reasons for confusing interpretations. The first is that we just don't want "normal for age." We want "optimal," which is normal for a youthful age. So a physician might tell him, you are normal for your age. But that may not be optimal, and he still could be suffering from low testosterone. You are referring to the second reason: To know the amount of testosterone that can reach the cells, you need to consider the total, free, and bioavailable testosterone. The third reason is that hormone optimization is a clinical specialty. That means that lab tests help us with a diagnosis, but as I like to say to my students, "When all else fails, look at the patient." Some patients are relatively resistant to testosterone and other hormones, and the physician needs to consider the medical history and physical exam. So the lab test could look okay but the patient does not.

The "bound up" situation goes like this: Total testosterone is the total amount in the blood, but the portion bound to a protein called sex hormone binding globulin (SHBG) cannot be used by the cells. Free testosterone is the amount floating free that the cells can use and so is a better measure of useful testosterone, but it does not consider the usable portion loosely bound to albumin. Bioavailable is the amount floating free plus the amount that is loosely bound to albumin that can be used by the cells. That is perhaps the most useful number.

As a doctor who specializes in testosterone replacement, I can read the labs and creatively determine what a man needs not only by his numbers but also by observing and listening to and examining the patient: his health, his energy, his symptoms. You don't want to bet the farm on one lab test. This is a clinical approach to medicine and labs can often be inaccurate. And remember that different patients feel best at different levels. Medicine is an art as well as a science. I want to stress that we should not "throw hormones at people." We should make a diagnosis of a deficiency disease, and if that is present, treat the deficiency with the hormone that is missing.

SS: Can you take too much testosterone? I know with women if we take too much estrogen or progesterone, we get very symptomatic, very easily.

RR: I always keep testosterone within physiologic ranges, the ranges that are present in young men. As you know, some athletes and bodybuilders overdose or abuse amounts.

SS: But what about abuse by athletes? Sometimes they use a hundred times more than what is considered optimal of steroid hormones like testosterone and human growth hormone, and, unfortunately, that is what makes the news—that is what creates the fear.

RR: With hormones there is too little, just right, and too much—which is abuse. If an athlete has a hormone deficiency, then I believe he should be able to benefit in replacement like anyone else. But sports have their rules (not mine, but theirs), and they say you can't use testosterone. Testosterone has anabolic (building muscle, bone, and cartilage) and androgenic (promoting male characteristics) actions. It is "bioidentical," and the right amount belongs in the male or female body. It is different from non-bioidentical anabolic steroids that are often used and abused by athletes. Testosterone can also be abused and can be taken in doses that are too high. In the general public and in the legislative world there is often confusion between replacement, as in the case of a hormone deficiency, and abuse. This is unfortunate because athletes are under enormous stress from their extreme situations, which can deplete hormone levels. As athletes get older, they may need replacement, but the rules don't allow it. So as a doctor, there is nothing I can do for these athletes in terms of hormone optimization because these are the rules of sports, and what is healthy is in conflict with these rules. They are two different concepts that don't meet.

SS: What about testosterone and prostate cancer?

RR: Since this is such a hot topic, let's look at the current medical literature. There is a landmark article by Morganthaler, from Harvard Medical School, called "Testosterone and Prostate Cancer: A Historical Perspective on a Modern Myth," published in 2006 in *European Urology*. This article examines why there is a myth that testosterone causes prostate cancer to grow. The key points include that there was one and only one case published in 1941 that implied testosterone caused prostate cancer to grow, since there was an equivocal rise in a blood test. Since then we have lots of cases that have shown that there is no progression of prostate cancer with testosterone administration.

So why do some doctors believe testosterone gives you prostate cancer? Where did this myth come from? Well, first we know that if you surgically castrate a man who has metastatic prostate cancer or if you use chemical castration with drugs like Lupron, the cancer will regress. But he may not have much quality of life at this point, and there are other increased risks like diabetes and heart disease.

This paradox is explained by a saturation model where there is already maximum stimulation of prostate cancer at very low levels of testosterone. Replacement of missing testosterone to youthful levels does not stimulate the cancer. Conclusion: There is not now nor has there ever been a scientific basis for the belief that testosterone causes prostate cancer to grow.

Another landmark article looks at the situation in a different way. The journal of the National Cancer Institute published an article in January 2008 that looked at data from eighteen studies and included more than three thousand men with prostate cancer and more than six thousand controls; it concluded that there was no association of the risk of prostate cancer with testosterone or free testosterone. So the scientific evidence is here now, but myths take a long time to die.

SS: So you are saying that testosterone doesn't fuel cancer—that we have cancer cells in us, but it's a matter of the immune system finding them and keeping them in check.

RR: Yes, testosterone does not fuel prostate cancer, and all cancers are less frequently seen in men with higher testosterone. A strong immune system is a determining factor—a strong immune system to keep the cancers that form at bay.

SS: Then my theory of building up my body with Iscador (which is a non-FDA-approved anthroposcopic medicine made from mistletoe that builds up your immune system to be so strong nothing can invade or attack) to fight my breast cancer was not such a crazy idea after all. I had always felt that building up was a better idea than taking poison (chemo). I took a lot of flack from the press for that one.

RR: Right. There is considerable medical literature on the benefits of mistletoe extracts as immune modulators, as well as reports of successful treatment of cancer. It is frequently used in Europe either by itself or along with conventional treatment. At this time I would not recommend treating men with active prostate cancer with testosterone, since it is so controversial, but let's follow where this goes over the next few years. You probably know my educated guess. In a basic science study reported by Gunawarden in *Cancer Prevention and Detection*, testosterone plus antioxidants promoted apoptosis (programmed cell death) of prostate cancer cells.

SS: Apoptosis is programmed cell death, as I understand it, the natural process all our cells undergo in our bodies. So that's a good thing, right? It is the normal function in each cell, and you are saying that this study says testosterone is the key factor in this process, that we all need testosterone for normal functioning.

RR: Right, apoptosis is programmed cell death, when cells take themselves apart in an orderly fashion, as opposed to necrosis, which is accompanied by inflammation. Apoptosis of cancer cells is obviously a good thing. This brings us to the inflammation connection. Chronic inflammation is associated with everything bad from heart disease to cancer to Alzheimer's. The "centerpiece" of inflammation is NFkB (nuclear factor kappa beta), and it is a factor in the cytoplasm of the cell that turns on inflammatory cytokines. Just about everything we do to stay healthy is involved in this process. What turns off NFkB and inflammatory cytokines?

- stress reduction
- exercise
- adequate sleep
- eliminating excess body fat
- keeping blood sugar low in order to stay away from diabetes

- avoiding too much animal fat in the diet
- keeping hormones balanced in the youthful range
- balanced antioxidant supplements
- omega-3 fish oil supplements
- vitamin D in optimal amounts
- resveratrol (the polyphenol in red wine)
- curcumin (in turmeric), milk thistle, and echinacea

There has been an avalanche of information in the past few years about taking resveratrol and vitamin D_3 as supplements.

SS: So, resveratrol is an important supplement, and you can find it in grape skins, right?

RR: Actually, resveratrol is found in red wine (the most is in Pinot Noir), but an optimal dose, which is much greater than you can get from wine, can be taken as a supplement. This is made from grape skins and is not the same as grape-seed extract.

SS: So NFkB *turns on* cytokines, which turn on prostate cancer, and supplementing with resveratrol *shuts off* NFkB, thereby preventing prostate cancer?

RR: I would say *helps* to prevent. It's very important. Also diet is the first step in disease prevention and health; my goal is to make my patients understand this and then make their daily regimen one with proper nutrition and exercise. Diet should be anti-inflammatory with lots of omega-3s and minimal omega-6s. Glucose and insulin should be kept under control, and in an ideal world just about all carbohydrates would be consumed in the form of vegetables. Also, no one really needs a lot of red meat.

Vegetables are needed for phase II detoxification performed by the liver. The liver doesn't get enough respect, because we could not live without it. The liver keeps us alive by removing toxins from the body that would otherwise cause cancer and inflammatory diseases. In order for the liver to perform phase II detoxification you must consume fruits and vegetables and healthy protein. If you eat organic food there will be fewer toxins and carcinogens delivered to the liver, and it will have an easier job of keeping you alive. It's a life-and-death struggle every single day. There are more potential health problems currently because of this toxic world, and it's an ongoing challenge. If you can afford it, why wouldn't you insist on organic food instead of contaminated food filled with insecticides and chemicals?

SS: But how do patients react to being "told what to do"?

RR: I try to get my patients to be more like partners in this; I don't want to speak down to them. But patients have got to want to follow an anti-inflammatory lifestyle, understand it, educate themselves, and make this their daily priority. I tell my patients, "You're in charge. I'm your consultant helping you to do this as safely as possible." I bring them information and guidance.

SS: When a patient comes to you, usually they don't have an illness. They are coming because they want to feel better to get their edge back. Where do you start?

RR: I ask them, "What do you want to do? How deeply do you want to get into this? What's your philosophy?" It's got to be in the patients' comfort zone. I never want to talk a patient into anything. They have to be completely comfortable with their preventive medicine program, with hormone optimization if it applies. If they are not sure, I say okay, think about it, and we'll talk about it later.

If they are ready to really make a change, then I have to start out with lifestyle and what improvements can be made. Saying platitudes like "eat a healthy diet" usually falls on deaf ears, so I have to get specific: Work out a nutrition plan, an exercise plan. We look at supplements and nutraceuticals based on their personal history, and we analyze the particular blood tests that would be specific to them, tests that would obtain information on their health status.

Then we talk about their hormones. I ask them about symptoms, and if what I hear from them indicates a deficiency of any hormones, I then explain what health benefits could be produced if the missing hormones were replaced. My objective is to try to get people feeling as good as possible as quickly as possible as long as it is completely safe. Right from the beginning I start with an educated guess of what will get that patient feeling right. I've been doing this awhile; based on science, based on research and lab work, I can pretty much pinpoint for each patient what their particular needs are, and then it doesn't take long to get it right.

SS: But what if a patient shows up and says, "I feel great, I'm not on any FDA drugs, I just want to stay this way." What do you do for them?

RR: In conventional medicine they call this kind of patient the "worried well." But I think that is a horrible term. I mean, what's wrong with wanting to be well? I love this type of patient because it allows me to go deeper into more cutting-edge medicine if the patient is open to it. This type of patient might be a candidate for stem-cell banking, which is a form of "biological insurance" on their future.

SS: What is an autoimmune disease?

RR: We are only as good as our *immune* systems. If you lose your immune system, as in AIDS, you can't defend yourself against all the common microbes in the world and against cancer. The other extreme is *autoimmune*, where your immune system reacts to tissues in your own body and looks at them as invaders and forms antibodies and attacks them. Autoimmune illnesses include lupus, rheumatoid arthritis, scleroderma, fibromyalgia, MS (multiple sclerosis), and Hashimoto's thyroid disease. Integrative medicine recognizes a connection between the gastrointestinal system and autoimmune disease as well.

SS: Why do so many menopausal women contract fibromyalgia?

RR: Fibromyalgia is an inflammatory state. Cancer, heart disease, dementia, and others are all inflammatory states. Fibromyalgia produces pain, especially at trigger points, and it is very much related to hormone levels. Women with fibromyalgia have more pain in the premenstrual and menstrual phase of their cycle. Pain is worse with menopause. Seems like a hormone connection—especially a progesterone deficiency, since progesterone helps women sleep naturally and decreases inflammation.

SS: Could this inflammation be rectified through replacing hormones?

RR: Very often. There are no 100 percents in medicine. But I find that more often than not it can be at least improved by hormone replacement. Thyroid is often the missing link, and thyroid resistance is associated with fibromyalgia even when the lab tests appear to be normal. Fibromyalgia, chronic fatigue syndrome, and Hashimoto's disease have overlapping symptoms and may all be part of the same condition.

A physician patient of mine came in with the complaint "I feel a hundred years old." I asked why and he said he had no energy, couldn't sleep, had no libido, had pain everywhere; he had lost his edge. This was in spite of the fact that he was doing everything he could; he was exercising, he had a low glycemic index diet, he was taking supplements. After testing, it boiled down to hormonal loss. When we put him on BHRT including thyroid, his energy came back, libido returned, pain was minimal—it was that simple.

SS: Could you catch an autoimmune disease before it had a chance to manifest, if you kept on top of your testing like CRP (C-reactive protein), which tests for inflammation?

RR: A CRP blood test is a good general measure of inflammation. But it is nonspecific. It tells you it is there, but you have to find it. Yet it is the best predictor of who's going to have a heart attack, and much more so than testing for LDL cholesterol.

But in answer to your question, which I think is "Could you prevent an autoimmune disease by staying on top of inflammation?"—I don't know. Would be nice, though. We can look for triggers of autoimmune disease with a functional medicine approach, especially gastrointestinal causes. We then can modify the patient's nutrition and lifestyle and may be able to prevent or reverse the autoimmune disease.

But now we have other tests that are "upstream" of CRP. Inflammatory cytokines: Interleukin-6 (Il-6), Interleukin-1 beta (Il-1beta), and TNF-alpha (tumor necrosis factor alpha). These are more advanced blood tests. In an advanced practice like mine, my patients are very knowledge-able (doctors, scientists, and self-taught wellness experts), and they will ask, "Hey, how about my Il-6?" These tests measure the chemical media-tors that tell the liver to make acute-phase proteins such as CRP. This test gives great insight and, as we know, if we can keep our inflammation down, it is our best bet to staying healthy. That's the exciting part of what I do; new medicine keeps advancing. Next year there will probably be an-other new test that goes even further.

SS: I find it exciting also; all of these progressive new measures are preventative and predictive, making it easier for the patient to know about a potential problem long before it becomes one. It's very clear to me that as patients we need to realize that we are the ones who have to be proactive. For the most part patients wait for the doctor to tell them what to do. This is a whole new way to approach health proactively.

RR: Absolutely. I take a deep personal interest in every one of my pa-tients, but no one will ever care as much as the patients themselves, and we docs are not mind readers (well, sometimes we are). Patients have to tell us what is going on, what they are feeling, and what they haven't mentioned. In conventional medicine the term "hypochondriac" is used a lot. Well, these often are patients who are frustrated because they want to go further in their health care but are not getting the right kind of un-derstanding. I like it when my patients communicate every symptom they are experiencing so that we can better get them to optimal health. I see people in my practice every day who understand that the only way to be and stay healthy is to constantly stay on top of their health and report everything.

SS: So you test for inflammation; then what?

RR: We test for fasting insulin. I want to see type 2 diabetes coming years before it shows up and head it off at the pass. In preventive/regen-erative medicine we watch for a gradual "creep up" of insulin levels and take steps to change the diet and lifestyle long before the numbers indi-cate any type of problem—you know, not wait until the numbers indi-cate disease. This is the most sensitive early warning.

We check for omega-3 levels. These omega-3s are building blocks for the good anti-inflammatory cytokines. Good numbers indicate someone who is going to be healthier, with less heart disease, dementia, cancer, and pain.

The evidence of taking supplemental omega-3s is dramatic.

In the GISSI Prevenzione Study in Italy, the sudden death rate of men who had previously had heart attacks was cut in half by an omega-3 sup-plement. No drug could do anything like that.

We also check for vitamin D levels. Since I began doing this, I have been astounded at how many people are dangerously low, even in south-ern California. Once again, low levels of vitamin D are associated with more cancer, heart disease, pain, osteoporosis, viral infections, and bad hair days (just kidding on the last one).

SS: Why would Californians be low in vitamin D? I mean, it comes from the sun, we get lots of sunshine in California. Is it because of sunscreen?

RR: Sunscreen does block vitamin D production. To produce vitamin D you need to sweat in the sun without sunscreen. But sun can cause photoaging (wrinkles) and skin cancers. Now, a little sun each day (about twenty minutes) is going to do you good, but if you are worried about wrinkling, then maybe you put a little sunscreen on your face. However, sunscreen applied to the skin may be absorbed into the body. My rule of thumb is, do not put anything on your skin you wouldn't eat. So you have to find that balance. Taking a vitamin D$_3$ supplement gets you the best of both worlds: the benefits of vitamin D without excess sun expo-sure. Another benefit of vitamin D is its antiviral effect. There is reason to believe that people get colds and flus in the winter because of low vita-min D levels. It's an important hormone (yes, hormone).

SS: So how much vitamin D should we take?

RR: When you spend a day in the sun in a swimsuit your body can make 10,000 to 20,000 IUs a day. A perfectly safe dose would be 10,000 IUs a day. This is much higher than what was thought safe a few years ago. The best way to know how much you need is to get the blood test for 25-hydroxy vitamin D. The reference range is 30 to 100, but health outcomes are optimal at the high end. Less cancer, less heart disease, less viral disease, less pain syndromes, more well-being.

SS: What else do you recommend in preventive medicine?

RR: I previously mentioned resveratrol, which is the polyphenol in red wine. It is thought to be the major player in "the French Paradox." That is not a movie—it is the paradox in which the French eat all those creamy sauces and other fun things, but have significantly less cardiovascular disease than Americans. This is another supplement with a wide range of benefits producing a healthier life.

SS: Please explain the mechanism of resveratrol.

RR: Here is the first question on your antiaging exam. What is the most consistent intervention that makes animals live longer and healthier? The answer is calorie restriction with adequate nutrition. Studies have shown this is effective for species that range from yeast to monkeys. If you get enough protein and vitamins and eat half of the calories, you'll possibly live to 150 years, but, of course, you will be very hungry for 150 years. Although there are "calorie restriction clubs," most people do not want to live like that and want more than a few snacks per day. But resveratrol turns on the same genes that control calorie restriction and they are called sirtuin genes, as in Sir1 and Sir2.

SS: Wait a minute. Are you saying that if you took resveratrol supplementation you would lose weight?

RR: No, sorry, not that easy. But, hey, this might even be better. You see, these sirtuin genes say, "Stay alive." What is the only way to stay alive? Don't die. Don't get cardiovascular disease, cancer, autoimmune disease, etc. This may be a way to duplicate the benefits of calorie restriction without starving.

SS: Okay, I'm not sure I am following.

RR: Resveratrol is an example of the coevolution of plants and animals. All life is in this big beautiful world together. Here is how it might have happened: Let's say the grape has a fungus on its skin and now this grape is in trouble because this fungus could kill the plant, so the grape makes resveratrol to stay alive. Resveratrol is a substance that "turns on" the same genes in a grape plant that are turned on in an animal who is starving to death due to enforced calorie restriction (no food available). This is the same gene that protects this starving animal from disease until the food supply is abundant again. The animals that got the message "The food supply is endangered; don't die or your species will be gone" are still here to tell the tale. The ones that did not get it are gone. So our mammal ancestor got the message and our genes respond to this day. When *we* take resveratrol supplements, they "turn on" the genes that protect us from disease even though we are not practicing calorie restriction. It is preventive medicine. By the way, we should not eat more calories than we need. If only I listened to my own advice.

SS: In other words, resveratrol turns on the gene in us that protects us from getting a disease such as cancer?

RR: Yes. It's a fantastic new breakthrough. Remember inflammation and NFkB that we talked about earlier? Guess what? Resveratrol turns off NFkB and inflammation. You can get it from red wine, but it's better to take it in capsule form. All of us should be taking this supplement.

SS: Let's talk about hormone replacement.

RR: I thought you'd never ask. The benefits of bioidentical hormone replacement in women are overwhelming. Once again, we are not "throwing hormones at you," we are treating a deficiency disease when present by replacing the hormones that are missing. Many excellent physicians are not aware of the current data supporting this medical intervention. The benefits include elimination of vasomotor symptoms such as hot flashes and night sweats, the reversal of bone loss, improved sleep, emotional stability, better brain function, increased libido, and improved quality of life.

SS: But everyone still seems to be worried about increasing the chances of breast cancer.

RR: They shouldn't be. In 2005, the Fournier Study in the *International Journal of Cancer* followed 54,000 women who were taking bioidentical estrogen and either bioidentical progesterone or *progestin*. *Progestins* are nonbioidentical fake progesterone. The women taking the bioidentical progesterone had a 10 percent *decrease* in the risk of breast cancer and the women taking the synthetic progestin had a 40 percent *increase* in the risk of breast cancer. An extension of this study, published in 2007 in *Breast Cancer Research and Treatment*, looked at 80,000 women. Those on bioidentical estrogen and progesterone had no increase in the rate of breast cancer, those on an artificial progestin had an incease of 69 percent in the risk of breast cancer.

SS: I know of this study and the information is significant and impressive. If this information were mainstream, it would eliminate the fear that doctors have due to lack of proper information. As a result of ignorance, patients get frightened away from hormones, which is truly unfortunate because it causes so many to suffer needlessly. I suspect the pharmaceutical companies have something to do with these significant studies getting buried. It is not in their interest for us to have access to inexpensive nonpatentable medicine. We only hear about the horrors of synthetic hormones from groups like the Women's Health Initiative, but that study and others never offer an alternative; they never do studies on bioidentical hormones and their tremendous benefits, so patients, and women in particular, are afraid and confused. As a result, women are suffering needlessly.

RR: Exactly. There is also another study, the de Lignières Study from *Climacteric* (2002), that concluded that the risk of breast cancer is not increased with bioidentical hormones but is increased with synthetic progestin. It's very clear to me that the problem is with synthetic progestin. Studies also show that the higher the progesterone levels over the course of a woman's life, including pregnancy, the greater protection from cancer. Real bioidentical progesterone prescribed properly is protective.

SS: Well, that would explain my scenario. I was estrogen dominant in my thirties and forties. I suspect it was brought on by the nasty birth control pills I took for so long that contained progestins. [Estrogen dominance, for my readers' sake, means that my body was not manufacturing enough progesterone.] I was diagnosed with breast cancer when I was in my early fifties, but was told that my tumor was ten years old, determined by the size. If only I had known two things: not to have taken birth control pills, and to *have* taken bioidentical progesterone to make up for what my body was not producing in perimenopause. When I think back on it, I had so many symptoms: irritability, depression, weight gain, lack of libido, tender cystic breasts. Progesterone replacement would have balanced out the ratio of estrogen to progesterone to levels dictated by nature in healthy women.

This is what excites me now: Young women, who are lucky to find qualified doctors such as yourself, have the opportunity to avoid this fate because you will know if a woman is estrogen dominant, and you can then simply rectify the matter before there is a problem by giving her bioidentical progesterone. Again, prevention!

Let's talk about stem-cell banking.

RR: When my patients who are hormonally balanced and taking the optimal nutraceuticals ask me "What's next?" I tell them, "Banking your own adult stem cells." This is so exciting because soon the stem cells will be cures for cancer, autoimmune illness, and heart disease. They have been used for years for bone marrow transplants for treatment of blood cancers like leukemia and lymphoma. Current studies are under way showing that heart function can be restored after heart attacks and heart failure.

What is new is the idea to bank your stem cells when you are perfectly healthy and have them stored as "biological insurance." They can be easily collected from the blood through an intravenous line.

SS: Are stem cells a treatment for autoimmune diseases?

RR: Regenerating bone marrow with transplanted stem cells can normalize the immune system and stop the autoimmune process. Patients with multiple sclerosis, rheumatoid arthritis, scleroderma, lupus, and type 1 and type 2 diabetes have been treated successfully in ongoing studies.

SS: Is there any way we can make more of these stem cells ourselves?

RR: When I lecture, I tell all the docs that they are already stem cell doctors; I tell them fish oil turns on stem cells in the brain, and testosterone turns on satellite cells, which are the stem cells in muscle. Optimal hormones and exercise turn on epithelial progenitor cells (EPCs). EPCs are the body's built-in system for repair of your cardiovascular system. They are a biomarker of wellness, meaning that the better the quantity and quality of your EPCs, the healthier you are. Exercise, nutrition, and nutraceuticals all can increase the quantity and quality of your stem cells. Blueberries, green tea, vitamin D_3, omega-3 fish oil, and resveratrol all increase your stem cells.

SS: What else? What about embryonic versus adult stem cells?

RR: There is a lot of confusion on this topic. There are two kinds of stem cells, those derived from embryos and those from other sources. Even if the stem cells are from umbilical cords or placentas or amniotic fluid, they are referred to as adult stem cells. All stem cells can divide and renew themselves; they are not differentiated into specific types, and they have the ability to develop into specialized cells. As of now, much more research needs to be done before embryonic stem cells can be used. There are currently no approved treatments or human trials using embryonic stem cells. Since adult stem cells do not come from embryos, there should be no ethical controversy. So the action right now is with adult stem cells, the kind that can be collected from your own blood. They have the potential to form all tissues as well.

SS: Everything, as in any body part?

RR: The potential is there, as well as the potential for rejuvenation treatments, to reverse aging. Also embryonic-like stem cells have been recently discovered in adult bone marrow, called VSELs, very small embryonic-like cells.

SS: This sounds fantastic for our soldiers returning with missing body parts. Have these VSELs been used yet?

RR: Not yet.

SS: But adults can bank their own adult stem cells as a biological insurance.

RR: Yes, and right now we've got all these FDA-approved uses such as for cancer, wound and bone healing, radiation emergencies, and experimental uses I mentioned earlier.

SS: Have you stored your stem cells?

RR: Oh yes, I banked them with the NeoStem Company, who I know you have interviewed for this book.

SS: Yes, and I, too, have banked my stem cells with the NeoStem Company. They are very excited about their company and the good it is doing. The future possibilities are mind-boggling. What will aging look like in the future?

RR: It won't look like much. It will be the ageless society. Someone who is fifty or sixty or seventy or maybe eighty won't look that different from someone who is forty. At least he won't feel that different. Of course, there will be more accumulated scars from surfboards and snowboards, but aging people will be able to do the same things they love both physically and mentally. The exciting part is that an aging person will have life experiences, hopefully some wisdom, yet they will have youthful bodies inside and out, kind of the best of both worlds.

It's all about energy and health, and the medicine we are able to practice right now is preserving energy and health. I see it every day: healthy, happy people. I never saw this before in my practice, especially in this age group. It's wonderful.

As I said earlier, a lot of my patients are docs and they were the ones who saw that *I* was changing when I started my antiaging preventive/regenerative program over ten years ago. They asked things like "Hey, what pill are you taking?" But it's not a pill, it's nothing you can just mention while casually walking through hospital corridors. It's a whole spectrum: nutrition, exercise, replacing hormones, detoxification, sleep, eliminating stress, taking advantage of the new cutting-edge approach to health. It's true health care. It's not about drugs, it's not about surgery, it's all of the above, and a true commitment to your health.

SS: You bet. How wonderful for your patients that you are so forward thinking. Not only are you taking advantage of the latest and greatest breakthroughs, but you also have your finger on the pulse of what's around the corner. I'm sure that is why so many of your patients are doctors. Thanks so much.

RR: You're welcome, Suzanne. I love what I do.

DR. RON ROTHENBERG'S
BREAKTHROUGH BREAKOUTS

- Geriatrics is the specialty of taking care of medical problems with elderly people—it expects the elderly will become sick and frail, and does its best to keep people alive, sometimes regardless of their level of function. Preventive/regenerative/antiaging medicine believes sickness and frailty are not inevitable, and works early to prevent the problems associated with aging.

- Low testosterone levels are associated with negative conditions from cardiovascular disease to diabetes to cancer; new studies conclude that men who have the highest free-testosterone levels live significantly longer.

- Testosterone replacement is critical for long life and good health.

- Testosterone does not cause prostate cancer.

- Resveratrol, the polyphenol in red wine, when taken in high doses as a supplement, activates the genes that protect against disease, promote extreme long life, and reduce inflammation.

- Vitamin D replacement is crucial to protect against breast, colon, and prostate cancers.

- To fight toxicity and free radicals, it is essential to supplement with antioxidants, omega-3 fish oils, vitamin D_3 in optimal amounts (10,000 IUs), resveratrol, curcumin, milk thistle, and echinacea.

- Keep hormones balanced with bioidenticals in optimal youthful ranges.

- Have a CRP (C-reactive protein) blood test to check for inflammation.

- Bank your stem cells when you are healthy and have them stored as "biological insurance." Stem cells have been used for bone marrow transplants to treat blood cancers like leukemia and lymphoma. And in the future we might discover how to use them to cure cancer, autoimmune illnesses, and heart disease.

4

WHAT I DO: MY REGIMEN

PEOPLE ARE ALWAYS ASKING ME, "What do you do? What is your regimen?" We are all unique individuals, and every "body" requires its own recipe for wellness. I will share with you my daily and monthly regimen as an example of how I live a breakthrough life. In the introduction you saw my vision of how I will be living my life in my nineties. This chapter shows you exactly what I do now on a daily basis so I can realize my healthy and alert future. You will need to find a qualified doctor, perhaps someone mentioned in this book or recommended in the resources section, and create with him or her your own wellness program. It doesn't take much time each day, but it does take diligence. If you are to embrace wellness, then you must be consistent. The payoff is huge. You will not believe how well you will feel. You will not believe the energy you will regain. You will not believe how your life and outlook will change while your health soars.

The 8 Steps to Wellness guide me as I put my regimen together with my doctor—they are my blueprint for what I want to achieve.

WHAT I DO DAILY

On most mornings I wake up, look at the clock, and think to myself, "How great," 6:30 A.M. I go to bed at 9:30 most nights, which means I had another good nine hours of sleep. Perfect. Just like the night before that and the night before that. In fact, most nights I sleep nine hours. Thank you, bioidentical hormones! It was never like this before. I had years of restless sleep, long before I recognized hormonal loss as the culprit. I never understood during those years when I wanted to tear my hair out that one day I could feel this good again. I felt like I was going crazy. I couldn't sleep . . . I just couldn't sleep!

FIRST REGIMEN OF THE DAY: human growth hormone (HGH) injection. I take 0.08 mg determined by my IGF-1 deficiency. I always take HGH alone and a half hour before I take anything else. The needle is so small I hardly feel it.

I look over at my sleeping husband. "I'm in the mood," I think to myself. Thank you once again, bioidentical hormones. I thought these feelings were gone forever. Now they are not only back but with a vengeance. Is my husband a happy guy! And so am I. How wonderful to feel this way again all because I got my hormones balanced.

I get out of bed to start my day and catch a glimpse of myself in the mirror. A few years ago, all I would see is my waist getting thicker and my thighs beefing up, and the vision was not a pleasant one. This morning's glimpse makes me think to myself, "Not bad!" Not bad for a female of any age. My waist is small, my stomach tight, my rear end has definition. Thank you, HGH, plus my yoga and my walking program and my good diet of real food. Somersizing is still working for me after fifteen years.

A half hour has passed and while Alan makes his incredible coffee, I rub on my daily prescribed amount of estrogen cream. Starting today, and for the next two weeks, I will also apply progesterone cream to my other arm.

I rub a little glutathione cream on the skin on top of my liver to stimulate it, and then I drink a glass of water with a fresh-squeezed lemon to get my liver ready for the onslaught of the day. Then I take my twice-a-day ½ teaspoon of resveratrol powder, mixed with a little water, for disease prevention.

The doorbell rings. It's my yoga teacher, Julie. I always look forward to yoga and love that Alan does it with me. I can't believe the difference yoga has made in both our bodies, with seemingly very little effort! It's something about the breath. Getting that oxygen deep between the spaces, you can feel the fat melting with each deep breath. Yoga also calms me; it gets rid of the "noise" that is constantly running through my brain. One hour of yoga is a treat. Just the act of breathing forces me to focus and concentrate. No room for all those other thoughts . . . just thoughts of health, and breath, and being limber, and healing.

After yoga Alan makes a fresh fruit smoothie—yum! Mangoes and papaya juice this morning, thick and smooth and sweet. Perfect for swallowing my supplements and vitamins. I space it out so that the last delicious sip coincides with the last vitamin. Okay, that's done. Taking vitamins is not my favorite activity, but I think of the benefits of each one as I take them. I find it helps if I read my personalized supplement vitamin readout while taking them. One at a time, I visualize each pill doing exactly what it promises. I know I feel better because of this supplementation. Whenever I have stopped my supplements in the past, for whatever reason, I lose energy. It makes sense, given the pollution and chemicals we are bombarded with on a daily basis. Our food supply takes the same beating. I feel we have no choice but to try to replicate what we should be getting if our diets were perfect and if the food supply were not contaminated. With my schedule I do the best I can, eating only organic when I am at home and cooking myself. When I'm on the road, it's pretty difficult to find organic food at the local Hilton, although I'd be happy to pay extra if they provided it.

Breakfast today is two fried organic eggs sitting on top of a nest of crispy browned fried onions, sautéed organic chicken sausage, and yummy sliced heirloom tomatoes topped with a drop of olive oil, basil pesto, and a little bit of crumbled feta. I don't fool around. I love my breakfast, and all this great fresh organic food is going to give me energy to get through the next few hours.

Today is a three-shot day . . . again. Do I love having shots? No, of course not, but once again it's part of the routine to which I have subscribed for perfect vibrant health. I am fine-tuning my health. I am trying my best to stay several steps ahead of the diseases that are trying to swallow all of us.

SHOT 1: Vitamin B_{12} and vitamin B complex mixed together in one syringe. I come from an Irish family; the Irish often have high homocysteine levels. High levels of homocysteine are responsible for heart attacks and stroke. My family has a tendency to die of stroke—both of my parents did. My blood work has shown I have a severe vitamin B deficiency. Knowing that I have a deficiency, and that vitamin B shots lower homocysteine levels, why wouldn't I do it? If this keeps me from having a heart attack, it's worth it. Plus it speeds up my metabolism, which makes the weight melt off!

SHOT 2: Iscador. Having been diagnosed with breast cancer in April 2000, and having chosen to treat my cancer by keeping my hormones at perfect levels and ratios instead of with chemo, I felt that augmenting my body with Iscador was a winning choice for me. Iscador is made from mistletoe extract and has been used in the Rudolph Steiner Clinics in

Europe since the 1920s in lieu of chemotherapy, producing the same results as chemo but without its nasty side effects. Iscador builds up your immune system to be so strong that nothing can invade or attack. Looking at my options for surviving cancer, building up made more sense to me than poisoning my body. So yes, I feel good about my every-other-day shot of Iscador. I have been cancer free for eight years and my health is perfect. Something's working. Since I have been injecting Iscador, I have not had so much as a cold. Yes, it's worth a moment of discomfort for this protection.

SHOT 3: Human growth hormone (HGH). As I mentioned previously, I take HGH first thing each morning. Oh me, oh my, why does this wonderful hormone get such a bad rap? It's because of overuse by athletes, who often take a hundred times more than what their bodies require. As you'll learn in this book, hormones are not to be played around with. Hormones should be replaced only if there is a deficiency and only in the amount each person requires. Not too much and not too little. As I said, I have an HGH deficiency, as indicated by my blood work and low IGF-1 levels. We make our maximum human growth hormone between ages twenty and thirty. After that we start to decline. You will learn in this book that the sooner you replace a declining hormone, the better health you can maintain.

Since I have been injecting HGH, my entire hormone composition has normalized and equalized. I have finally found the missing piece to the entire "hormone song." Now with the addition of HGH I truly feel "perfect." And it's never been easier to be and stay as thin and energized as I was at my optimal prime. It is fantastic to be able to "fill the tank," as they say. Top it off . . . when the gas tank in your car gets low, you top it off. Do the same with your body. That's it. The hormones and vitamins take about twenty minutes. Yoga is an hour. Breakfast, a half hour. On the days I don't do yoga I try to walk for forty minutes.

The thing is, I enjoy all of it—the great sleep, the satisfaction of replacing real hormones, my happy mood, the great libido, the enjoyment of finding a type of exercise I love to do, and eating a wonderful, delicious, nutritious breakfast. I'm ready for the day . . . a long day, full of energy and vitality, with a brain that is working at optimum. I feel a spring in my step, a joy. I have love in my life. Life is good and I'm privileged to be living it.

I can understand that when you are reading this it all sounds like too much work. When you realize what is available to you, that you can fine-tune your health by taking advantage of this breakthrough medicine and achieve perfect vibrant health, the results are worth the effort. Remember what your grandfather used to say, "As long as you have your health." He was right. Without health we have nothing. With vibrant health, we are living at optimum. Nothing is free. But taking these steps promises a better, healthier, happier, fuller, satisfying life.

WHAT I DO ON A MONTHLY BASIS

Every month I go to Dr. Michael Galitzer for my tune-up. He tests me for fatigue and to see that all my organs are working optimally. Any gland or organ that shows weakness or fatigue is the one we target with appropriate intravenous treatments.

If I have been traveling a lot during the month, which usually involves airplanes, changing time zones, restaurant food, more wine than usual, coupled with the stress that is part and parcel of my lifestyle and work, I find it comforting to go to the doctor to stay well and build up with vitamin C and glutathione intravenously. Sometimes we do chelation if I have been performing or around people who are smoking. I go "on" for a living, and enjoyable as it is, it also taxes my nervous system and wears me out physically and emotionally. In essence, it breaks me down. Anti-aging medicine builds me up. Makes sense, doesn't it?

If I have been having a glass or two of wine after my nightly show, my body reacts. Wine affects my liver and weakens it, so I promise my doctor to do better next time and then we "feed" me homeopathic liver-stimulating drops and usually an IV of glutathione and vitamin C. When I leave his office, I feel great. Energized . . . uplifted . . . healthy.

During the year I look into treatments that are in the future. I have been using nanotechnology patches, which I will explain in this book, for energy, pain, and sleep. It's so great to regenerate energy without drugs, to eliminate pain without drugs, and to sleep without drugs. I have also banked my stem cells for the future. I explain this later in the book. All I know is if, God forbid, I ever need a new organ or eyes, or teeth, or skin, or limbs that I can have my own banked stem cells injected. When you get turned on by this new medicine, you will, like me, keep digging deeper to take advantage of the newest nondrug technologies.

My daily and monthly plans pull together everything I need to live the breakthrough life. In the following chapters you will find out more about the 8 Steps to Wellness and how you, too, can live the breakthrough life. Because of this new medicine I truly believe I will live out my long life in good health and enjoyment. Living to 90, 100, or 120 is the new possibility.

Why, you ask, would we want to live that long? You don't have a choice. Technology has provided MRIs, CAT scans, sophisticated blood tests, and antibiotics, to name a few, all of which prolong our lives. This is a good thing. But, like it or not, you often are coerced by fear into taking advantage of these advances. This is the way medicine is presently conducted in our country. No one is ever told anymore to go home, drink lots of fluids, and get plenty of rest. Instead we are given a host of pharmaceuticals that usually create side effects and dependencies. The patient is left with a body that has been cut up, poisoned, drugged, sewn together, in pain, leading to a general overall deterioration of quality of life, yet this person is kept alive with machines and feeding tubes.

By embracing your good health now while you are still in good shape, you will protect your long future. You can't enter your older years with a weak body and expect to be vibrant and healthy. You must begin now—it does take some effort, but the payoff is tremendous.

The medicine practiced in America today is fifty years behind the times. We are the best when it comes to surgery, but we must ask ourselves, why is so much surgery being done? If we truly practiced health care, we could prevent many of the conditions requiring surgery. Proaction is the answer to prevention; surgery is the end result of decline. Decline is preventable if you are willing to put in the effort. It's up to you.

5

BILL FALOON

Anything one man can imagine, other men can make real.

–Jules Verne, *Around the World in Eighty Days* (1873)

IT IS IMPOSSIBLE to discuss the thrills and benefits of an antiaging, break-through approach to medicine and health in this new millennium without being introduced to Bill Faloon.

In many ways, Bill Faloon is able to do what no doctor is capable of achieving. When doctors take a radical stand against the establishment, they risk being ostracized, ridiculed, shunned, and marginalized. Both Bill Faloon and I have nothing but admiration for the brave and courageous doctors in this book who fearlessly declare that a change is necessary and essential if mankind is to survive. It's that serious.

Bill Faloon is fearless. He is knowledgeable, and doctors respect him; he is known and recognized by doctors as a true font of breakthrough medical information. Bill, through his remarkable magazine, *Life Extension*, is able to give voice to the most cutting-edge doctors and new thinking. His nonprofit organization has been able to scientifically prove the benefits of supplementation, bioidentical hormones, and natural approaches to health and healing. He also focuses on prevention, which in so many instances is the answer to our health problems.

I first became aware of Bill Faloon more than a decade ago. I know of no one more dedicated to the truth. He and his company spend countless millions on research every year, looking for the answers to extending life and substantiating the efficacy of quality supplements. Indeed, people are living longer, but it's by jumping on this fast-moving train and embracing prevention—by recognizing that the old ways are no longer relevant—that we can now expect not only a long life but also robust health and supreme quality of life.

In 1980 Bill Faloon and the Life Extension Foundation joined together to uncover pioneering approaches for preventing and treating the diseases of aging. Bill is passionate about living longer with health, and is the editor of *Life Extension* magazine, a journal that is printed monthly and is arguably the most impressive gathering of cutting-edge medical information in the country. In 2003 Bill Faloon compiled a 1,500-page medical reference book titled *Disease Prevention and Treatment*, dedicated to enlightening the world about lifesaving therapies.

Where I once eagerly awaited the arrival of my monthly *Elle* magazine, I now await *Life Extension*, because I know I am going to learn something new that will change my personal approach to health and wellness. Every month it is filled with information that will improve the quality of your life, and in many instances, it will save your life.

If I could recommend one thing to you, it would be to subscribe to this wonderful magazine. Bill Faloon is remarkable in his grasp of the newest lifesaving therapies. This interview was very eye-opening and impressive.

SS: Thank you for your time, Bill. I know putting out a monthly magazine does not give you much breathing space. Tell me about *Life Extension* magazine. I know it is part of a nonprofit organization dedicated to slowing the process of aging, but how did you get started?

BF: Back in 1980 a man named Saul Kent and I gathered together a group of people who wanted to slow aging and who didn't want the typical odds of contracting disease to affect us. There were about three hundred of us who wanted to improve those odds, so we worked together in a loose-netted confederation: talking on the phone, corresponding by regular mail, and exchanging information. We had doctors, research scientists, and plenty of interested passionate laypeople who just didn't like the odds that they were supposed to contract cancer with a one-in-three chance in their lifetime—and if not cancer, certainly some vascular event if they lived long enough.

None of us liked these inevitabilities, so we wanted to see how we could prevent these age-related pathologies; or if we did contract these diseases, what could be done to better treat them.

SS: That was pretty cutting-edge thinking for twenty-eight years ago.

BF: Well, we knew that there was an abundance of information that was being ignored by the conventional establishment. Back in the 1970s people had more respect for conventional medicine than they do right now, so we were very much revolutionaries. We didn't believe that conventional doctors had all the answers. For instance, when we would go into a hospital and look at the chart of a member in our network, we would see, for instance, a patient who was anemic and obviously malnourished. Simple problems like this, if corrected, could result in patients getting *out* of the hospital, as opposed to continuing their downward spiral until they no longer lived.

SS: So, how has medicine changed today?

BF: It's not changed a lot. There is a substantial increase in scientific knowledge about what can be done to better prevent and treat disease. Unfortunately, that knowledge is not being translated into clinical settings. It's shocking that we've got all this good science and so little of it is being translated into clinical medical practice.

SS: Why?

BF: You have to understand that economic motivation has been a big factor for the last twenty or thirty years for a lot of our doctors. That has been regrettable. Being a great doctor is a calling to treat people better, to discover new ways of curing disease—but today, you get a lot of doctors who are in it for the money. Of course, there are many other well-meaning doctors who are very sincere, but we find they are usually overwhelmed by the bureaucracy that has occurred with HMOs, Medicare, and insurance regulations that constrain what today's dedicated doctors can do for the patient.

SS: So, has medical practice transformed over the last thirty years to the *detriment* of the patient?

BF: Yes. Patients are suffering in a major way, and they are not getting individualized care. They're not being paid attention to as individuals. They are pretty much put on an assembly line. If a cardiovascular doctor is treating heart patients, he'll probably prescribe the exact same dose of a statin drug to every single one of his patients.

SS: Interesting. Much like the way hormone treatment has been for women.

BF: It's exactly the same. The doctor will often write the same prescription for every patient. In some cases, it lowers their cholesterol so much it puts them in a danger range. In other cases, it causes all kinds of side effects that weren't ever necessary if the patient's individual response was closely followed and dose adjustments were made.

SS: Here's a question you may not want to answer: Is there any kind of incentive for doctors to write prescriptions for certain pharmaceuticals?

BF: Oh, major incentives. In the past, "high prescribing" doctors were often given incentives like free vacations. Today, the incentives are more indirect, but the drug company influence is still very strong. For example, doctors can get their continuing education medical credits taken care of by being flown to seminars where paid speakers talk about the benefits of specific drugs, and they get taken out for nice dinners where salesmen talk about the benefits of brand drugs. For physician-scientists, pharmaceutical companies offer to support their research. This creates tremendous pressure on doctors to publish good results on a pharmaceutical company's drug. If your research funding is from a pharmaceutical company selling a drug, and your research suggests the drug doesn't work as well as advertised or the drug causes a bad side effect, how objective can you be?

SS: Then for many doctors and the patients who place their trust in them, the "art of medicine" has been compromised.

BF: In a major way. There is no economic incentive for doctors to treat patients better. They don't get paid more for saving lives, and as a result, they have fallen into an assembly-line mentality where the more patients they can treat in a given day, the more money they make. If they do try to spend some extra time with patients, they wind up not making as many dollars.

SS: Hopefully, a magazine like yours, *Life Extension*, will educate patients as to what they should be doing in case they realize their doctor or doctors have deficiencies; then the patients themselves can fill in the gaps. That is not a bad thing. I believe it is crucial that patients take control of their own health and not leave it up to someone who could never know their bodies as they know themselves.

In the twenty-eight years that you've been involved in this cutting-edge medicine, what have you yourself embraced by being around all these brilliant medical minds?

BF: *The most valuable knowledge I have acquired is understanding that consuming the wrong kinds of foods increases my risk of contracting lethal disease, while eating a healthy diet promotes youth and longevity. When it comes to cancer, eating the wrong foods can enable existing cancer cells to propagate in a way that can overwhelm the patient, whereas healthier dietary patterns can help eradicate the disease.*

Because of these basic understandings of the mechanisms involved in age-related disease processes, it enables us at Life Extension to see what foods cause disease and what foods keep us healthy. We have prepared flowcharts that show what happens when too many of the wrong foods are ingested. These charts demonstrate how toxic foods adversely affect our bodies, so that people can understand the critical importance of eating a healthy diet.

SS: Give me an example.

BF: All right, take a basic dinner: steak, baked potato, with omega-6 fats in your salad dressing, and dessert. What happens is that a horrendous process goes on in your body: You dramatically increase your cancer and vascular risks.

People are not aware of how many omega-6 fats are in our diets. When you eat in a restaurant, you can be sure the vegetables are not organic; they've likely been sprayed with pesticides. The steak most likely isn't organic, and it is very often tenderized with MSG, a nerve toxin. And a typical salad dressing—even if it says olive oil—often is diluted with other vegetable oils loaded with omega-6 fats. Yet you think you are eating something healthy. With their high-glycemic load, potatoes and most desserts facilitate a surge in your blood sugar level, and this in turn prompts excess insulin secretion. When you add up the effects of the high-glycemic load and the omega-6 fats, you are building up arachidonic acid in your body—a precursor to many inflammatory mediators, including those involved in atherosclerosis and cancer. The glutamate toxicity from the MSG is a major assault on your health. Glutamates are damaging and dangerous, and people must be educated to understand this.

SS: So how do we protect ourselves?

BF: You avoid ingesting toxic foods. You can supplement with a type of vitamin B_{12} called methylcobalamin, which is the neurologically active form of B_{12}. It has a remarkable effect of protecting against glutamate toxicity. The most important factor, however, is learning that many foods you think are okay are really quite dangerous.

SS: Let's talk about polyunsaturated oils. Many people believe they are heart-healthy oils.

BF: The problem is that most polyunsaturated oils—be they safflower oil, soybean oil, corn oil, or sunflower oil—are loaded with omega-6 fatty acids. People today are ingesting way too many of these omega-6s in their diets and relatively little omega-3 fatty acids. This imbalance leads to a host of problems, including an excess production of arachidonic acid in the body, which can be converted into the toxic inflammatory mediators responsible for most of the diseases that people encounter today. The charts here reprinted from *Life Extension* magazine provide a striking look as to how excess dietary consumption of refined vegetable oils rich in omega-6 fats, high-glycemic foods, and foods high in arachidonic acid can increase the risk of cancer, vascular diseases, arthritis, and a host of other degenerative conditions.

SS: Explain to us, what are omega-3s?

BF: We get omega-3s primarily in coldwater fish, but the *Perilla* and flax plants also provide omega-3s. You have to intentionally introduce omega-3s into most diets. The most efficient way is to use coldwater fish as your protein source and then take fish oil capsules to make sure you are getting enough. You want to avoid saturated fat–containing foods like red meat and full-fat dairy products. You also want to avoid foods that contain arachidonic acid like egg yolks, poultry skin, and organ meats. In response to excess levels of arachidonic acid, certain enzymes that pro-

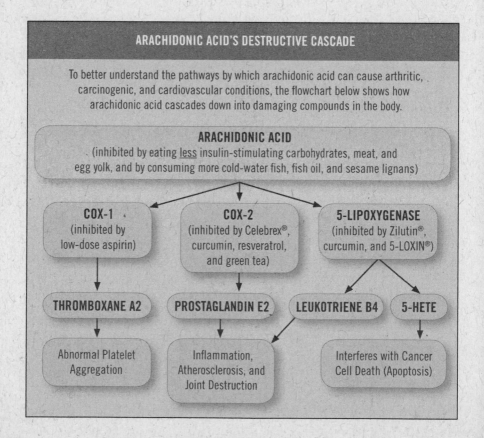

ARACHIDONIC ACID'S DESTRUCTIVE CASCADE

To better understand the pathways by which arachidonic acid can cause arthritic, carcinogenic, and cardiovascular conditions, the flowchart below shows how arachidonic acid cascades down into damaging compounds in the body.

ARACHIDONIC ACID
(inhibited by eating <u>less</u> insulin-stimulating carbohydrates, meat, and egg yolk, and by consuming more cold-water fish, fish oil, and sesame lignans)

COX-1
(inhibited by low-dose aspirin)

COX-2
(inhibited by Celebrex®, curcumin, resveratrol, and green tea)

5-LIPOXYGENASE
(inhibited by Zilutin®, curcumin, and 5-LOXIN®)

THROMBOXANE A2

PROSTAGLANDIN E2

LEUKOTRIENE B4

5-HETE

Abnormal Platelet Aggregation

Inflammation, Atherosclerosis, and Joint Destruction

Interferes with Cancer Cell Death (Apoptosis)

mote inflammation and fuel cancer cell propagation increase in your body, predisposing you to serious age-related disorders.

SS: As for flax, I put flax oil in my morning smoothie. And of course, olive oil is so delicious; I just never realized that it might be diluted with cheap, omega-6-rich vegetable oil to keep the price down. This is one place you don't want to cut corners.

BF: Olive oil is a very important food constituent to include in your diet; it's monounsaturated. You just have to be careful and read labels.

SS: Cancer. It's everywhere. Are there any natural breakthroughs you've come across that protect or help reverse?

BF: Cimetidine, which is the generic name for Tagamet. You can buy it over the counter. If you have the most common form of colon cancer and you've had surgery to remove the primary tumor, most antiaging doctors recommend 800 milligrams of cimetidine each night for a year. A study published in 2002 showed that overall your chances of surviving for ten years are 85 percent if you take cimetidine, compared to only 49 percent if you don't take it. The study also showed that in colon cancer patients who expressed high levels of a specific protein on the surface of

CANCER-PROMOTING EFFECTS OF 5-LOX		
Tumor Growth Factor	Cellular Effects	Inhibited by
Epidermal Growth Factor (EGF)	Stimulates tumor cell proliferation	5-LOXIN®
Vascular Endothelial Growth Factor (VEGF)	Stimulates angiogenesis, tumor growth, and metastasis	5-LOXIN®
Tumor Necrosis Factor-Alpha (TNF-α)	Induces matrix metalloproteinases, increases invasiveness and metastasis;	5-LOXIN®
	induces NF-kappaB, increases cell adhesion molecules (I-CAM, V-CAM)	5-LOXIN®

5-lipoxygenase (5-LOX) acts as biological fuel for cancer cells by stimulating EGF (epidermal growth factor), VEGF (vascular endothelial growth factor), and other growth factors. Tumor growth factors that enhance cancer cell proliferation, invasiveness, and metastasis can be inhibited by a natural product called 5-LOXIN®.

their cancer cells the ten-year survival benefit was 95 percent for the cimetidine group, compared to only 35 percent for the group that did not take cimetidine. Cimetidine interferes with cancer cell progression via multiple pathways, costs very little, and is relatively side effect free.

Our magazine has been publishing this kind of information going back to 1985 about the benefits for many types of novel cancer therapies, yet oncologists have routinely ignored this lifesaving data despite its being published in their own medical journals.

SS: It's ignored because it's over the counter?

BF: It's ignored because there is no drug company recommending it to the oncologists. The doctors don't hear about it at their seminars; they seldom have the time to read their own medical journals; and when they do read them, they fail to translate that material into the patient setting. There is just a lot of apathy in the medical profession these days.

SS: Because it's easier to do it the way they've always done it?

BF: It's easier and more profitable. Back in 2000, Suzanne, we set up a medical center, and we put a lot of money into the infrastructure of the place. The idea was to treat cancer the right way. The problem was we could not get a qualified oncologist in there. The really good ones had their own practices, and when we sought oncologists from the large establishment cancer centers and tried to persuade them to work at our new treatment facility, they all flunked our interview test.

SS: What do you mean?

BF: These doctors were looking to treat high-volume cases and administer lots of chemotherapy. In fact, the first thing they asked us was about their chemotherapy "bonuses." It turns out that a big part of these doctors' salaries comes in the form of how much chemotherapy they administer. Chemo is big profit.

SS: If the public knew this, they would be shocked. I'm shocked. When you are diagnosed with cancer, you are so vulnerable and trusting.

BF: When Life Extension tried to open a world-class cancer center in 2000, we had all these doctors telling us how much money we could make if we just set up the assembly line. We kept telling them, that's not why we are doing this. Interestingly, most of these doctors confidentially told us, "If someone in my family had cancer, I would send them here." That's how little confidence they had in their own practice.

The most shocking call I received was from someone who had the most efficient moneymaking business of all. He had an "in home" chemotherapy setup. He felt with Life Extension's credibility we would be sending his nurses all over town administering chemo to hundreds of cancer patients. He was talking to the wrong person, of course, but he really thought he was going to share gigantic profits with me by us recommending his in-home chemo services. So it's very clear that cancer treatment has become a huge assembly-line business. We're challenging that in major ways, and as you can imagine, the "establishment" doesn't appreciate that.

SS: How many other therapies are being overlooked by mainstream oncology?

BF: The September 2007 edition of *Life Extension* magazine was dedicated to exposing lifesaving cancer drugs being unfairly suppressed by the FDA. These are not so-called alternative therapies, but conventional drugs that have been shown in human clinical studies to save cancer patients' lives, yet are still rejected by FDA bureaucrats. For example, back in 2002, we published favorable data about a prostate cancer drug called Provenge and questioned why the FDA had not approved it for advanced cases. Here we are in 2008, and the FDA has still not approved it. Some prostate cancer support groups are involved in litigation against the FDA. They feel this is out-and-out murder, denying terminally ill prostate cancer patients access to a drug with proven efficacy. It may be several years before that drug comes up for approval again.

SS: A friend of mine was given massive doses of chemotherapy in this country. The cancer came back three months later, so she went to a clinic in Germany where they did a chemo-sensitivity test and found that the chemo she was given in this country had had no effect on her cancer; it's terrible, all that torture and violence thrown at her body for nothing. Why don't we do chemo-sensitivity tests in this country? It seems so logical.

BF: We've been recommending chemo-sensitivity testing for twelve years now. Dr. Robert Nagourney is the pioneer. He's in southern California, and we've referred many patients to him. The idea is that you take a living sample of the patient's tumor and you expose it to different chemotherapy drugs to see which ones are actually effective against that person's cancer cells. But the reason it's not done more often is because this process interferes with the "assembly line." These doctors don't want to have to go through that extra step of doing a biopsy and a culture to keep those cells in a living condition, then have to send them by Federal Express to another laboratory, then wait for that laboratory's test results to come back. That's all extra effort. These doctors just want to be able to administer standard-dose chemo—which is essentially cookbook medicine—to their cancer patients. This enables them to do the large volumes of business that provide the big profits.

Just recently, Life Extension has identified a much more effective method of evaluating individual tumor cells in order to determine what the optimal conventional and natural therapeutic approaches should be. A laboratory in Germany can take a blood sample and test for the presence of circulating tumor cells. This data can enable a patient and his oncologist to better decide whether chemotherapy is necessary. If there are no circulating tumor cells, for example, the patient may elect to avoid chemotherapy. This test of circulating tumor cells, however, provides even more important data. By analyzing the genetic makeup of the circulating tumor cells, this German laboratory then uses a validated computerized model to calculate which specific chemo drugs and natural agents are most likely to eradicate an individual's circulating cancer cells and metastatic tumors. The reason that analyzing tumor cells circulating in the blood is so important is that these metastatic circulating cells are often quite different from a genetic standpoint from the cancer cells removed from the primary tumor. The detailed individual reports from this German laboratory provide the treating oncologist with tremendous data to determine the specific treatments that are likely to be most effective.

Of course, for all of this to come together, you need a compassionate and knowledgeable oncologist who is willing to take you off the assembly line and utilize these avant-garde circulating tumor cells' assay reports.

SS: I can't tell you how disheartening it is to hear this. Doctors take this pledge "to do no harm." We, the patients, believe that; we trust them. It saddens me to know that there are some doctors out there who are unethical and lazy. It's hard to imagine that a doctor wouldn't go whatever distance necessary to be sure that if you were to have to take this violent treatment, that at the very least it would be the right fit.

BF: It's not just chemo—it's radiation. So often we hear of a patient who has undergone radiation treatment when it was totally inappropriate. Can you imagine a patient with metastatic disease in every part of his body and the radiation oncologist says, "Well, let me try to treat your primary tumor." They then bill Medicare tens of thousands of dollars! Not only does this do no good for the patient, but it weakens them further—it does put a lot of dollars into the clinic's pocket, and that's the problem. You've got these big centers set up to administer radiation to cancer patients, and, of course, the more cancer patients they run through, the more money they make.

SS: Shocking, sad, disillusioning, disheartening, wrong.

BF: As I said before, the way cancer treatment is administered today is via assembly-line medicine. It often involves a repetitive "all cancer patients are the same" process that's very profitable. There are actually well-substantiated allegations that mainstream oncology centers don't want to introduce better therapies *because* that would take away from the profits of existing therapies.

One of the causes of action in the lawsuit on the Provenge drug is that there were supposed conflicts of interest within the FDA, based on the fact that if Provenge were approved, then some other popular cancer drugs wouldn't be used as much.

There are very strong suspicions, if not factual events, that you can point to indicating that the pharmaceutical companies don't have a strong interest in actually curing the disease. The really disheartening fact is that the pharmaceutical companies have such strong lobbying influence over both the FDA and Congress that they can restrict what Americans are allowed to have access to. This is something that Life Extension has been battling our entire existence; the fact that we don't have free choice in health care. We have to battle to gain access to what we consider better therapies. But sometimes people end up dying because they are not able to get the therapy in time.

SS: Well, we are a litigious society and doctors know that if they follow standard of care—even if the patient ends up dying—they cannot be sued. So even if they could think outside the box, they aren't able. It's a mess, Bill. This is why I admire the alternative doctors, such as the doctors I have featured in this book and others. They are truly courageous.

BF: Interestingly, alternative doctors are almost never sued. The patients and their families see that these doctors are making heroic efforts attempting to save the patient, and if they don't work, they understand that the patient was in bad shape to begin with. Standard of care, pathetic as it is, is protected by judges who can base a dismissal of a wrongful death malpractice case on the fact that this is just the way medicine is practiced.

SS: What do you think of hospitals today?

BF: Do you realize how prevalent malnutrition is in hospitals? Hospital environments are noisy and disruptive, and it all has a wonderful appetite-suppressing effect. If you're looking to lose weight, check into a hospital. You won't eat as much. The food may be bad, but what's even worse is the commotion, the lack of privacy, the lack of an orderly schedule, and it all conspires to cause a patient not to want to eat a lot. There's also an increase of inflammatory response when you are in a hospital setting. You are under extreme stress, and a lot of inflammatory cytokines are running through your body, which will absolutely kill your appetite. So, because of all these factors, most patients don't want to eat in a hospital setting and normally come out looking like they lost a lot of weight—because they have.

SS: What's the number one cause of death?

BF: Medical ignorance. Absolutely. There's no debate on that. If you were to eliminate the ignorance—meaning if you were to take the scientific knowledge that exists right now and apply it universally—you would see a dramatic decline in morbidity and mortality. Hospitals would go bankrupt. Radiation centers would have to simply shut their doors. It doesn't mean that people are going to live forever, it just means you would dramatically postpone when these people are going to contract these diseases.

SS: So where is the weak link? Is it the medical schools?

BF: Medical schools are part of the problem. They focus on disease, not health. The Western model of medicine is disease focused. Contrast this with traditional Chinese medicine. The Eastern model of medicine is health focused. You go to a practitioner of traditional Chinese medicine to stay healthy. Our medical schools are also heavily influenced by the pharmaceutical industry in what they teach medical students. Our medical schools focus on drugs to treat disease, not strategies to prevent disease in the first place. The weak link, though, is across a very broad spectrum and includes the pharmaceutical industry, the health insurance industry, and government regulations that stifle medical innovation and progress.

When a person does come down with a disease, the fact that the doctor may only treat a couple of the underlying factors and ignore the rest is what I refer to as "absolute medical ignorance." A person, for instance, with coronary artery disease needs to be under the guidance of a physician who realizes there are a number of reasons why that disease developed. Just to prescribe a statin drug and low-dose aspirin and tell the patient that he or she is okay is not serving the patient well. Statins and aspirin may postpone the event by a couple of years, but much more must be done to comprehensively address the underlying processes that caused the coronary artery disease in the first place.

SS: I would think addressing the underlying causes would be automatic. It seems basic.

BF: You would think it would be automatic to check the underlying causes. At Life Extension we *did* the work for the doctors and for our readers to educate themselves. It's all there in our publications. We identified fourteen major risk factors, and we even have a diagram with fourteen daggers aimed at the heart, showing how all these factors conspire to cause the endothelial dysfunction that results in coronary atherosclerosis.

The underlying factors involved in atherosclerosis that result in coronary artery occlusion (i.e., heart attack and congestive heart failure) also apply to the cerebral vessels that result in the epidemic of stroke.

The well-known causes of atherosclerosis are elevated total cholesterol, LDL, triglycerides, and low HDL. Some of the other independent risk factors involved in the development of atherosclerosis include:

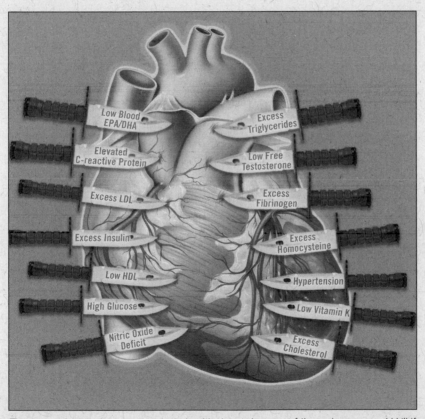

This image depicts daggers aimed at a healthy heart. Any one of those daggers would kill if thrust deep into the heart. In the real world, however, aging humans suffer small pricks from the point of these daggers over a lifetime. The cumulative effect of these dagger pricks (risk factors) is arterial occlusion and, far too often, angina or acute heart attack.

- excess homocysteine
- excess fibrinogen
- high glucose
- low testosterone in men
- high C-reactive protein levels
- nitric oxide deficit
- low EPA and DHA (omega-3 fatty acids)
- oxidized LDL

All of these are proven risk factors for coronary artery disease; unless the doctor corrects every one of these factors, the patient is going to progress at a faster pace than if medical ignorance weren't there.

SS: Can you reverse atherosclerosis?

BF: Yes, there are a couple of different plant extracts that can do this. Pomegranate was shown in a 2004 study to reverse arterial wall thickness over a one-year period. Those who drank 8 ounces of the juice per day *decreased* arterial wall thickness by 30 percent as opposed to a 9 percent *increase* in arterial wall thickness in the group who did not drink the juice. Another impressive study tested a melon extract (called GliSODin) that boosts SOD (superoxide dismutase) in the body. That, too, was able to reverse carotid artery stenosis.

These nutrients seem to work by reducing oxidant stress and free-radical damage. Pomegranate juice also helps protect and enhance the biological benefit of nitric oxide on blood vessels.

As we get older, we have less nitric oxide in our arteries and the result is that we suffer from endothelial dysfunction. As our endothelium becomes more dysfunctional, that is when atherosclerotic plaque will accumulate to the point where the blood flow is restricted or completely blocked.

SS: And that is not a place we want to be. So by these simple preventative measures you are able to *reverse* a condition, rather than simply keep it from becoming worse. This is exciting. Most Western medicine works by keeping the disease at bay.

BF: Yes, this is an absolute breakthrough. In the past we would recommend garlic and fish oil, and that is still important, but something as simple as pomegranate juice has been documented to actually reverse atherosclerotic disease. The drug companies have not figured out a way to do that yet, but the nutritional supplement companies have put enough money into research to develop natural compounds that work much better than prescription drugs.

SS: As a layperson at home watching TV, one would think all the answers lie in pharmaceutical drugs. They have commercials for everything, and when you listen, you can actually hear yourself saying, "Well, I have that. I didn't know that was a disease. I better get this pharmaceutical."

For instance, ED (erectile dysfunction)—long ago it was called impotence, and it wasn't a disease; it was usually stress and/or emotional problems. I mean, all guys have occasional impotence, but now it has taken on respectability in the form of ED. Instead of asking himself, why am I stressed, or why am I not feeling the connection to my partner, this man runs to the doctor (money for the office visit) and asks for the prescription (more money). Same thing with Viagra when maybe it's not a disease—just that the man needs testosterone replacement.

BF: Well, a good rule of thumb is if you see it advertised on TV, don't use it. Especially food—food that is advertised on TV is not the food you want to be eating. For most of the drugs advertised on TV, unless you have a very specific medical condition, there are often much safer and more effective alternatives in the natural field. Of course, you never see these advertised because, for instance, many of the makers of pomegranate juice don't have the money to run national TV ads.

The FDA allows pharmaceutical companies to advertise but makes it illegal for companies that sell dietary supplements to make the same claims. So, you've got government restrictions against the natural supplement industry, and you have the pharmaceutical companies who pretty much own Congress and the FDA. So, yes, as an average consumer, if you're going to rely on TV to dictate what you do, you are condemning yourself to a premature death.

SS: On another subject, my friends laugh at the amount of supplements I take daily. I feel it's necessary for the world we live in today.

BF: It is necessary, based on a preponderance of scientific evidence showing that these supplements interfere with the pathological processes involved in the development of age-related degeneration. If we succeed in documenting that taking the right supplements can help prevent us from contracting horrible diseases, guess what? We're going to swallow these pills every day, and more and more people are following our plea—especially when it comes to fish oil, which has had wonderful publicity over the last five years. There are a lot of other equally important supplements, like vitamin D and magnesium.

SS: Let's discuss magnesium.

BF: There's a magnesium organization run by one of the most dedicated people I know, named Paul Mason. He's put his whole life into educating the world that if they just consume more magnesium, heart attack risks would go down. He's collected over eighty scientific studies that show that even small amounts of magnesium in drinking water, often just 5 to 20 milligrams per liter, lower the risk of heart disease.

SS: How much should one take?

BF: At least 400 milligrams a day, but 800 milligrams would be even better. Some people get diarrhea, so you take as much as you can without inducing diarrhea.

SS: Curcumin?

BF: More and more research shows that curcumin may prevent every common disease we can think about. There are very few nutrients that have that broad-spectrum effect, but curcumin may prevent Alzheimer's disease, cancer, atherosclerosis, and chronic inflammatory disorders. It seems to have a beneficial effect on just about every medical condition that we can name, and it costs very little.

SS: Zinc?

BF: You need about 30 milligrams a day of zinc. You don't need a lot of zinc, but 30 to 50 milligrams a day is fine.

SS: Vitamin E?

BF: Vitamin E appears to protect against prostate and breast cancer if it is taken in the form of gamma-tocopherol. Most commercial supplements contain only alpha-tocopherol vitamin E. While there are benefits to taking the "alpha" form of vitamin E, it is critical that the "gamma" form of vitamin E also be taken. Most people need around 200 milligrams a day of gamma-tocopherol. The gamma form of vitamin E appears to suppress the cyclooxygenase-2 enzyme better than alpha-tocopherol, so it has broad-spectrum, anti-inflammatory benefits, and it seems to help protect against vascular disease.

SS: Probiotics?

BF: Some people really benefit from them. I've heard remarkable testimonials from people who take them who have complained of digestive upsets, and three weeks later they have no more problems. Yet for others it doesn't work at all. So it's a very individualistic thing.

SS: But it seems that so many of us were overprescribed antibiotics. I now no longer will take an antibiotic unless it absolutely cannot be avoided; but even antibiotic use in your earlier life could be responsible for a continuing imbalance of the bacteria in the gut, right?

BF: It's important, but once you recolonize, if you don't take antibiotics, those bacteria may not need to continue replicating. You're not going to overdose on friendly bacteria, but it may not be critical to continuously take a probiotic day in and day out if you don't need it. Now, some people really do need it; their bacteria aren't replicating for whatever reason, and in this case it becomes an important supplement for these individuals to consume.

SS: The first time I ever heard of the high-sensitivity C-reactive protein test was in *Life Extension* magazine. Explain inflammation to my readers.

BF: Inflammation is something that occurs in response to an injury, and we know what that looks like—the pain, swelling, and reddening. As we grow older, unfortunately, a chronic inflammatory state sets in our bodies, which sometimes is not even noticeable, though you might feel some pain and stiffness in your joints. What's going on is that a lot of toxic, inflammatory by-products are being produced that are damaging the linings of your arteries. These toxins are causing inflammation in a way that damages the DNA, so your risk of cancer increases or your risk of heart disease and stroke increases dramatically, because the inflamed arteries are not functioning the way they should.

The good news is that curcumin specifically inhibits a dangerous inflammatory mediator called nuclear factor kappa beta (NFkB). Curcumin is one of the most effective ways to suppress the expression of this common inducer of chronic inflammation. As people grow older, curcumin is something to include as part of a daily regimen. It will assist tremendously in reducing chronic inflammation that can be measured by testing for levels of C-reactive protein in the blood. If you want to know if you are suffering from a chronic inflammatory state, just have your blood tested for C-reactive protein. The ideal levels we recommend are no more than 0.55 mg/L for men and 1.5 mg/L for women. If these levels are elevated, then soluble fiber, curcumin, fish oil, and antioxidants like vitamin C will help, along with healthy changes to one's diet. Weight loss can also reduce elevated C-reactive protein.

SS: I recommended to a friend of mine to have this C-reactive protein test because of her chronic coughing. Her test came back at a level of 15. What's going on?

BF: If a person has a chronic C-reactive protein level of 15, she has a serious underlying inflammatory problem that needs to be corrected. It could be a metabolic problem, prediabetes or diabetes, or arterial inflammation, or a systemic (whole body) state of chronic inflammation. This patient would benefit from curcumin, fish oil, and antioxidants to lower the inflammatory expression. She should also be taking nutrients that protect against glucose toxicity in the body, such as an amino acid dipeptide called carnosine and a fat-soluble form of vitamin B$_1$ called benfotiamine. If your friend does not significantly reduce this chronic high level of inflammation, she will most likely become sick and prematurely die.

SS: It's exciting to think that a simple blood test could give you the information to reverse the situation and save your life. I think anything chronic—coughing, choking, stomach pains, stiffness, elevated blood pressure—are signs that all is not well. Our bodies talk to us. Inflammation is the red flag, the warning that needs to be heard . . . or else.

I am not a fan of statins, yet most adults I know are taking some form of them. Isn't there an alternative nondrug, nonharmful way to lower cholesterol and reverse arterial plaque? What about niacin? What about nattokinase, or red yeast rice supplements, or curcumin?

BF: Niacin is much more effective than statins in protecting against heart disease, particularly in people with low HDL and high triglyceride levels. Statins don't raise HDL very well, whereas niacin raises HDL and lowers triglycerides. Niacin is also an excellent way to decrease the number of small, dense LDL particles, which reduces the propensity of LDL to induce atherosclerosis. Niacin is a wonderful alternative except most people can't tolerate it because of the uncomfortable flushing it causes.

SS: I take it—500 milligrams in the morning and 500 milligrams at night. I have no problems at all, and I like that it has been shown to actually reverse and flush out arterial plaque.

BF: You are lucky. I think most people eating Western diets need niacin, fish oil, and sometimes a low-dose statin drug. If one changes to a healthier diet, they can often stop taking the statin drug.

SS: Let's talk about hormones. As I sit in my office today in 2008, yet another report has come out on the dangers of hormone replacement. Of course, the report is talking about Prempro, which we know puts a woman at risk for cancers, but there was no "however"—meaning, however, we are not talking about bioidentical, real, natural hormones. I think of all the women who threw away their hormones today after hearing this. Why are bioidenticals ignored by virtually every study that has been done?

BF: We know that you can take all the vitamins you want, you can follow a very good diet, but if you don't balance your hormones and get yourself into a youthful hormone profile, you're going to feel lousy, you're going to age prematurely, you're going to contract diseases that all the other good things you are doing for yourself aren't going to prevent. In other words, hormone balance is the cornerstone of an antiaging program. You balance your hormones and then you add on all these other ways to protect yourself against lethal age-related disease. We've had members suffer from horrendous chronic inflammatory conditions; they've tried every imaginable remedy: natural, conventional. It hasn't worked, and then they come to us and we look at their hormone levels. They might have virtually no testosterone, virtually no DHEA, they've got estrogen imbalance; we get them balanced, and the pain goes away. Most of them do not need drugs anymore.

SS: That would be my scenario. "I was lost and now I'm found" . . . today with perfect hormone balance, I take no pharmaceutical drugs. Not one. I am not the patient the drug company wants. Maybe it's that simple. Maybe that is why bioidentical, real, natural hormone replacement is met with such resistance; if we all got as healthy and as well as I am and feel, then we wouldn't need their drugs.

BF: With a lot of people, once we get their hormones balanced, they no longer need sleep medications, anti-inflammatories, and statin drugs. We've seen cases of high cholesterol disappear once testosterone is restored and hormone balance is achieved in both men and women. We published a study four years ago showing that if sex hormones are restored in aging people to youthful ranges, in each and every case they were able to get the LDL and cholesterol down to a safe range, and, in turn, each of these people got off the statin drugs. That was a controlled study.

SS: Then why the ignorance?

BF: Because the drug companies educate the doctors. The drug company can't treat heart disease with testosterone, because the FDA has not approved it. The other reason is that many doctors lack curiosity to look at the medical literature to see hundreds of published studies that document the critical need of the vascular system and the heart muscle itself for adequate testosterone levels. Doctors are inundated with pharmaceutical companies touting all kinds of medications, but testosterone just isn't one of them.

SS: When was the FDA put in charge of our health, and how did the pharmaceutical companies get this power?

BF: I will say it in one word . . . corruption! The drug companies have lobbied the FDA to keep competitive products out of this country. We at Life Extension almost went to jail for life because we were promoting European medications—some of which were later approved in this country as being highly effective—but they wanted to incarcerate us. Those drugs would have competed with existing products.

Life Extension understands that we have a very corrupt regulatory system in our country, which wants to keep out competitive but more effective products and keep their less effective products on the front line. The criteria for a pharmaceutical company to seek FDA approval are not predicated on whether the new drug is particularly safe; it is not about the new drug being significantly effective. It's all about "can we patent it?" Is the patent strong enough for the pharmaceutical company to risk spending all this money to see if it is barely safe and effective enough to receive FDA approval. If the drug doesn't have strong patent protection, it's not even considered.

SS: So something like my cancer treatment, Iscador, an anthroposcopic drug made from mistletoe extract that builds the immune system, will never see the light of day?

BF: Never. We must change the law to tear down the barriers that keep safe and effective therapies out of the hands of Americans. Since its inception, Life Extension has devoted enormous resources to trying to install a free-enterprise approach to medicine, the way it has been with the computer sciences and the communications industries. It's frustrating because we have identified all these wonderful scientific discoveries over the last thirty years, but somehow these have not been translated into medicine because of today's quasi monopoly that is protected by the federal government. Competitive forces, i.e., doctors who are making these breakthrough discoveries, are frightened out of business or put in jail so they cannot provide a better product, that is, a better approach to prevent or treat disease.

SS: How did the hormone melatonin slip by as an over-the-counter hormone? You can buy it at any health food store.

BF: Melatonin was introduced by Life Extension back in 1992. We risked (again) going to jail for bringing it in, but we saw so many published studies substantiating the anticancer, antiaging, and sleep-inducing properties of it, plus so many free-radical-suppressing benefits that extended beyond those of any other antioxidant. I went on national TV shows to tout melatonin as something every aging human should consider taking. Melatonin has been shown to extend the life span of animals, reduce cancer risks, boost the immune system; it seems to do just about everything that is good in a young body. As we get older, we don't produce as much melatonin. There is no apparent toxicity risk for melatonin. I had a member call me at home one night because her child had taken an entire bottle of sixty 3-mg capsules. She was very concerned, and I told her not to worry, that the child may wake up a little groggy but there will be no problems whatsoever. Melatonin is a natural hormone that produces remarkable beneficial effects in the body and does not have druglike side effects. You take the dose that makes you feel most comfortable.

SS: I take 20 milligrams nightly and I sleep eight to nine hours, like a baby. What I feel is sorely lacking in alternative medicine is, for lack of a better term, "the alpha dog." Meaning I would like to find the one doctor who oversees all my other doctors and keeps track of all the therapies I am taking to be sure I am not overlapping and doubling up when it is not necessary.

BF: At Life Extension we do have consultation services for members with cancer who want to have that one-on-one planner essentially overseeing their entire program. People hire a wedding planner to make sure everything is going right—in a way it's kind of the same thing. But at the moment you are right, Suzanne, you (the individual patient) are the person who has to be in charge.

SS: Right, and I am okay with that because of all the research that I do for my work and my books. But not everyone is as involved in all the latest therapies and antiaging discoveries. The other problem, of course, is cost. These therapies are expensive and the tragedy is that most people cannot afford to partake in antiaging therapies, because very little of it is covered by insurance. Supplements, hormone replacement, going to the doctor when I am well for "building up therapies," HGH, Iscador, and vitamin B . . . it all adds up. Yet, I am not sick; I am a productive person in society. I do not, as I said, take a single drug. I am not a drain on the system. On standard of care and the Band-Aid theory, people get sick, require hospitalization, require massive amounts of expensive drugs, and it all pulls the system down. It's too bad our regulatory agencies are so weak, because it seems to me that if everyone were as healthy as you and me, medical care costs would shrivel.

BF: I'd like to think that with the individual health adviser service that Life Extension offers, people can call us and we can help a little bit or at least help them understand something that doesn't make sense to them. It's a free service for anybody. We feel it is part of our nonprofit philosophy to be available to make sure people have the accurate information they need, not just from our Web site, or our *Life Extension* magazine, but just to educate those who might not have the background that they need to help themselves overcome a problem.

SS: Bill, if you were running things, where would medicine be today?

BF: Medicine would be the number one priority instead of where it is right now. We've got defense spending at record-setting high levels, and I know that's a debatable issue, but hundreds of billions of dollars are often spent on weapons systems that are never used. If money were directed into real health care research, we would probably find a cure for every disease we can name. Human beings would live much longer and suffer far less. I look at what happens to humans as they age, and I think it's a horrendous calamity. Aging should be the national priority and not so low on the federal-funding food chain that it doesn't receive adequate attention or funding.

I've been in enough businesses that involve death and dying, or trying to save terminal patients' lives, to realize that when a person is diagnosed with a serious medical condition, all the peripheral political problems of the world become meaningless. The only concern that person has is trying to get better. If we could all put ourselves in that mind-set where nothing matters except one's own health—which is deteriorating rather rapidly with aging—then maybe we would think, "Let's put the priority into saving lives." At Life Extension we spend an enormous percentage of our revenue on scientific research projects.

SS: It seems to me that the answer is rather simple: Think about every single piece of food you put in your mouth and what effect it is going to have on your health. Avoid toxins to the best of your ability. Sleep, love, eliminate stress. Am I being too simplistic?

BF: Diet is the problem and the answer. And, yes, we need to consider food as a medium to grow and maintain a healthy body. When you think that way, you can plan your eating so that it reduces your risk of disease. Regrettably, most Americans eat foods that substantially contribute to common age-related disorders.

Consuming a healthy diet enables one to postpone the dying process and extend his or her productive years. If you look at the Japanese living on the island of Okinawa, they are still productive in their nineties and one hundreds. You look at the way they practice calorie restriction and the types of foods they eat, and their real life example shows us that it is absolutely possible right here and now to reduce our risk of degenerative disease and extend our healthy life spans.

SS: How does calorie restriction slow aging?

BF: It does so by several well-documented methods, such as dramatically lowering fasting insulin and glucose blood levels. This slashes risks for most common age-related diseases. As far as slowing the aging process itself, we at Life Extension focus our research on the effects of calorie restriction on gene expression. There are basically two types of genes involved in aging. There are genes that enable us to function in youthful metabolic patterns, and then there are genes that are expressed as we grow older that are detrimental to healthy cellular metabolic processes. We are learning, through our own research, ways to control gene expression using specific nutrients that mimic the effects of calorie restriction. By doing that we are able to take older cells and enable them to express the beneficial genes so that they then behave more like youthful cells. Ultimately that will be a genetic engineering mechanism by which people are going to be able to control the rate at which they age and potentially reverse the aging process itself.

SS: Are you talking about genomics?

BF: Yes. We've already proven that resveratrol is one of those nutrients that has a positive effect.

SS: Resveratrol, as in red wine?

BF: Yes, but you can also get it in supplement form. Resveratrol positively affects many of the genes involved in aging. Certain red wines don't have much resveratrol, but most do, and red wine is very healthy for you to drink in moderation. Resveratrol is good, but not the panacea; I don't want people to think resveratrol is the magic bullet. Life Extension is evaluating other natural compounds that may produce even more favorable improvements in gene expression than does resveratrol.

We know that our diet greatly affects genes, for the good and bad. And we know if we take in enough vitamin D, we're going to control our genes in such a way that we're less likely to get cancer, and we're less likely to suffer a lot of age-related problems. It's clear that a lot of what we eat (and don't eat) favorably (or negatively) affects our gene expression; but some of the more definitive compounds that we've identified, such as resveratrol and other natural substances, have enough of an impact that I personally am taking them. Our hope is that we will continue to identify compounds that will essentially enable us to control our gene expression the way we can control a computer program nowadays.

SS: Sounds like science fiction.

BF: No . . . just the future—and in some cases, the future is now. The other way this could happen is that if we could access the type of embryonic stem cells that are necessary, theoretically we could regenerate just about every tissue and organ in the body.

SS: The future is exciting. I am very interested in keeping my insides young and being in my optimal prime. But I would be lying if I told you that manifesting a youthful appearance along with a youthful interior wouldn't be thrilling also.

But my real interest at the moment is my right as an individual belonging to the greatest country on the planet to be able to practice the kind of medicine I choose without interference from the government. If I choose to live a nondrug life, and if I choose to replace my hormones with bioidentical hormones, I want to be able to do that.

BF: There's no question that our conventional medical system, weakened by regulation and the influence of the insurance and pharmaceutical industries, has failed many people. It's like putting a Band-Aid on a gaping wound. But I do think the American public is smarter than we think, and they have, in fact, made some positive changes in their dietary patterns already. People have started eating their fruits and vegetables. They are eating fish a couple of times a week, and most of them are taking fish oil capsules.

People are recognizing that they can do something right now, and they are not accepting aging as an inevitable consequence of growing old. That's a very radical change. Back in the 1980s when we started this magazine, we got a lot of publicity because it was so unusual for a group of people to want to actually do something about aging. Now it's pretty commonplace—people are eating differently, taking supplements, replacing hormones—so we've made a major step forward. But as far as the medical profession, they haven't advanced very far at all. That's where we as individuals have to take charge of our own health care and educate ourselves. Fortunately, the information is out there to make good rational decisions with the risk of side effects virtually nonexistent.

SS: I think when people say, "Getting old sucks," what they are really saying is, "I have no energy." When I look at aging people, they are "out of gas." Antiaging to me is reinstating vitality.

BF: If you don't want to make it to sixty, then indulge in all kinds of bad habits. A sixty-five-year-old person today is, on average, healthier than a sixty-five-year-old was thirty years ago. That means the message about healthier lifestyles is getting out there.

SS: You've had a lot to do with that.

BF: Well, I'm proud of our work. I've had a personal mission to accomplish my entire life; it didn't just start at a certain age. When I was told you're going to get old and die, I didn't accept that. I told people, "I'm not going to die." I'm going to figure a way around this. I have a unique advantage because I'm not practicing medicine day in and day out like these doctors. I spend fifteen to eighteen hours a day either in e-mail communications, on the phone, or reading scientific papers. I have a very unique advantage over a physician who's out there from seven in the morning until late at night, sometimes taking calls at night so he can't even get to sleep. I feel good that people are recognizing that they can do something right now and not accept aging as the inevitable consequence of growing old. This thinking is a very radical change, and I do feel that all of us involved in this mission have made that impact.

SS: Most definitely. Thank you.

My readers are offered a free copy of Life Extension *magazine by calling the toll-free number 1-888-884-3666 (twenty-four hours a day) or visiting www.lef.org/goodhealth.*

BILL FALOON'S
BREAKTHROUGH BREAKOUTS

- Supplement a healthy diet with a type of vitamin B_{12} called methylcobalamin—the neurologically active form of B_{12}—to protect against glutamate toxicity, which is the result of ingesting MSG.

- For healthy omega-3s, eat coldwater fish as your primary protein source, and then take fish oil capsules to make sure you are getting enough. Avoid saturated-fat-containing foods like red meat and full-fat dairy products, and foods that contain arachidonic acid like egg yolks, poultry skin, and organ meats.

- Drink 8 ounces a day of pomegranate juice to help reverse the arterial wall thickness that leads to atherosclerosis. Pomegranate juice also helps protect and enhance the biological benefit of nitric oxide on blood vessels.

- Even small amounts of magnesium can lower the risk of heart disease.

- Curcumin may prevent Alzheimer's disease, cancer, atherosclerosis, and chronic inflammatory disorders.

- Vitamin E appears to protect against prostate and breast cancer, if it is taken in the form of gamma-tocopherol.

- Niacin is more effective than statins in protecting against heart disease, particularly in people with low HDL and high triglyceride levels.

- Melatonin has anticancer, antiaging, and sleep-inducing properties, plus many free-radical-suppressing benefits that extend beyond those of any other antioxidant.

- Calorie restriction slows aging by dramatically lowering fasting insulin and glucose blood levels.

PART II

8 Steps to Wellness

We live in a toxic, stressed world; it is working against us, and to ignore the obvious is asking to be sentenced to poor health. This whole new approach is a slow educational process. It takes time for patients to understand that we are going to restore their body to its perfect natural health, and that we are going to use their own body to heal itself, and put back what has been lost through stress and aging. The end result will be a quality of life they have probably never known.

–Dr. Andy Jurow, Burlingame, California

6

8 STEPS TO WELLNESS

We are now at the threshold of the Superlongevity Revolution, the radical extension of the human life span that will shake society to its very foundation. Its impact will be felt by every person, institution, and organization.

–Michael G. Zey, Ph.D., *Ageless Nation*

YOU CAN BE WELL; you can fine-tune your health to perfection and prevent disease if you understand the triggers that make us sick. Sickness is not a normal state, and those who are chronically ill have not been exposed to information that could prevent the conditions they are now suffering. New breakthrough medicine believes in building up the body to optimal health and strength. Even chronic illness can be reversed.

The best part of this news is that breakthrough medicine makes it possible for us to be healthy at any age if we choose to take *charge* of our health, and that's the good news; wellness is achievable for *everyone*.

My quest for health in the past several years has manifested in my following 8 Steps to Wellness.

To achieve optimal health, it is essential to understand the profound impact of adapting these eight steps. If you change the way you take care of yourself and use these principles, you can expect a long life as a well person and avoid the present template that most often ends in the nursing home.

You may think you have heard some of these steps before, but this is different. Breakthrough medicine understands how the parts of our bodies work together and are connected. Breakthrough medicine understands that whatever we put in our body has a direct impact on our health. There are ramifications to everything you eat, good and bad. You will learn the value of detoxification through intravenous nondrug treatments. You will realize that our damaged food supply leaves a nutritional void; therefore, daily supplementation is a necessity. By embracing these 8 steps, you will be amazed at how quickly your health and energy will turn around.

THE 8 STEPS TO WELLNESS

1. Get Bioidentical Hormone Replacement Therapy
2. Avoid Chemicals and Detoxify Your Body
3. Take Nutrition Seriously
4. Create a Healthy GI Tract
5. Avoid Pharmaceuticals Unless Absolutely Necessary
6. Supplement Your Diet
7. Exercise Regularly
8. Get Proper Sleep

1. GET BIOIDENTICAL HORMONE REPLACEMENT THERAPY

Real bioidentical hormones are the backbone of breakthrough medicine, and any cutting-edge doctor will tell you that is where it starts. Doctors say they can't even begin to try to influence a patient on the next seven steps until they get the hormone issue on track.

This step explains all the hormones, the different stages of hormone loss, and why replacing your lost hormones with bioidentical hormones is absolutely vital.

So many are "toughing it out" due to all the negative publicity surrounding hormone replacement, which is always about synthetic hormones, not bioidentical hormones. Synthetic hormones are the harmful hormones that do not replicate what our bodies produce.

When you experience the joys of real hormone replacement, you will understand that replacing lost hormones reinstates your health and vitality, plus it gives you back your edge. Without hormones you can expect a slow but steady decline in *you*.

2. AVOID CHEMICALS AND DETOXIFY YOUR BODY

We truly are what we eat, and it has never before been as important. We are experiencing an environmental assault unlike anything human beings have ever known in the entire existence of mankind. Toxins are everywhere: in our homes and offices, in the air we breathe, the water we drink, and the food we consume.

We are able to control this exposure to some degree. We will never again be able to live an existence that is devoid of chemicals and toxins unless we move to the most remote part of the globe and eliminate all modern conveniences and technologies from our lives, and even then acid rain and chemical clouds would be passing overhead. But making simple changes in your lifestyle and diet will not only add up, it will create an internal environment predominantly made up of healthy cells rather than unhealthy cells; this ratio is key to beating the present unavoidable environmental assault. Simply eat clean, real (organic if possible) food and try at all costs to avoid chemicals in the foods you consume. Eat at home more often so you know the exact quality of your food. Switch to clean, chemical-free cosmetics and take steps to eliminate as many pollutants from your home as possible.

You don't have to do this cold turkey; start with baby steps. It won't take long before the idea of eating chemically laden food will seem outrageous. Each doctor in this book stresses the need for detoxing patients through different modalities, including:

- homeopathics
- energy medicine
- intravenous treatments
- chelation
- cleansing diets
- infrared saunas
- colonics
- hyperbaric oxygen chambers

Read the Step 2 section to learn about all the latest advances available that assist us in undoing the effects of our polluted, unhealthy environment. When you change the way you eat and the way you live your life, and switch your household cleaners to natural products, your health will get better. This is your choice to make, and it determines whether your health will soar or spiral downward. By making these simple changes, you will restore your energy, and good health will become who *you* are!

3. TAKE NUTRITION SERIOUSLY

Nutrition goes hand in hand with good health. Seriously embracing the quality of the food you consume will save your life. Toxicity is no joke. Diet sodas are creating havoc with our health and our brains. According to Dr. Russell Blaylock, a renowned neuroscientist, "Young people are experiencing dementia and mental problems on a scale never before seen." Alzheimer's is epidemic and the most feared of all possible conditions.

Autoimmune diseases, GI problems, cancers, mood control, and happiness are all seriously affected by the food we consume on a regular basis. Good, real, healthy food is delicious, and it does not mean that you have to abandon wonderful flavors like olive oil, sea salt, butter, herbs, spices, or flavorings; meals like roasted chicken, meat, or fish; delectable vegetables flavored with olive oil and lemon, or sautéed in butter; potatoes of any kind, peppers, fresh garden salads; fruits like mangoes, papayas, and all the berries you can consume. Eating correctly is a joy; each meal provides an opportunity not only for pleasure, but also a chance to build up and create an environment that will strengthen your body.

4. CREATE A HEALTHY GI TRACT

Most everyone I speak with has trouble with their stomach—when I say "stomach" here, I am including everything from the mouth to the anus. The GI tract is called the second brain. It is vital for our overall good health to keep this beautiful, ingenious organ intact and working well.

Sadly, most of us rush through our meals, hardly tasting and rarely chewing properly. We fill ourselves with chemical-laden foods; we overeat, abuse sugar, abuse alcohol, and expect to be well. Couple this with hormonal imbalances, throw in cigarette smoking and pollution, and it's no wonder we are always holding our stomachs in agony.

When you follow the pathway of the GI tract, you will understand why chewing your food is the first change you can make toward wellness; then by also eliminating toxins, you will understand how you can turn your food into superfood, build up your body, build healthy cells, and keep malfunctioning cells at a minimum.

Once you understand the function, importance, and workings of your GI tract, you will have a new and profound respect for this ingenious body part. You cannot be healthy without a good working gut, yet it is the most abused part of our bodies.

5. AVOID PHARMACEUTICALS UNLESS ABSOLUTELY NECESSARY

Antiaging medicine, longevity medicine, alternative medicine, energy medicine, cutting-edge medicine, or what I refer to as breakthrough medicine, are all saying the same thing—*we are taking too many pharmaceutical drugs!*

Please know that these doctors are not antipharmaceutical, nor am I. As I will state over and over in this book, when you need a pharmaceutical, it is a godsend—particularly for pain, infection, mental illness, and other conditions outside my scope of knowledge—but whenever you can treat a problem or a condition without pharmaceuticals, it is always the better and safer way.

This new shift in medicine is exciting; these doctors are making patients well. They are healing; they are thinking outside the box and practicing the "art of medicine." Imagine cleaning out arteries without statins. Imagine being able to restore hearing and to prevent the continued deterioration of macular degeneration, in many cases actually reversing the condition. Imagine healing the GI tract and eliminating the stomach problems that have plagued you all of your life. Imagine taking away pain without drugs, imagine sleeping nine hours a night without drugs, and imagine not having acid reflux. It goes on and on. Today's new medicine heals rather than manages, and eliminates this Band-Aid approach to which we have become accustomed.

Imagine the possibilities if you are willing to embrace change. Imagine not ending up in the sorry state so many people are now experiencing: drugged out of their existence, sick, crippled, and in nursing homes with dementia or Alzheimer's. This does not have to be your fate if you embrace the new breakthrough medicine that is available now and being practiced by Western-trained, highly credentialed doctors, all of whom collectively realized that the way they were approaching medicine (allopathically) was, in fact, not only no longer working but also working against us. Today's new medicine is life changing and lifesaving.

6. SUPPLEMENT YOUR DIET

Our food supply is horribly depleted and supplementation is more important than ever before. To get all the proper nutrients we need to build healthy cells, it is vital we supplement our already good diets. There are several new breakthrough supplements that have surfaced and are spoken about by the doctors in this book. Resveratrol is certainly discussed with extreme enthusiasm. There are other new and exciting supplements available such as turmeric, vitamin D_3, zinc, niacin, rhodiola, cinnamon, and omega-3 fatty acids. The more antioxidants we can load up on the better. Supplementation is necessary to be truly well, even if you are eating only the best of foods.

7. EXERCISE REGULARLY

We have all heard it over and over, and yet it mostly falls on deaf ears. I always take the example of a brand-new car left in the garage for weeks, just sitting there. Of course, when you finally go to start it up, the car will sputter and choke from lack of use. Our bodies are the same in that they require usage to operate correctly. Walking forty minutes a day is miraculous for the frame, and free weights stimulate bone growth and give beautiful definition to our muscles.

My exercise of choice is yoga. I look forward to it three to four times a week, and in between I use free weights and I walk almost every day. Breathing is an important part of yoga, and oxygen is what makes our cells breathe and stay supple and healthy. No matter our age we want to be flexible and fluid, and it is possible throughout our lives by making a commitment to the type of exercise that makes us feel best. Yoga is low impact, so it allows for an ageless approach to exercise. Choose something that you know you will stick with and make it an enjoyable activity, like taking a beautiful walk each day and deep breathing.

8. GET PROPER SLEEP

You cannot be healthy if you cannot sleep, and here is where hormones kick in. With imbalanced hormones sleep is impossible. I will explain in chapter 30 the medical value of sleeping and why chronic sleeplessness may lead to heart attack and weight gain. In order to be thin, you must sleep. In order to be happy, you must sleep; to be healthy, you must sleep; to be hormonally balanced, you must sleep.

Sleep is nature's way to restore health, yet most American adults get no more than five hours of sleep a night (if that). Inadequate sleep is a recipe for disaster. The good news is that you can retrain yourself to sleep again, but it won't happen until you replace the missing hormones lost through the aging process, or if you have hormonal imbalance due to great stress (this pretty much includes everyone), or if you are consuming toxic chemicals.

Dear Suzanne,

I wish I could explain to you the profound impact your book Ageless *has had on my life. At thirty-seven years of age, I had no idea the symptoms I was feeling were related to perimenopause. Who wants to believe we are anywhere near menopause at only thirty-seven? I was having problems sleeping, waking with hot flashes, carrying extra weight, and moody as all hell. I would hear voices coming out of me, shrieking at my kids, and wonder who was the horrible woman overreacting to them. I had no interest in sex. My doctor did the "typical" checkup and told me I was fine—probably a little stressed.*

It wasn't until I read Ageless *that I understood how hormones affect every part of my physical and emotional well-being. I sought out one of the doctors in your reference guide and I am happy, so happy, to tell you I am on bioidentical hormones. I now sleep like a baby, with no hot flashes. My moods are even—everyone in my family thanks you for that! Plus, I am back to my "wedding date weight" and enjoying my husband like we are honeymooning!*

Thank you for your guidance. I know I will live a long, healthy, and happy life thanks to all the work you have done in bringing this information to us. You have opened the door to this kind of medicine and helped millions to see a better way of life. I will be forever indebted to you.

Sincerely,
Becky G.

7

STEP 1: GET BIOIDENTICAL HORMONE REPLACEMENT THERAPY (BHRT)

Replacing lost hormones is crucial to feeling good. You need to plan for the rest of your life if you want to keep up with your health. The old ways no longer work.

–Dr. Candice Lane, Westlake Village, California

THE FIRST STEP TO WELLNESS is bioidentical hormone replacement. This is the backbone to health, longevity, and a better quality of life.

Any book on antiaging must address the importance of replacing lost or declining hormones with real bioidentical ones. It is the crucial first step that leads to all new advancements as laid out in this book. These new breakthroughs go beyond the traditional "standard of care" box and zoom you into the next millennium of forward-thinking advancements.

It is difficult to understand why bioidentical hormone replacement has created such a stir between the traditionalists and those who follow cutting-edge medicine. Whether you want to call it "alternative," "anti-aging," or as I do, "breakthrough medicine," conventional doctors push aside these treatments because they are not rooted in double-blind studies (what traditional doctors use to measure effectiveness). These doctors don't see, instead, that countless other studies do exist that prove bioidentical hormone replacement therapy is safe and effective. It seems because we are mostly dealing with nonpatentable, nonpharmaceutical medicines, the motive must be big business—pharmaceutical companies are not making huge amounts of money from these hormones. Bioidentical hormones do put a kink in the bottom line of drug companies, but ask the people who actually take them, and they will tell you they are ecstatic. Ask any of us who have experienced the joys and well-being of true natural hormone replacement and the unanimous response is, we love our treatments and they are lifesaving. I hear this all the time from women who learned about this from my other books. They say they would not, could not, live without them. I feel the same way.

In order to make an informed choice, you need information. I have been practicing breakthrough medicine with my antiaging doctors for over a decade and I love each day; I feel good all the time. Bioidentical hormone replacement is truly the backbone of new medicine. It is crucial you understand this. Every doctor I have interviewed for this book, no matter his or her specialty, knows the importance of replacing the hormones that have been lost in the aging process. All adults from middle age on need to put back the hormones they have lost through aging, stress, and the environmental assault. If you can grasp this concept, then all will fall into place.

Hormone replacement is restoration. *Restoration stops the* deterioration.

The next few chapters will help you understand hormone replacement therapy so you can start down the path of breakthrough medicine. I have written two other books that cover hormone loss and bioidentical replacement—if you have read *The Sexy Years* and *Ageless*, you will be somewhat familiar with these topics. However, I will fill you in on the latest advancements with "breakthrough" moments that bring you up to speed on what is happening in the exciting world of hormone replacement. In the next chapter, "Know Your Hormones," you will learn the difference between the major and minor hormones and how they work within the body. Even though it is a lot of information, refer to this chapter often so that you can truly grasp what each hormone is and what functions each one performs in the overall "song" of good health in your body. Every hormone is crucial, and having even one that is low or missing will throw off the entire system. Once you understand your individual hormonal requirements, you will have a greater appreciation of the following chapters, which explain what happens to our bodies as we lose our hormones and how we can best go about replacing them with bioidentical hormones that replicate what nature has given us versus synthetic hormones that do not.

Dear Suzanne,

I am forty-three years old and went into menopause three years ago. That's when things crashed here at home (and at work). My incredible husband of twenty-one years stopped telling me I was the most beautiful woman in the world and my two teenagers spent their "at home" time hiding from me.

I felt awful. No interest in sex. No interest in cooking (although I am famous for my Sunday dinners), lack of focus at my work, always exhausted because I couldn't sleep more than a few hours each night, and bitchy as hell to those I love the most. And my rear end was as big as Kansas; I have always been a size 4 to 6.

Then I read your book Ageless, and there I was . . . the seven dwarfs of menopause were living in my bed and in my kitchen and even in my car; I experienced road rage for the first time in my life and almost got socked.

Now that I am "Mrs. Bioidentical Hormone Replacement" (and so are all my girlfriends), I am happy all the time, my husband can't stop touching and kissing me and saying "Thank God for Suzanne." My kids are back and I just got an important promotion at work. I am one very happy camper.

Thank you very, very, very much, Suzanne. You and your book arrived just in the nick of time and my family is extremely grateful.

Very sincerely,
Dorothy P.

8

KNOW YOUR HORMONES

It's not enough to add years to one's life ... one must also add
life to those years.

–John F. Kennedy

AS I'VE SAID, the cornerstone of breakthrough medicine is bioidentical hormone replacement. The key is to first understand what hormones your body produces and what happens when you lose them. This chapter will explain the different minor and major hormones in your body.

THE MINOR HORMONES

ESTROGEN

Estrogen is primarily a female hormone, though both men and women make estrogen—women have high levels of estrogen and low levels of testosterone, and men have the opposite. It is one of the most powerful hormones in the human body and can affect many of our tissues and organs, including the brain, liver, bones, and skin, as well as the uterus, urinary tract, breasts, and blood vessels. When women have estrogen deficiency, they can suffer from many problems, including unexplained weight gain, bloating, itching, sweating and hot flashes, bladder infections, depression and fatigue, heart palpitations, and more.

Estrogen is also one of our sex hormones, along with progesterone and testosterone. When you have no sex hormones, you cannot "feel" sex. Sexual feelings are restored when the sex hormones are put back into the body in the proper balance.

What is generally called "estrogen" actually comprises three classical components:

- estradiol
- estrone
- estriol

There are also about thirty other estrogens, and researchers are regularly finding more and more different forms.

Here are some things you need to know about estrogen:

Estrogen must be balanced with progesterone, and each woman has completely different needs. There is no "one size fits all" in determining what these needs are and how every woman must replace her lost hormones.

Estrogen in females is made primarily in the ovaries. In the first thirty-five years of a woman's life, estrogen, progesterone, and testosterone pulse through her system, maintaining a healthy equilibrium while she is reproductive.

A reproductive woman naturally makes estrogen every day of the month and progesterone two weeks of each month. No woman has ever made estrogen exclusively, yet Premarin, the synthetic so-called hormone (made from pregnant mare's urine), is estrogen only. If a woman takes only this, not only is she taking a hormone made from a substance alien to the human body but she also is not taking progesterone to balance the estrogen. This can be dangerous . . . a possible cancer setup.

No woman ever made estrogen and progesterone every day of the month. If that were true, then your body would always be pregnant. The only time a woman makes high levels of estrogen and even higher levels of progesterone at the same time is when she is pregnant.

Once your hormone levels begin to decline, you will need to replace the estrogen and progesterone in the exact amounts for you, usually determined by a blood test.

PROGESTERONE

Progesterone is primarily a female hormone, but it is also found in males in small amounts. It is made in the ovaries and the adrenal glands, and in pregnancy it is produced in the placenta. Progesterone has a calming effect; it repairs and maintains a healthy brain, builds bones, is a natural diuretic, burns fat, and helps to prevent cancer.

Progesterone also helps balance estrogen. It is vital that the ratio is correct and individualized for each woman. Progesterone never poured every day in nature the way it has been given to so many women in the form of Prempro, the synthetic hormone. With Prempro (*Prem* stands for Premarin and *Pro* for progesterone), women are given a daily dose of horse estrogen that is not compatible with what we make in our own bodies, plus a daily dose of a *progestin*. Progestin is not progesterone, no matter what the pharmaceutical brochures say. It is a synthetic replica of progesterone with no compatibility in a woman's body and has possible terrible side effects, cancer being one of them.

In other words, synthetic *progestins* are dangerous. Bioidentical *progesterone*, which mimics what our bodies make, is good for you. Remember this difference; it could save your life.

People who take progestins such as Provera have shown an increased risk in breast cancer. In fact, progestins are *antiprogesterone* in their effects. It is that serious. Nature gave us progesterone for a reason. Nature did not want us to try to make something "not as good," such as a progestin. Stay away from progestins for your health's sake.

We do not want pregnancy-level progesterone and estrogen pouring continuously at the same time, all the time—our insulin levels can rise in this state. This isn't dangerous when we are pregnant, as most women these days are pregnant only two or three times in their lives, but we do not want to mimic the hormonal state of pregnancy when we aren't.

I am speaking not as a doctor here, but as someone who has talked to many doctors, who has immersed herself in the study of hormones, and who takes them herself. Some women ask their doctors to give them continuous combined hormone therapy—that means they are getting a steady stream of estrogen and progesterone, mimicking pregnancy, which means they do not get a period every month. By taking hormones like this, your insulin will go sky high, you will gain weight, and it will be dangerous to your health. It also is not good to fake a "pregnant state"; the body will eventually get confused because *no* woman was ever meant to be pregnant her entire life.

If you cycle your hormones, taking estrogen every day and progesterone two weeks every month, you will get a period. This is nature. This signals to the brain that all is well. This is your healthiest state. Even if you haven't had a period in a long time, it will reactivate once you start taking hormones. It might take a couple of months. Once it comes, you are on track again. You are protected from the diseases associated with hormone loss. Young healthy women are protected because they make a full complement of hormones and are at their healthiest—this is what we are aiming for with bioidentical hormone replacement.

If progesterone levels are too low with regard to estrogen levels, a woman will experience sleep disturbances, irritability, anxiety, weight gain, breast swelling, breast tenderness, itching, bloating, sweating, loss of memory, and loss of libido.

The reason is because *there is no balance!* There has to be a balance of the correct ratio between estrogen and progesterone. Only a qualified doctor can help you find this. Hormonal balance is the goal at any age to not only feel good, but most of all to be healthy. Be patient, you'll get there. It took a long time to get this imbalanced, so you need to give it time to get it just right. The good news is that some relief is immediate. You will start to feel better right away, but perfection will take time, a few weeks, or months. For me, because I was completely drained of estrogen (which feels awful), it took a whole year to reach perfection, but along the way I was feeling better and better.

A lot of young women become "estrogen dominant" and start feeling imbalanced. Estrogen dominance doesn't mean you have too much estrogen, it means you don't have enough progesterone. So, for younger women sometimes it's normal to start out with just progesterone to balance things because they already are making enough estrogen.

If there is too much estrogen in the mix and not enough progesterone, the lining of the uterus becomes thicker than normal. This scenario can make for a heavy buildup of the uterine lining, which causes excessive bleeding, and it could increase the risk for uterine cancer. Progesterone prevents this buildup if it is given in the correct ratio for you, which will stop the excessive bleeding and will also protect against uterine cancer. Progesterone also protects against breast cancer, decreases fluid retention, helps maintain normal blood sugar levels, assists in lowering LDL cholesterol levels, and has a sedative effect on the central nervous system. Progesterone depletion is also implicated in postpartum depression. Doctors can rectify this depression by replacing bioidentical progesterone until a new mother feels "right." So often a woman is instead handed an antidepressant, which is a drug and does not put back what she is missing.

TESTOSTERONE

It is important to understand the role of testosterone not only in the male body but also in the female body. Let me explain both.

To be female, we naturally have a ratio of high estrogen to low testosterone. This ratio is crucial to balance. This ratio is what makes us women.

To be male, the ratio is exactly the opposite: Men have high levels of testosterone and low levels of estrogen.

The ratio is the key in both men and women. When either ratio is off, the brain signals the alarm bell that all is not well . . . and you can feel when you are "off." Men lose their edge; they lose their muscle definition and mass. Their shoulders start to slope downward, they sleep more, and their erections finally go when the ratio reaches the point where the man has lost so much testosterone that he now has more estrogen than testosterone. It is also the time when he starts to get the diseases of aging. You name it, most every disease starts with hormone decline.

Recent reports have come out that testosterone levels in men have been gradually declining over the past fifty years. Dr. Ron Rothenberg says it aptly: "We are just half the men that our fathers were." In a certain sense, that is true. Men of our grandfathers' age had testosterone levels and sperm counts that were much higher. I find this alarming; I mean, how will the next generation be affected? If this continues, our very existence is at risk.

For women it is the opposite . . . we have high levels of estrogen and low levels of testosterone. But the ratio of both is what keeps us looking and feeling good. We need a certain amount of testosterone—it is produced in the ovaries and is known to improve clitoral and nipple sensitivity, increase libido, improve the quality of orgasm, and can increase muscle strength and bone density. Loss of testosterone leads to fatigue, a feeling of being imbalanced, memory loss, abdominal fat, and weight gain. Testosterone replacement in women decreases the risk of breast cancer (Dimitrakakis, 2004.)

But more than that, it's part of the "hormonal song." It is the whole complement that nature has given us in different ratios to differentiate woman from man. Testosterone makes us feel good. Bioidentical testosterone can decrease inflammation, which protects the heart (Grodstein, 1997), improve energy, protect bone density, lower LDL cholesterol levels, raise HDL cholesterol levels, enhance blood glucose levels, improve muscle strength, improve brain function, and decrease body fat.

Too much testosterone can bring about excessive (and embarrassing) chin hairs; it can cause oily skin, acne, scalp hair loss, unwanted body hair, aggressive behavior, and salt or sugar cravings.

Testosterone can "rev up" a waning sex drive. Sometimes when you have been without your sexual feelings for a while, you need to add testosterone to wake things up again. Most doctors recommend that you put a little bit of it right on your clitoris. Oh my, that does wake things up.

Testosterone deficiency is determined by a blood test. If you find that your skin is getting oily, or you see acne bumps or the beginnings of a "beard," then you are taking too much. Always remember, with hormone replacement, never too much, never too little—like Goldilocks's porridge, it must be just right, but you will know this from your symptoms. Chin hairs are your body talking to you.

Testosterone is an anabolic steroid, meaning that it builds bone and muscle. To have your youthful, fit body, you need to have adequate testosterone. Without it you could work out at the gym all day and see no results. Testosterone also feeds the heart muscle, which is the largest muscle in the body and has more testosterone receptor sites than any other muscle. This is your pumping power. Without testosterone your heart muscle loses its strength. Convinced?

PREGNENOLONE

Pregnenolone is the memory hormone. In animal studies it improves memory one hundred times more than DHEA. According to Dr. Thierry Hertoghe, it "improves memory because it clarifies thinking and stimulates concentration, prevents memory loss, reduces fatigue, fights depression, protects the joints, relieves arthritis, and speeds healing."

Progesterone and pregnenolone are hormones manufactured in the adrenal glands, as well as in the ovaries and testicles, before they are metabolized into DHEA, which is another important hormone (more to come on that).

In the adrenal cascade, pregnenolone is the first hormone to be made from cholesterol, and progesterone is the second. Both can be converted into several other adrenal hormones besides DHEA, including the sex hormones, aldosterone, and cortisol.

Taking replacement hormones like pregnenolone and progesterone that occur early in the adrenal cascade lets your body's wisdom choose which other hormones it will make from them, according to your body's needs. This is especially important if you are under stress. With adrenal fatigue, the sex hormone levels often fall because your adrenal glands are not able to manufacture adequate levels of hormones. One function that sex hormones serve is to act as antioxidants that help prevent the oxidative damage caused by cortisol. So the lower the sex hormones, the more damage there is to tissues, especially when you are under stress.

This oxidative damage is one of the key factors of accelerated aging. Either pregnenolone or progesterone can better be used to raise the hormonal levels in both men and women and decrease some aspects of adrenal fatigue. Pregnenolone and progesterone work by bypassing the very complex and energy-consuming steps required of your adrenals, so that they do not have to work so hard to keep your hormone levels balanced.

These are important hormones and can be administered in your individual requirements by cream or sublingual drops.

DHEA

DHEA (dehydroepiandrosterone) is called the "mother hormone" of the body. It is made in the brain and in the adrenal cortex and is one of the most plentiful hormones in the body. Just as you need cholesterol to make pregnenolone, you need pregnenolone to make DHEA.

Hormone replacement is like a song: In order to be in tune, you need to understand how each hormone is affected by the next. They all work together. For instance:

- from progesterone, we make cortisol
- from DHEA, we make the hormone androstenedione, which turns into estrone and testosterone
- estrone is then converted into estriol
- estradiol can be made from testosterone

It's a lot of science, but you get the picture. All the steroidal hormones are interdependent. That's why embracing hormone replacement needs to be understood in its entirety. Just "throwing in" DHEA without replacing all the other hormones won't work.

Adequate levels of DHEA can increase testosterone levels, increase muscle mass, decrease body fat, improve memory, decrease depression, and improve the immune system by controlling cortisol levels and adrenaline levels.

DHEA is protective against arteriosclerosis because DHEA lowers cholesterol levels and insulin levels, protecting against diabetes, if you are eating correctly. Enhancing the immune system decreases the risk of malignancies or cancer and helps prevent the decrease in mental function that could be a precursor to Parkinson's or Alzheimer's since it protects the neurons in the brain.

Nature thought it all out for us, but we figured out how to outlive all of our hormones. That is why replacement is so fantastic. When you see all the protection provided to us from our God-given hormones, you realize that in order to stay in the game, in order to keep our edge, in order to take advantage of this long life we have been afforded, we must replace all our hormones with bioidentical equivalents to stay healthy.

MELATONIN

Melatonin is the sleep hormone. Without it you cannot sleep soundly or deeply. Melatonin is what makes you yawn and want to go to bed at night—it also creates the day/night rhythm that is so important to your body's balance.

Melatonin is also a powerful antioxidant and captures potentially damaging free radicals. It protects the heart and arteries and reduces the risk of cardiovascular disease. Its antioxidant properties help reduce the risk of cancer, and in the lab melatonin has been shown to slow down the growth of cancer cells. It has also been shown to inhibit the proliferation of the AIDS virus. Plus, melatonin protects the pancreas and the organs and the immune system.

Melatonin is a wonderful hormone, available in the United States over the counter. I get mine from Life Extension because of their quality reputation. It is always important to get good-quality hormones and supplements.

Melatonin relaxes muscles, relieves tension, reduces stress and anxiety, especially at night, and lowers blood pressure. Without adequate melatonin you will get poor sleep deprived of dreams and full of agitation. Without melatonin you don't know when to go to bed, and when you do, you will have a hard time getting to sleep and staying asleep.

Without enough melatonin you will often feel tense, anxious, irritable, and aggressive. You will age more quickly, with prematurely graying hair and bags under your eyes.

There are ways to supplement declining melatonin. In chapter 31, "The Future Is Now," I talk about sleep patches created with nanotechnology. They are quite remarkable because they reduce the time it takes for the melatonin to pour and you go to sleep quicker and easier. I take melatonin supplements plus I wear the sleep patch nightly to ensure I get my nine hours. I take my sleep very seriously, and I love that I do not have to take a sleeping pill or a drug for any reason when I have nature's tools to work with, such as that provided by melatonin supplementation. I take 20 milligrams nightly. To understand this wonderful hormone even better, read Dr. Thierry Hertoghe's interview in chapter 9.

At some point in our forties our melatonin levels decrease drastically because the pineal gland runs out of gas. We also need the amino acid tryptophan, which is found in many of the foods we eat (turkey is a good source), to produce melatonin. With these foods, tryptophan is converted into serotonin, which then turns into melatonin. So a healthy diet continues to be the stuff of good health, and the foods we consume have a major effect on our bodies' abilities to manufacture the hormones we need.

HUMAN GROWTH HORMONE (HGH)

Human growth hormone gets a bad rap, which is unfortunate and unjustified. The bad rap on HGH is that athletes overuse it and take (usually) a hundred times more than the human body ever requires. That's why athletes can bulk up by taking superhuman doses and end up looking deformed from doing so. Taking those amounts can and often does lead to cancer and heart attacks. This is the definition of HGH abuse.

I inject HGH daily on a "need" basis, as I have a deficiency as determined by my IGF-1 levels. In fact, since I started two years ago, my needs have increased, which makes sense because each year as we age chronologically, our bodies make less and less of all of our hormones. And I would suppose that I am at an age where I'm not producing much of anything on my own.

No need to worry; I restore my normal human growth hormones with HGH, and I have never felt better. It's as though I finally found the missing piece of the song. Now my body is playing like a finely tuned instrument. I love the way I feel with the addition of HGH. The added benefit is that weight is no longer a problem. I eat right, exercise daily, take my supplements, avoid chemicals if possible, and my weight is a nice 127 for my five-foot-five frame.

Human growth hormone is released by the pituitary gland under the direction of the hypothalamus gland. Most HGH is released during deep stages of sleep each night, while lesser quantities are released during daytime hours. Though it remains in circulation only a few minutes, the effects of HGH are profound, delaying many of the manifestations of the aging process. With age most people lose muscle mass; fat accumulates around the stomach, thighs, and elsewhere; hair turns gray; wrinkles appear; and organs such as the heart diminish in capacity.

HGH and IGF-1 affect all the organs and tissues of the body; they improve the cognitive function and mood of the brain; improve blood flow to the heart and cardiac output; promote less atherosclerosis and narrowing of the carotid arteries; increase lung function; promote less fat (especially abdominal fat); promote more muscles and stronger bones; increase exercise capacity; and increase immune system function.

The decline in HGH is called "somatopause" (all hormones have a pause). The decline begins at around age thirty and the depletion is usually completed by age forty-five. Before modern civilization, the maximum life expectancy was around age forty-five. So nature had it all figured out. It gave us just enough to last through our reproductive years, but we have learned to trick our bodies into living longer. At present we are expected to live the second half of our lives with a real disadvantage. Sorry, not for me.

Without HGH you have decreased memory, mood, well-being, quality of life, intelligence, sleep, muscle, lung function, joint cartilage, sexual function, capacity to exercise, immune function, and heart function. Without HGH, fat and insulin resistance increase, cholesterol becomes worse, skin wrinkles, and you have trouble healing.

We need to understand the importance of replacing this wonderful hormone, and when this is understood, it will no longer be expensive. In reality it should not cost more than insulin, but because of all of the scare tactics and the media "gloom and doom," people are scared off, turned off, and misinformed, thus keeping the prices high.

How can something that our own body once made in abundance be bad for us? Maybe it can be the same with all the hormones: If we find out that we can feel so well, and be so healthy by replacing natural HGH hormones daily, then we will not need to resort to pharmaceuticals.

HGH is a major part of the antiaging movement. These qualified doctors know that we can reverse the inevitabilities of aging, including the diseases that are now accompanying old age, by replacing all the missing hormones. HGH is one of them.

However, you can't look at HGH as a magic bullet. You must exercise, you must eat right, you must sleep. But if you do these simple things, HGH will reward you handsomely. HGH, in combination with replacing all the other missing hormones, is truly the fountain of youth.

HGH heals in so many ways. It has the capacity to improve many illnesses and medical conditions. HGH replacement has produced a significant improvement in illnesses such as fibromyalgia and Crohn's disease, in burns, and in other injuries. It has become clear that HGH promotes healing.

The physical changes that occur with HGH therapy are obvious: more muscle and less fat, including abdominal fat. Up to 50 percent of abdominal fat can be lost in six months, especially when HGH therapy is combined with exercise and complete hormone replacement. HGH therapy is built on a foundation of exercise, diet, and supplements. Cosmetic changes also happen: more than 50 percent of the patients will experience a decrease in facial wrinkles, a decrease in graying of hair, and even a decrease of hair loss in men.

Energy changes with HGH. Some people describe it as limitless energy, both physical and mental. With HGH there is a reversal of depression, a positive outlook on life, and increased memory.

From my own standpoint, I know that when my house burned down, I was able to stand there looking at the smoldering ashes of what was once my home and feel positive about the future. It wasn't fake, it was just a feeling of balance and that I could handle this tragedy and move on and look forward. I often wonder if I hadn't been on full hormone replacement how different I might have handled the situation. My balanced hormones had a positive effect—I had people writing me from all over the world saying they were inspired by my reaction to the loss of all my material belongings . . . I hadn't thought of that. However, I do feel that energy does have a ripple effect, and then I couldn't help but think if everyone was in perfect hormonal harmony, what a different world this would be.

It's important to know that you cannot think you can just start injecting HGH and the world (and your body) will be a better place. HGH is just *one part of the missing "song."* For better health you need to start with lifestyle changes including diet, exercise, and supplements, while also balancing all the key hormones. The results can be profound if you truly embrace the entire program. You will be able to re-create the physiology you had in your twenties but with the wisdom and the experience of your chronological age.

THE MAJOR HORMONES

We are the age of our oldest organ.

–Dr. Thierry Hertoghe

THYROID

The thyroid is a *major* hormone, meaning that if it is high or low for too long a period of time, you are at risk of death. Take your thyroid seriously.

The thyroid gland is butterfly shaped, situated just below the Adam's apple. The hormones produced from this endocrine gland are responsible for our metabolism, which is the sum of all physical and chemical processes. In other words, the thyroid hormones control the efficiency and speed at which all our cells work. If your thyroid is low, you will notice rapid weight gain. When my thyroid gets "off," I can gain as much as five pounds in a week with no change in my good diet.

Of all your hormones, the thyroid is the most important! According to Dr. Mark Starr, in his book *Hypothyroidism Type 2*, "Without the crucial influence of the thyroid hormones, proper maturation and function of the other hormone glands is not possible." I agree with Dr. Starr. The thyroid stimulates the cell energy production that is necessary for life, as well as maintains our body's relatively constant temperature. That is why a major symptom of hypo (low) thyroid is extreme sensitivity to hot and cold. The thyroid orchestrates the development of our brain and sexual maturation. Without a well-working thyroid, harmful cell waste accumulates, and the immune system is dependent on normal thyroid function. Low thyroid leads to susceptibility to infection. If your thyroid isn't working properly, it doesn't matter how well you eat or how much you exercise; your health will suffer.

How do you know if you have a low thyroid? Swelling is one way to tell. Swelling usually begins around the face. Upper arms become thickened, and this swelling and thickening eventually spreads throughout the body's connective tissues. Connective tissue helps hold our bodies' organs together—this is kind of important! We have connective tissue in the lining of the blood vessels, nervous system, muscles, mucous membranes such as the sinuses, the gut, and each cell in our glands and organs. Most doctors don't know to examine for thick skin as related to low thyroid, so you must do this on your own, and tell your doctor you want to have your thyroid tested.

Thyroid imbalances can manifest as either physical or mental/emotional symptoms. Any organ in the body can be affected by the thyroid. Every cell between and including the hair on the head and the toenail depends on proper thyroid function for development.

There are many other symptoms of low thyroid, including chronic pain, fatigue, dry skin, high blood pressure, a slightly irregular heartbeat, sleep apnea, sensitivity to hot and cold, unexplained weight gain, missing outer third of eyebrows, constipation, repeated infections, brittle nails, hair loss, intolerance to heat, muscle weakness, low blood pressure, osteoporosis, joint/muscle pain, cystic breast/ovaries, chronic sinusitis, slow movements, slow speech, hoarseness, slow heart rate, cavities, TMJ syndrome, swollen gums, rotting teeth, mitral valve prolapse, joint pain, headache, and increased cholesterol levels. The list just goes on and on.

Growth disturbances, mental disturbances, and abnormalities in genital development are chiefly governed by the thyroid gland. Textbooks are filled with literature about low thyroidism and short stature.

Low thyroid causes our metabolism to slow down. This explains the weight gain and the constipation. The low energy output is why a low thyroid patient gets so cold. The centers of our cells are called "mitochondria" and do not function properly with low thyroid, which causes fatigue and energy loss. You see it around you, older people who seem to be out of gas. Some people literally cannot stay awake because of the lack of energy from low thyroid.

Low thyroid also causes asthma, which gets worse in the winter, causing frequent infections such as colds, sinus infections, and pneumonia. Decreased circulation from low thyroid also causes dry, itchy skin. Puffy eyes, eczema, psoriasis, cellulitis (deadly skin infection), and teenage acne are all symptoms of low thyroid. Absence of or diminished perspiration is a symptom, and skin cancers and melanomas are also symptoms of low thyroid.

Even hair is seriously affected by low thyroid, resulting in premature baldness and hair loss. This is important because 40 percent of American women are suffering from significant hair loss related to low thyroid hormones. Redheads are particularly at risk.

The reason you need to be concerned about all of this is that hypothyroidism, or low thyroid, gets worse with the passing of time. Occasionally there may be a sudden change for the worse, such as the autoimmune disease known as Hashimoto's disease. For some unknown reason, the body decides to destroy its own thyroid gland. This syndrome often runs in families but not always.

Are you getting the picture that the thyroid is involved in *everything*?

The good news is that low thyroid can be easily corrected by augmenting the body's own production with bioidentical thyroid hormones.

Thyroid function gradually slows down as we age. Many doctors prescribe thyroxine, which is T4, and triiodothyronine, which is T3. Approximately 93 percent of the hormones being secreted by the thyroid are T4, with only 7 percent being T3. In healthy people almost all thyroxine is converted to T3.

You can diagnose your thyroid needs by a simple blood test. Low levels of T4 and T3 are signs that you do not have enough thyroid hormones.

An elevated TSH (thyroid stimulating hormone) is a sign of thyroid deficiency. When your TSH is high, it means the pituitary gland is trying to produce more hormones. Your doctor must test for both T4 and T3. Both forms of the hormone are needed to regulate the body's metabolic rate. One without the other will not work.

Armour dessicated thyroid, which is derived from porcine thyroid tissue (in other words, from the pig), is a natural form of thyroid hormone. Armour is best tolerated in patients whose bodies cannot properly convert thyroxine into the active form of the hormone, but for many patients thyroxine (also a natural form of the hormone) works as well or better. Dr. Broda Barnes stated more than fifty years ago that patients taking thyroid replacement therapy have much better improvement of symptoms with natural desiccated thyroid hormone than with synthetic hormones.

ADRENALS

If you have ever flatlined your adrenals, you remember the feeling—you have a complete absence of energy, depression, rage or crying, and an inability to sleep, all brought on by constant stress, poor nutrition, and consumption of chemicals, particularly diet soda.

That's most folks at some point in their lives. When stress continues over a long period of time, the adrenal glands deplete the body's hormonal and energy reserves. It's no fun. This prolonged stress weakens the immune system and inhibits the production of white blood cells that protect the body against foreign invaders, in particular lymph node function. Adrenal dysfunction causes weakness, fatigue, and a feeling of being run-down, which is accurate because you are run down. It also interferes with sleep patterns and rhythms, making you feel even more worn out. Allergies, infections, low blood sugar, and low blood pressure can kick in with weakened adrenals. Thyroid problems may overlap with weak adrenals for some people.

If weak adrenals continue, the levels of other hormones, namely cortisol and aldosterone (which affects hearing, among other things), are affected. The adrenal glands regulate the body's metabolic rate, meaning they regulate the metabolism of proteins, fats, and carbohydrates. Adrenals also regulate nerve energy, physical energy, glandular energy, and the oxidation process.

Many hormonal imbalances are the direct result of adrenal insufficiency. When the adrenals become too tired, adequate levels of cortisol and DHEA cannot be produced. Long-term stress can have a serious impact on the adrenals and cause them to shrink and reduce production. This causes cell damage, which sets off a chain reaction accelerating the aging process.

The adrenals are the orchestra leader . . . the Zubin Mehta of the body. The adrenals direct the rest of the endocrine system to keep all the hormones normalized. Knowing that their function is so important, you can then appreciate why you feel so absolutely awful when they are out of whack. Body rashes, pimples, and weight gain are bad enough consequences of burned-out adrenals, but adrenal dysfunction can cause an overall hormonal change affecting the entire system—it is essential to normalize function.

So, how do we do that? Sleep is the best remedy, but because sleep is impossible when your adrenals are shot, you need to reregulate them by changing your lifestyle. Dr. Michael Galitzer (see chapter 24) suggests relaxation, going to bed early, and regular laughter. As for supplements, he recommends 2,000 to 4,000 milligrams per day of vitamin C, because the highest concentration in the body of vitamin C is in the adrenals, vitamin B_5, pantothenic acid, 500 milligrams twice a day, or licorice tea.

For severe adrenal dysfunction, supplementation with bioidentical cortisol is recommended.

I have burned out my adrenals from overwork four times in my career, and now I need to supplement with bioidentical cortisol, perhaps for the rest of my life. May this be a warning to all those workaholics—there is a big price to pay. I take my cortisol replacement seriously because I do not want to have a heart attack. I have burned out my adrenals so often, my adrenal glands are shot and just won't rev up again. I wish I'd known what I was doing to myself when I took on all that work.

Too much work, unhappiness with your life or choices, a lack of confidence, and, most significantly, a lack of sleep all help contribute to adrenal burnout. By meditating and getting therapy, sleeping more, eating better, cutting out diet soda, and, if necessary, taking bioidentical cortisol (hydrocortisone), you can restore your adrenal balance, get back your energy, and repair conditions like age spots, constipation, dark circles under the eyes, mood swings, dizziness, impaired respiration, poor concentration, edema (swelling), and hypoglycemia.

CORTISOL

Cortisol is another *major* hormone, meaning it is vital to life. You cannot live without it; if it is too low or too high for too long a period of time, you won't live very long. Cortisol is secreted in small amounts from the adrenals. If your adrenals are burned out, guess what? Your cortisol is going to be high until eventually your adrenals are completely shot. High cortisol is no fun. Sleep becomes impossible, and then a vicious cycle is in place. Whenever any hormone is out of balance in your body, it will affect the way you feel. Hormonal imbalance causes discomfort, irritability, and a feeling of not being well.

Too much cortisol plagues people who seem to thrive on stress, particularly because high cortisol is a sign that your adrenals are overstressed. People with burned-out adrenals are energized and invigorated by the continuous flood of cortisol that stress produces. If the cortisol-producing adrenal glands are *too active* it can translate into euphoria or excessive activity or even disabling mania. We all know someone like that, those manic types . . . after a while it's just too much to be around them. We're actually watching them burn out. Burnout is not pretty.

With appropriate amounts of cortisol, stress doesn't depress you. Cortisol is a mood hormone. If you experience anxiety at the end of the day, are irked by small things, or feel unable to confront or escape from a situation; if you feel pessimistic and defeated, or have excessive sensitivity to stress, or have trouble organizing thoughts, or become paralyzed by stress and feel exhausted afterward, or have suicidal thoughts at night . . . you need to have your cortisol levels checked.

As we age, our cortisol levels don't go up, they decline, and then we get adrenal fatigue caused by chronic stress; whether it's psychological or physical—from overexercising, chronic pain syndrome, joint-muscle aches and pain, chronic allergies, or asthma . . . these are all symptoms of low cortisol. This is why doctors are always advising their patients to manage their stress. It's lifesaving advice that few heed. We know stress is bad for us, but our adrenals can be the deciding factor in just how bad. If stress gets to a breaking point, then heart attack or stroke is inevitable.

The average person naturally makes 20 to 30 milligrams of cortisol daily. But if you are stressed, your adrenals get rocked like a boat. It can knock you out for a week or a month because you just don't have the energy to bounce back. At this point patients are often advised to take a vacation, sit on a Caribbean island—and all of a sudden they feel great again.

Cortisol helps the body respond to stress. The problem with the lives we live today is that we are bombarded with stress day in and day out. Once cortisol gave us superhuman strength to deal with a saber-toothed tiger attack. Now we deplete our cortisol by releasing it all day as we deal with the common stresses of modern life, leaving us little in reserve. Depletion of cortisol levels leaves us feeling depressed and fatigued. Again, it is a setup for a heart attack and it won't take long for it to happen.

Antiaging doctors take high cortisol very seriously. When you have high cortisol, you are definitely not sleeping, you are padding around the house all night long. The next day you are exhausted but run around like a maniac because your cortisol levels are so high; this syndrome very clearly is a recipe for disaster. A lot of "A"-type men have those sudden heart attacks and no one can understand it because "Gee, he was on the tennis court yesterday and now he's dead."

Cortisol does so many wonderful things for us: stimulates appetite, boosts energy levels, improves digestion, eases movement in the joints, eases inflammation and pain, and enhances the immune system. Even though cortisol is associated with stress, in actuality it is the antistress hormone when it is balanced.

Cortisol also stimulates the brain, muscles, heart, and circulatory and respiratory systems. It fights certain cancers like leukemia and some lymphomas.

There are certain characteristics you can actually see or feel if your cortisol is high: if you have a swollen face, a buffalo hump of fat on your upper back, disappearing hair from the top of your head, or too much hair in general; if you are underweight, have low blood pressure problems, lupus, fibromyalgia, or osteoarthritis; if you crave salt or sugar to the extent of bingeing; if you have digestive problems and allergies; if you are stressed out, easily confused; if you have eczema, psoriasis, urticaria (nettle rash), skin allergies or other rashes; if you have difficulty getting aroused for sex or trouble concentrating. All these symptoms indicate high cortisol.

Cortisol can be replaced as determined through blood testing or twenty-four-hour urine testing. The remedy is to replace according to your particular needs indicated by lab work, but you must take your replacement diligently four times a day, spread out the way it once poured in nature: sunrise, midday, midafternoon, and sunset.

Cortisol responds to light, even the tiniest bit—computer lights, phone lights, or night-lights—and could be the impairment that keeps you from sleeping. I put black tape over all the lights in my bedroom and sleep in complete darkness. There was a study done of one hundred subjects put into a completely dark room, with the exception of a pin light on the back of their knees, and each subject's cortisol level went up as a result.

Cortisol reads light, which is why it pours at sunrise until sunset. After sunset our cortisol levels are supposed to go down naturally, allowing for sleep, but because we are leading such stressful lives, cortisol levels now stay artificially raised, triggering an unhealthy vicious cycle.

I had to retrain myself to sleep. I started by going to bed at 10:00 P.M., which was difficult because I had gotten into a routine of going to bed quite late, 1:00, 2:00, or 3:00 A.M. I guess all those years of being a night-club performer trained me to stay up (or, most likely, my adrenals were totally shot). After a while I tried going to sleep at 9:30. I put the TV on a timer so it would (hopefully) bore me to sleep and then turn itself off rather than my old way of sitting up clutching the clicker like it was the most important thing in my life (what we do to ourselves . . . geez).

By taping the small lights, by forcing myself to go to bed early, by taking melatonin supplements, a hot bath, and a nanotechnology sleep patch, I finally did it. I now go to bed at 9:00 or 9:30 nightly. I go out only two nights a week; I eat right and stop eating after dinner.

I try not to watch news about the war in Iraq before I go to bed, and I have finally succeeded. I sleep a good eight to nine hours nightly, and it has improved my health, my looks, my energy, my libido, and my mood. In fact, everything is better since I started sleeping.

Also, I faithfully take my bioidentical compounded cortisol four times a day, and I will until something else comes along. I am quite interested in what Dr. Jonathan Wright (see chapter 2) says about cell therapy, that I might actually (through adrenal cell injections) be able to rejuvenate my adrenals and get them to rev up and start working again. He is doing this in his clinic in Washington State, called the Tahoma Clinic. I'm seriously thinking of starting the therapy.

The other real bummer of high cortisol induced by stress or poor diet is weight gain. People with adrenal fatigue with resulting high cortisol frequently overeat in their attempt to bolster their lagging energy and then end up gaining weight.

The temporary increase in cortisol levels produced by driving the adrenals with too much fast food and caffeine causes people with chronically low cortisol to put on weight, because even a temporary excess of cortisol causes fat to be deposited around the middle (spare tire). The extra weight adds to their lethargy, making them eat more and more of the wrong foods to get through the day. Knowing how to eat properly can keep energy steady without resorting to this destructive pattern.

If you are going to use cortisol, you will need the help of a qualified physician. In physiology, hydrocortisone is the name of one of the hormones in the adrenal cascade. Antiaging doctors will give you hydrocortisone, compounded by a compounding pharmacy. It is bioidentical and has nothing to do with the steroid called cortisone. Conventional doctors get this mixed up. A friend of mine was given hydrocortisone by her gynecologist, who is also versed in all bioidenticals and bioidentical cortisol.

When this same person went to her ENT (ear, nose, and throat) conventional doctor, he was appalled that she was taking what he thought were dangerous steroids. This illustrates the confusion that is out there. This woman had all the symptoms of adrenal burnout, including nettle rash all over her body, and bioidentical cortisol replacement was an appropriate treatment that would have brought her relief.

Remember, it is important for you to understand how your body works if you want to stay healthy in this stressed-out, crazy world.

The doctors that you choose need to have an in-depth knowledge of adrenal function and understand how to use adrenal extracts and cortisol together for optimum benefit. Don't be afraid to ask your doctors if they know what they are doing. This is your life and your body.

INSULIN

Insulin is the last of the *major* hormones. Again, if any of your major hormones (insulin, thyroid, adrenals, or cortisol) are too low, too high, or missing, you may not live very long. The major hormones are the leaders of the pack. They govern the body. We all know the seriousness of high insulin as it relates to diabetics. The eating patterns of most Americans are constantly testing the body's ability to cope. If you consume chemicals and large amounts of sugar (bread, white rice, pasta, high-starch vegetables, too much fruit), you are putting your body at risk. A doctor once told me, "I would rather have cancer than diabetes." That gives you an indication of the seriousness of elevated insulin.

Insulin is a hormone manufactured by the pancreas and has profound effects on aging. Low insulin levels can be due to diabetes, or malnourishment from not eating or not consuming enough carbohydrates, or overexercising. High insulin levels can be due to smoking tobacco, stress, overeating, low estradiol, chronic yo-yo dieting, and drinking alcohol.

Some foods that are digested enter the bloodstream as the simple sugar glucose, which the body uses as an energy source. Insulin directs glucose, which is then able to pass from the bloodstream through the cell membrane and into the cell, where it is burned as fuel.

Elevated insulin can cause:

- high blood pressure
- blood fat abnormalities
- abnormal immune system functioning
- accelerated biological aging
- acne
- ankle swelling
- burning feet
- constipation
- decreased memory or concentration
- depression
- fatigue
- fluctuating high blood pressure readings
- fuzzy brain
- irregular menstrual cycles
- irritability
- loose bowel movements, alternating with constipation
- sugar cravings
- water retention
- weight gain, especially around the middle

High insulin levels cause a woman's body to shift hormone production away from estrogen, which is unfortunate because estrogen protects against osteoporosis, heart disease, and Alzheimer's. Also, estrogen pushes the production of testosterone. So now you have an imbalance. Low estrogen and high insulin alter body composition and shape, causing unhealthy weight gain, which is then a risk factor for high blood pressure, heart disease, and further hormone imbalance.

9

DR. THIERRY HERTOGHE

And now we are on the brink of the can-do era, when the leopard will be able to change its very spots.

–Robert Ettinger, *Man into Superman* (1972)

YOU CAN'T GET TOO FAR into learning about bioidentical hormone replacement without hearing of Dr. Thierry Hertoghe.

He comes from four generations of hormone therapists and was fortunate to inherit the great skills of astute observation of hormonal problems from his father and grandfathers. The most respected doctor in his field, Dr. Hertoghe is known all over Europe as the "father of bioidenticals." He is the president of the International Hormone Society (over 1,900 physicians) and of the World Society of Anti-Aging Medicine (over 4,500 physicians). He is a member of the International Advisory Board of the American Academy of Anti-Aging Medicine. He lectures regularly to medical professionals and laypeople in the United States and abroad on the subject of hormonal deficiencies.

He is most content working with patients, but because of his depth of knowledge, much of his time is now spent in courtroom settings explaining to government officials and medical boards all across Europe the tremendous health benefits of replacing declining hormones with bioidentical hormones and offering compelling evidence for the efficacy of bioidentical hormones. He explains that by doing this, it will unburden their governments from the health expenses that accompany the present pharmaceutical approach to maintaining disease.

Dr. Hertoghe understands that when a person practices bioidentical hormone replacement, his or her health improves drastically, and it becomes a win/win situation: The patient feels great and the government is not responsible for the enormous, mounting health care expenses that have become part and parcel of aging.

Dr. Hertoghe's argument with the heads of the European government medical boards is to ask them to take a commonsense approach: "Put back what our bodies once made with nondrug, nonpatentable bioidentical hormones and people will feel well, get better, conditions will clear up, moods will normalize, marriages will stay intact, and overall the population will be healthier."

When the population is healthy the burden of health care costs on the government diminishes. Pharmaceutical companies do not have the same hold over government officials in Europe as they do in the United States. This is too bad for us. We are at a disadvantage. Nonpatentable medicines get more and more difficult to obtain. We are, for the most part, being forced into taking chemicals. Thank God for doctors like Dr. Hertoghe.

Dr. Hertoghe's team of doctors and professionals see patients at his offices in Belgium, treating both men and women for hormonal disturbances. I have had the pleasure of getting to know Dr. Hertoghe and, as you will read in his interview, the man is passionate about health and life. His book is called *The Hormone Solution*.

SS: Good evening, Dr. Hertoghe, and thank you for giving me your time, especially since it is so late where you are in Europe. You are known as the "father of bioidenticals" in Europe. Why are you so passionate?

TH: Because hormones do so much for the body. Your body contains more than one hundred different types of hormones, and they pour into your bloodstream at the rate of thousands of billions of units a day. Hormones regulate your heartbeat and your breathing. Hormones make men men and women women. Hormones put you to sleep at night and they wake you up in the morning. They control your blood pressure, build up bone, maintain muscle tone, and lubricate joints. Hormones govern growth; they make the body produce energy and heat. Hormones burn fat. Hormones govern the menstrual cycle and allow pregnancy (and birth) to occur. They fight stress, prevent fatigue, calm anxiety, and relieve depression. Hormones make and keep memories. Hormones maintain the correct level of sugar in the blood and tissues. They resist allergic reactions and infections. They soothe pain. Hormones control your sex drive, virility, and fertility. They stimulate your brain and your immune system. For all those reasons I am passionate about the subject.

SS: I get it. It's amazing when you realize the overwhelming importance of hormones and the hormonal system that there is still such resistance to replacement.

TH: For the last seven years I have been working with the medical boards to give them information. You see, I come from a tradition of doctors. All of them before me were attacked verbally on a regular basis for their beliefs. My father, grandpa, and great-grandpa used to ask, "Why don't other doctors see this?" So when I became a doctor, I realized that you have to give people the information. It's become a mission for me. A duty. And when you are giving information that you truly believe in, you get passion. I mean, hormones are crucial to every single function of the human body. You can't live without them. But in today's world, with all the stress, pollution, and chemicals, rarely do our bodies have the optimum levels of hormones, particularly as we age.

SS: And that's when we start getting sick. It is commensurate with hormonal decline.

TH: Yes . . . so people don't enjoy optimum health, whether that means arthritis or heart disease or flagging sex drive or gray hair and wrinkles or out-of-control weight gain. But I have a dream that it will only take another two to four years for people to get it . . . to understand. When people begin to understand that you don't have to forget things, or that you can sleep all night long, or that you don't have to be depressed or anxious. When people can accept that there are ways to avoid aging as we know it, or at least to delay its occurrence far into the future. When people finally understand that you don't have to have osteoporosis or cancer, things will change. We've accepted aging as inevitable; we didn't like it, but we accepted it, but we've been wrong.

SS: Do all hormone levels drop with age?

TH: Of course, your endocrine glands cannot maintain the same production of hormones they did in your younger days. And that loss is the most crucial and correctable underlying process that causes the signs and symptoms of aging as well as a host of other health problems.

When all our hormones are at optimal levels, our bodies are healthy, efficient, resilient, flexible, and strong. But even a small drop-off can create havoc. This can happen as early as our thirties. I experienced this. I was in my early thirties, tired all the time and having difficulty recovering if I went to sleep late. The sleep I did get was restless, my face was pale, my body was starting to lose its tone and firmness, I had trouble focusing, and I could no longer manage multitasking. I was often cranky and supersensitive to stress and it was interfering with my work, my relationships, and my family life. Even though I was experienced in nutrition, hormones, and longevity, I thought I was too young to be affected. My hormones were shifting and needed to be replaced and corrected. I needed to heed my own advice relative to nutrition and value a good night's sleep.

SS: What about synthetic hormones. How do you feel about them?

TH: Synthetic hormones differ by an atom or two from the chemicals the body makes. This might not sound so bad until you consider that the difference between testosterone and estrogen (the difference between a man and a woman) is a matter of just a couple of atoms.

Natural bioidentical hormones in amounts as close as possible to what your younger body made for itself can re-create the same state of health and well-being you once enjoyed.

SS: Most people don't know where the hormones in the body are produced. Can you tell me?

TH: Well, the *brain* produces pregnenolone, DHEA, ACTH (adreno-corticotropic hormone); the *pineal gland* produces melatonin; the *pituitary gland* (the anterior part) produces growth hormone (GH), ACTH, TSH (the posterior part produces vasopressin); the *thyroid gland* produces the thyroid hormones, calcitonin; the *adrenal glands* produce DHEA, cortisol, aldosterone, and pregnenolone; the *kidneys* produce EPO (erythropoietin) and convert thyroid hormone T4 into active T3; the *liver* produces somatomedin C, and converts thyroid hormone T4 into the active T3; the *pancreas* produces insulin; the *ovaries* produce estrogens and progesterone and some androgens; and the *testicles* produce testosterone and dihydrosterone.

SS: Was it automatic that you would become a doctor, being that your father, grandfather, and great-grandfather were doctors?

TH: Well, we talked about hormones, health, and aging at the dinner table. It was there I learned the secrets of good health even before I was an adult. But I have to say I didn't start medical school with much enthusiasm. My chosen field at that time was psychiatry, but as I began working in the hospital, I couldn't escape the feeling I was working with the wrong medicine. In many of the psychiatric patients, all I could see were signs of hormonal deficiencies. They were clear as day but had been overlooked by many medical professionals. Endocrinologists, the doctors "officially" in charge of hormones, seemed mostly to specialize in diabetes and only occasionally ventured into other therapies. Most of them were very traditional and spent their time on disease treatment rather than prevention. The medicine I knew from my father was aimed primarily at achieving and maintaining total health. So finally I switched to general medicine and the success I had with a surprising number of endocrinological cases finally lit a fire under me.

SS: What happened to your patients?

TH: One female patient I had was forty-nine and losing her hair. She'd also gotten flabby muscles and dry skin, felt tired and stress sensitive all the time, and had bouts of nervousness, depression, and upset stomach, none of which bothered her until she reached fifty. We got her hormones balanced with natural estrogen, progesterone, cortisol, and DHEA, changed her diet to support them, and she looked and felt better within two months. Her hair even stopped falling out and grew back. I had many cases like that, and I discovered I could help people understand what their bodies were telling them in order to zero in on the most appropriate treatment and that gave me a sense of mission.

SS: You are very well known for your work with thyroid.

TH: Well, thanks to my father, I started taking thyroid hormones to correct hypothyroidism when I was very young. This disease typically goes undetected in young people, especially in young men.

SS: Thyroid is pretty easy to spot even without blood tests, right?

TH: Yes, dry skin, constipated, stiff joints, fatigued, sensitive to hot and cold, and very tired . . . exhausted. When the thyroid is working correctly, it energizes cells and organs by stimulating the mitochondria (known as the cells' little powerhouses), freeing heat and energy. Thyroid hormones warm the body, especially the extremities, and prevent sensitivity to hot and cold. They prevent morning fatigue. Thyroid hormones provide a quickness of mind, because they protect not only the brain, but also the kidneys and the digestive and immune system organs along with other body tissues, the heart and arteries among them. Thyroid stimulates fat-burning and dissolves cholesterol, thereby opening up the arteries and moderating blood pressure as the hormones encourage the elimination of waste from the cells and around the cells of the arterial walls, making them more supple. They prevent constipation by activating smooth muscle cells of the intestinal walls and eliminating swelling, and they help you avoid diffuse headaches, also by eliminating swelling and improving blood flow through the brain. Thyroid also reduces the risk and severity of heart disease, cancer, and other conditions with otherwise high mortality rates. The thyroid is a major hormone and a major player in your health.

SS: Are there any other symptoms?

TH: Well, without sufficient thyroid hormones, the body bloats. You'll have a particularly swollen face, with puffy eyelids and thicker lips . . . especially the lower lip. If that's not enough to make you want to ensure proper levels, you might also want to know that that effect is thanks to waste materials that accumulate between the cells. Without thyroid hormones you'll also have dry, rough, brittle, and sparse hair, lifeless eyes, a pale face, cold hands and feet, constipation, and dry skin.

SS: Whew . . . other than that everything's okay [laughs]?

TH: No, there's more . . . you'll have problems with memory and concentration. You'll get fat, without changing anything about the way you eat or how you exercise. You'll feel tired, especially in the morning and when you are resting. You'll feel cold, especially in the evening and when you are resting. You'll have stiff and painful joints, especially in the morning and after resting. Some people get slowed down in their movements and their thoughts, while others get agitated, hyperactive, and hyperkinetic, moving constantly, probably in an unconscious attempt to accelerate blood circulation to supply nutrients and hormones to the tissues.

SS: So how does a person test for thyroid?

TH: In the blood, high levels of TSH [above 4mIU/ml (micro units per ml) and, in some cases, even above 2 mIU/ml], can indicate low thyroid activity. You'd also want to make sure you keep your free triiodothyronine level above 1.8 ng/dL and your free thyroxine above 0.8 or even 1.2 ng/dl. If your numbers fall below those, supplements are indicated. We check for T3 and T4. That's very important to get both.

SS: So when the levels come back and supplementation is recommended, what do you give them?

TH: I was just defending a doctor in the United Kingdom who was being attacked for thyroid hormone therapy use, which is one of the basic therapies of antiaging medicine. This guy had a world expert testifying against him and there was absolutely nothing the expert said in his attacks that was correct.

It was about Armour thyroid (desiccated thyroid) versus Thyroxin. The attack was on two levels. They said Armour was not a good product, which is incorrect. They said there was no evidence to prove it was better than the synthetic Thyroxin, which is incorrect. The studies proving the efficacy of Armour thyroid and similar medications containing both thyroid hormones (thyroxine and triiodothyronine) is on the International Hormone Society's Web site at www.intlhormonesociety.org.

SS: What hormones do you take?

TH: Well, I am fifty-one years old, so I know my glands are not making hormones on their own anymore. I take thyroid hormones, melatonin,

DHEA, testosterone, pregnenolone, cortisol, a derivative of aldosterone, and growth hormone on a daily basis, and I have taken these for years. I need and depend on these replacement hormones to maintain my mood, energy, and physical fitness. I eat a healthful diet, which I believe is crucial, and I also take vitamin and mineral supplements to support the hormonal balance I'm after.

SS: How do you know it's working?

TH: If I don't take thyroid, I'm tired, stiff, and cranky in the morning and I don't think clearly. If I don't supplement with enough cortisol, I have powerful sugar cravings. I also feel drowsy and I can't concentrate. Every stress feels like too much to handle. On the other hand, it's important to know that too much cortisol leads to an unhealthy feeling of euphoria, so you don't want to take too much.

Growth hormone is the supplement I'd be the least willing to give up for any reason. I started taking it over ten years ago for reasons of vanity. I was starting to have jowls. Taking growth hormone stopped and reversed that process, but I found I also reaped other amazing benefits. I'm calm and cordial even in the midst of conflict. When half my house burned down only days before a huge conference presentation, everyone thought I would lose it, but I was able to keep going, deal with the fire, comfort my wife, and deliver my speech without a hitch. This is all thanks to the growth hormone.

SS: You know, my house burned down this year, all of it. Lost everything, including my first seven books, which I had written longhand. But I too was calm, and reflective, and grateful not to have been in the house when it happened. I attribute that sense of calm to the full complement of all my other hormones that I am replacing and also to growth hormone.

TH: That's a typical growth hormone effect. There is an unfounded fear of growth hormone. It is thought to increase cancer, or increase diabetes, or increase cardiovascular disease, but there is no proof. There was a study on people with severe growth hormone *deficiency* who had a 50 percent *increase* in cancer . . . in overall cancer.

SS: Why would no or low growth hormone increase cancer?

TH: Growth hormone is protective. It has powerful immune-stimulating effects.

SS: You mean it's part of the "song"? That we need to replace *all* the missing hormones?

TH: Yes, for sure. And we decline in growth hormone at age thirty. It's one of the fastest-declining hormones in our body. Only DHEA declines more quickly. All the major characteristics of aging are due to growth hormone deficiency. Growth hormone is such an important hormone that it makes a person stay tall and strong and with good muscle strength and definition. When an adult does not have enough growth hormone, the amount he has may actually be comparable to that of a dwarf. You will develop a crumbling back, you will develop atrophy of the organs, and your body becomes flabby. Without GH you will develop more fat and less muscle. Small wrinkles are due to sex hormone deficiency, but when you have big wrinkles, like sagging cheeks, that's a growth hormone deficiency.

Without growth hormone you sort of have a collapse physically, but you will also have a mental collapse if you become severely deficient in GH; for instance, I didn't take GH between the ages of thirty-one and thirty-eight and I started having anxiety for no reason. Once on GH therapy (I started at age thirty-eight), I lost the anxiety and started spending a lot of my time battling for justice for this type of medicine. I challenged the National Medical Board because the court was attacking antiaging doctors in Belgium. For example, seven thousand physicians were sent a booklet saying that all antiaging doctors were charlatans, bad doctors, and crooks. At that time no one ever dared to challenge the medical boards. I've challenged them thirteen times, eventually by helping other physicians, and won almost every court trial. GH makes me less anxious, calm, and it's a hormone that makes you see things more clearly.

SS: I know of the physical ramifications (which are tremendous), but I've never heard of it as an antidote to anxiety.

TH: I was elected as a full member of the medical board and came to the medical board meetings for seven years. All the medical board members were against me because I strove for human rights, and they were angry because I was garnering so much press. But I was always calm. That's growth hormone.

SS: Then wouldn't growth hormone be a good thing for menopausal women who are going through such anxiety and depression?

TH: Yes, absolutely, but you can't just take growth hormone, you have to replace all the other missing hormones or it won't work. It's very important to understand that. If you are missing your female or male hormones, or if you are cortisol deficient and you are not replacing these hormones properly, then growth hormone won't work. In fact, it will even worsen the situation. If a person has low cortisol or low adrenals, for example, or if a person is under a lot of stress and has burned out their adrenals, and then you give them GH, it lowers both cortisol and adrenal levels, further aggravating the condition. On the other hand, the lowering of cortisol by GH treatment may have a healing effect when cortisol levels are too high. Excessive cortisol will cause tissue wasting (it burns up too much tissue to provide energy) and makes sleep impossible, and it's not good for the heart or the muscles. We should strive to find the right balance of cortisol, but it is important to avoid excesses.

SS: How do you feel about bioidentical hydrocortisone, which is cortisol replacement?

TH: I'm for bioidenticals as a first choice of treatment. If you take it, you must take it twice a day.

SS: Some doctors say four times a day to mimic nature. That, in nature, it pours in "peaks," and so to replace it properly you need to take it at sunrise, say at 7:00 A.M., then again four hours and forty minutes later, say at 11:40 A.M., then again at 3:00, then the last dose at sunset at 7:00 P.M.

TH: You are correct. Most people need to spread it out that way, if the deficiency is severe, but some people can take it twice or just in the morning.

SS: Well, my deficiency was severe, so I take it as I mentioned above even though it is a huge pain in the butt to remember. But I feel better, my breast tenderness calms down, and I sleep better. I just feel I need it.

TH: But know that you lower your cortisol by taking melatonin at bedtime.

SS: So GH is part of the "language" that every hormone must talk to all the other hormones.

TH: Correct. GH works in concert with all the other hormones. You don't just take one hormone; you replace all of them for optimal health and well-being.

SS: How important is the lymphatic system?

TH: Very important. It's the fluid that surrounds all the cells that have to be washed away and renewed. If you don't have a good working lymph system, you have a disadvantage. Do you have a problem with your lymphatic system?

SS: Yes, after my house burned down, I got a lot of lymphatic congestion from the stress. That's when I got interested in the job of the lymphs. I was surprised to find out that there is no lymphatic "pump." Our blood is pumped, but the lymph just sits there if you don't move, and if you get stressed, it becomes congested. Then it can't do its job to wash away all the debris.

TH: If you interrupt the drainage through sickness or stress, the drainage has to be diverted from other lymphatic vessels where you do have some lymphatic estrogen. Each time you straighten your muscles or get out of bed, you move the lymph vessels.

SS: So the Rebounder (small trampoline) has benefit, or yoga, or really any exercise, like swimming.

TH: Anything that stresses your muscles assists in lymphatic drainage.

SS: You know, you can buy growth hormones online. I have many male friends who purchase it that way, but they are not doing any other supplementation. What's going to happen?

TH: Well, first of all, the GH you buy online doesn't work very well. You don't want to buy an inferior product, especially when it comes to hormones. And secondly, if you are not replacing correctly you will gain weight.

SS: But here's the problem. Athletes are taking ten to twenty—sometimes one hundred—times more GH than they need and they get that "Andre the Giant" look. So GH gets a bad rap because people and the media see this misuse and then condemn the whole notion.

TH: Yes, but it's not so terrible to get bad press. It gets people thinking about it. They hear about the product, and that there are intelligent people defending the proper use and its benefits, and that if you take it correctly you look better and have more energy. And then the truth comes out.

SS: Is human growth hormone something that once we begin we stay on it for life?

TH: Well, you can always stop and return to how you previously felt, but honestly, once you realize how good you feel replacing all the hormones, you won't ever want to stop because you feel much better. Not only is your body weight better, but your body composition improves. Muscle tone improves and fat goes away. At present, my body fat is 4.8 percent. Not even athletes have that composition at my age.

SS: I presume you eat correctly.

TH: I'm not tempted to eat poorly because I feel the consequences when I do. It's not worth it. I spend all this time working at hormonal balance and the well-being that comes with it and then I could ruin everything with sugar or alcohol. Not worth it. People have to understand the effects of diet. The two most common causes of high estradiol are drinking coffee and drinking alcohol. A Greek study showed that two cups of coffee a day or just one glass of alcohol a day increased estradiol levels by 60 percent.

SS: Why do coffee and alcohol raise estradiol levels?

TH: The study doesn't say why, but I can speculate that it increases the conversion of testosterone to estradiol. Alcohol certainly does that, as do caffeine and caffeinated beverages like Coca-Cola; drinking large amounts of tea also increase the conversion. So we have to go back to the diets for which our bodies were intended—drinking lots of water or herbal tea and not excessive caffeine. When people do that they feel better. Coffee not only increases female hormones, but it also decreases growth hormone—this was proven by a study—and caffeine also increases insulin, which, as you know, is the hormone that makes you fat.

SS: You must not be very popular in Europe. That's the coffee-drinking Mecca of the world [laughs].

TH: Well, people have a hard time in the beginning, but after a while they feel grateful because they feel so good.

SS: What do you think about the long-term effects of the chemicalization that's happening to all of us, not only globally, but especially in the United States where the eating habits are beyond poor? What do you think is going to happen to us?

TH: I think it's already happened. When we go to the U.S., from the moment we arrive at the airports, we're astonished. You have incredible obesity, like nowhere else. The only other place where this is happening with such astonishing rapidity is in the rich Arab countries. This is all the effect of chemicals. Chemicals divert the endocrine system. They lower some hormones and increase others. Many of the chemicals like pesticides have a female hormone structure.

SS: So there's an estrogenic effect on us?

TH: Yes, and very strong. That includes the drinking water that has been taken and tested from regions where female hormones—in particular birth control pills—have entered the water source.

SS: So, you are saying that as individuals we must go out of our way to pay attention to and think about every single thing we put in and on our bodies?

TH: Yes. You see, America is always ahead of all the other countries, and in this case for the first time we are not envious.

SS: Are you talking about weight, because we are the fattest?

TH: Yes, but the world is going to catch up, because the globe always follows your example.

SS: Hopefully, you will continue to make an impact through your books, your practice, and your lectures. So, aside from all the doom and gloom, what are you excited about relative to medicine in the future?

TH: The most exciting prospect of all is stem cells. They can now make stem cells that can grow new teeth; they can put stem cells in the retina of the eye of blind mice and they can see again, not perfectly, but they can see. The possibilities are fantastic. I have a patient (who is a doctor) who has had five heart attacks and is now in Thailand receiving stem cells to regenerate his heart. This is an amazing new breakthrough in medicine. They are also making great progress with Parkinson's and Alzheimer's by injecting stem cells into the blood. About 30 percent of people with degenerative disease appear to reverse their disease to some degree. Eventually we will be able to totally reverse disease. You see, *we are the age of our oldest organ;* so if, for instance, your heart is your oldest organ, that would be considered your real age.

SS: Yes, I've heard of this. In fact, Dr. Eric Braverman of New York City (who is mentioned in chapter 15 of this book), is doing that; it's called AgePrint. Through testing he can determine the oldest organ in a person's body.

TH: Yes, we are doing that at our office also. This is going to allow us to live a very long time. Once we can reverse and regrow that which is damaged or diseased, through stem cells and new advances, we will change medicine forever. For instance, in the future we'll probably be able to inject stem cells into the endocrine glands to rejuvenate glands so that people will begin to make their own hormones again.

SS: That is an exciting thought.

TH: The frontier of medicine is truly hopeful and exciting. It's unfortunate I must spend so much of my time fighting preconceived notions of hormones and progressive treatments. But I must; I feel that it's a duty. As I said, I come from a tradition of doctors. They were always on the forefront, being criticized and attacked. So I feel it's up to me to present the information based in studies and my own personal experience not only with myself, but also with my patients. I have accepted that I may not accomplish my dreams, but that my mission is to accomplish what is necessary to educate the medical community about the advantages of this type of medicine. My patients get better. I see the results. I have energy and passion, and I give hormonal balance the credit. That's why I do what I do, and I don't think about the fact that there is a force against this medicine and that it is unfair and unjust. I don't think about it. I just keep pushing on. I am not burdened by the hard feelings that paralyze people. Because I am so well, I feel I have an easier life than others. The stresses are not so stressful because of the way I take care of myself. I approach all of it with calm, passion, and purpose. That's what gives me happiness.

I have a dream about the changes I anticipate. The World Society of Anti-Aging Medicine and the International Hormone Society are growing in extraordinary leaps and bounds. I imagine two years from now we will have the biggest medical organization in the discipline. Then we will become mainstream. We are currently holding a course in endocrinology with four hundred hours of lectures and instructions, to teach all the interested doctors in the world about the efficacy of this kind of treatment. This is the way to treat patients to get better.

SS: That's what the patients want. Not to be on harmful drugs for life, not to be on drugs that are merely a Band-Aid and weren't designed to heal. Doctors take an oath "to do no harm."

TH: That's what we do in this kind of medicine. We heal. We make patients feel good. We give them back their energy. We give them back their sex lives; we change their diets and put them on a road to good health. It requires that the patient and the doctor do their part together. When that happens, it is magical.

DR. THIERRY HERTOGHE'S BREAKTHROUGH BREAKOUTS

- When all our hormones are at optimal levels, our bodies are healthy, efficient, resilient, flexible, and strong. But the right amounts are essential. Growth hormone, when taken in concert with the right levels of other hormones, keeps your body healthy.

- Thyroid hormones at the right levels have a variety of benefits, including protecting the brain, the kidneys, and the digestive and immune system organs, along with other body tissues, the heart and arteries among them.

- The lymph system washes away all the debris and waste fluids. Any kind of activity that stresses your muscles, such as exercising and stretching, assists in lymphatic drainage.

- Avoid coffee and alcohol. Both raise estradiol levels, which prevents you from feeling good. Coffee not only increases female hormones, but also decreases growth hormone; caffeine also increases insulin, the hormone that makes you fat.

- Stem cells are an amazing new breakthrough in medicine. With the regenerative properties of stem cells, eventually we will be able to totally reverse disease.

Dear Suzanne Somers,

My wife and I have been together since high school in east Texas and have enjoyed a thirty-five-year love affair that produced four great kids. Last year, she suddenly became this other person I did not know who complained a lot about the smallest things, was sharp with our children, and on top of all that, the "love" disappeared from our love affair. We were sleeping in the same bed, but were not together. And her up and down all night, with the Harlequin books and the refrigerator door opening and closing, led to her packing on about twenty-five pounds. She was a petite little gymnast in school.

Our oldest daughter saw you talking about your book Ageless and ordered it. There was some resistance from my wife at first and then she sat down and read your book start to finish without a break; she was really into it.

Next thing I knew we were on our way to Houston to consult with one of the doctors you mentioned. I don't know what he gave her, but within a couple of days, things started getting better and now four months later, we are once again one happy family. The weight is dropping off, the love has returned, and I can now look forward to many more wonderful years with the girl of my dreams.

Now it's my turn. I have an appointment with the doctor next week.

Thank you, Suzanne Somers. You have given our family the greatest gift of health and happiness and we toast you at every opportunity.

Sincerely,
Dustin R.

10

HORMONAL PASSAGES

WHEN I BEGAN MY decline of hormones, no one talked about it, no one understood it; my mother's generation toughed it out and never spoke of it. It was called the "change of life" and the connotation was "dark." It meant the end . . . over, done, finished, useless. No wonder no woman wanted to admit she was in this passage.

Men didn't understand the passage—all they knew was there was a change coming over Mama and it didn't look good. She no longer felt like having sex, she started getting fat, and her good cheer was masked by what seemed to be a new and not so enjoyable personality.

And Mama felt bad about herself. Who was she now that she was no longer able to make and take care of children? Her job was over. Women of my mother's era didn't have careers, and their lives were devoted to raising their families. But now the children were grown and gone and life with Dad was not like it seemed on TV.

I officially went into menopause on my fiftieth birthday. I was hot-flashing, bloating, and uncomfortable as the toasts were being made at my lovely party. The decline had started long before this; I just didn't realize that the changes in my body, and the feelings, energy loss, and out-of-control emotions, had to do with hormone loss. After all, I was only in my early thirties when my hormones started going into decline. It never entered my mind that hormonal decline had begun. I was on top of the world . . . the star of the number one television series in America, a show that people around the world watched. Every week I was on yet another prestigious magazine cover. I ran from one place to the next: photo shoots, feature films that were produced during my hiatus, TV specials, a successful Las Vegas show, talk show appearances, all while juggling my personal life as a wife and full-time mother of my son and two stepchildren. I stayed away from Hollywood parties to try and find some balance, did not accept movies that would take me out of the country, tried my best to "be all to everyone."

The first change I began to notice was sex. I just didn't feel like it. I loved my husband deeply, passionately, but I don't know . . . was I just worn out? It was one more thing at the end of the day when I really wanted to sleep, when I wanted to have some time to take care of myself, plus I didn't want to admit that I couldn't "feel" sex. I couldn't figure out what had happened. My husband and I had always shared a wonderful intimacy, but now I felt like an outsider.

As women we can still participate even if we're not totally in the mood, and I did a good job making sure my husband didn't have a clue, but I began to ask questions of myself: What was wrong with me? It didn't help that I was considered "America's Sex Symbol"! There it was, screaming at me from every magazine cover. I could not connect with the girl in those photos. I felt like a fraud.

The next thing I noticed was inexplicable weight gain. Strange, especially since weight had never been a problem in my entire life—I grew up being called "Bony Mahoney" (my maiden name). Why were my hips suddenly spreading? I was eating less and less and exercising hours daily with constant new dance routines, always in preparation for Las Vegas or the next TV special. It didn't add up.

Then my moods changed. I could get angry easily (not usual for me), cry often for reasons that didn't make sense, and felt that no one understood me. My sleeping became jumpy and erratic, my health deteriorated— coughs, colds, flus—and I felt an overall exhaustion. My diet was good, I thought; I never consumed chemicals, thank God, so the food I was eating was real food, but sugar was a big part of my diet. I loved cakes, pies, and cookies. At the craft table at *Three's Company*, there were morning donuts and bagels with cream cheese, and cookies and pastries in the afternoon. Who knows how many of these I grabbed without thinking, shoveling them in my mouth to fill me up. If you think there is not much attention being paid to nutrition today, you wouldn't believe the ignorance that existed just a short twenty-five years ago.

I didn't feel good, but why? I had an enviable life. I was "the Queen of

Jiggly," I was on the cover of *Newsweek*, and featured on *60 Minutes* and a *Barbara Walters Special*. I was in my thirties . . . what was wrong?

Little did I know that much more was going on with me than the outward manifestations I was experiencing. Little did I know that I was deep in the initial throes of hormonal decline and that I was in a perfect setup for cancer. How could that be? I was so young.

One of the most important things to get from this book is that we are never too young. Hormonal changes start early, and we can throw our bodies into change even faster with stress, a poor diet, by consuming chemicals, or by messing with our bodies' natural systems with things like birth control pills. The earlier we understand this the better able we will be to take care of ourselves and replace the hormones that we are losing. I'll explain here the various stages our bodies go through as we age—and it's not just women, men experience this loss, too!

PMS

PMS is a by-product of low progesterone and can be mild to severe for women in their teens and twenties. Young women suffer and think it's all part of being a woman, but if they had a qualified doctor who understood they were losing progesterone, they could enjoy the benefits of progesterone replacement. They would feel better and they would be protected later on from cancer.

You see, low or missing hormones are at the base of cancer. Young women with perfectly balanced hormones do not get cancer unless there's a genetic aberration or an environmental cause. A perfectly hormonally balanced woman is reproductive and the brain recognizes this template. Once we begin hormonal decline, our problems start. That's when we get our first cancers, heart problems, dementia, etc., so if our hormonal imbalances begin at an early age, such as in our teens or twenties, our brain senses that all is not well and we are not going to be able to reproduce. This is not good for us. At this point the brain would like to eliminate us (biologically speaking) because we are only here for one reason and that is to perpetuate the species. The job of the brain is to sense when we can no longer reproduce and then get rid of us to make room for the young, strong, healthy ones. I know this is harsh, but it's simply the reality of biology.

Women today are losing their hormones earlier and earlier, which is why we are having problems such as PMS and teen rage. This early loss is exacerbated by poor diet, excessive use of chemicals (diet sodas, Doritos, Splenda, etc.), environmental assault, and stress, stress, stress!

To think it's as simple as replacing lost, low, or missing hormones with real natural bioidentical hormones and everything goes back to normal. Your mood is better, the pain is gone, plus you are protected from cancer, but only if you clean up your diet—you can't consume a diet of chemicals!

Diet is so important in regulating mood swings and keeping our brains healthy. Dr. Russell Blaylock feels that young people are destroying their brains with their chemical diets—we know that kids would rather eat a bag of chemically laden chips than eat a piece of broccoli.

The real problem here is ignorance on our parts as well as the doctors'. We are living in a new world of stress and chemicals. We are under the greatest environmental assault in the history of mankind and we wonder why people are doing such crazy things to each other. Balanced hormones are a huge part of our health, physically and emotionally. When one hormone is off, all the other hormones are off. So, if you have a progesterone deficiency early in life, it is a predictor of your future emotional and physical health. It's that serious. No kidding.

PERIMENOPAUSE

Perimenopause affects women from their early thirties on and is the most dangerous passage we experience. Dangerous because it is not understood nor taken seriously by physicians as a general rule, and dangerous because you are surging: one day your estrogen is sky-high, the next day it plummets. The same goes for your progesterone levels—most young women become estrogen dominant, meaning they are no longer making adequate supplies of progesterone. This is dangerous because it is a setup for cancer. The usual age that perimenopause began used to be forty to forty-five, but today's lifestyle has accelerated this process, so that young thirty-year-old women are now often in the initial throes of perimenopause.

All women are different, but if you have a high-powered job, or experience stress in your life now or did in your childhood, or if you consume a lot of chemicals in your diet or are exposed to them around your household, you will experience accelerated perimenopause.

Perimenopause is often brushed off as insignificant, but the reality is that you are nearly running on empty. Women are losing their hormones earlier and earlier due to the environment and stress. It is a passage that can last as long as fifteen years, and the process is a slow drain, like loosening the plug in the bathtub and letting the water slowly seep out. It is not until menopause that the plug is pulled out completely. Then you can't ignore it anymore.

But the slow drain of perimenopause is confusing and upsetting to young women who don't understand why (like me) they are not feeling right. They are beginning to gain weight for no reason. Sleep is interrupted. It's frustrating because at this age most women have spent their twenties rubbing their children's backs to sleep, and getting up with them when they are scared, sad, or sick. Now finally Mom can sleep through the night uninterrupted. And then . . . she can't.

What's wrong? And why doesn't sex feel the same anymore? And why does she feel emotional, or quiet, or sad, or depressed, even when there is no reason to justify feeling this way? And Dad's not too happy, either. He's been patiently waiting for his turn. To have her back to himself again, but she's not in the mood. Or she's crying again. What's wrong?

It's your hormones!

Hormones, hormones, hormones! They regulate everything. Your perimenopausal gal is out of balance, but she can't put her finger on it. It couldn't be hormones, she thinks, she's too young. Hormones are her mother's domain. Hormone concerns are for old people. And then she goes to her unqualified doctor (a doctor who has not studied the hormonal system, and that means most of our doctors), who brushes it away. No one taught them much about this passage in med school.

Women—pay attention to perimenopause! This is the passage where we women get our cancers! I got my cancer in perimenopause, but it didn't really rear its ugly head until menopause. By the time it was found it was a fairly large tumor. And, yes, I did have mammograms every year since my fortieth birthday, but mammograms missed it every single year for *ten* years. Why? Because it was on the back of my chest wall, and mammograms did not pick it up. Not until my doctor suggested an ultrasound for my cystic breasts (most likely provoked by twenty-two years of synthetic birth control pills) did they find it. Another year and it would have been "good-bye, Suzanne."

This is also the time that we lose our feel for sex. We lose our feel for sex because we lose our *sex hormones*! Without sex hormones we can't *feel* sex. We can participate, but we lose interest because our physical feelings are not there. In times past, women accepted this and participated without enjoyment for the rest of their lives. It became somewhat of a duty. Women of those times were taught that men need sex. We were there to provide it for them. But today we have the power and privilege to actually enjoy this wonderful activity, but without hormones the feeling goes away.

You do not have to live this way! Perimenopause needs attending to and treatment by a qualified doctor. You do not have to wait until menopause to talk to a doctor about replacing your hormones. If you are not with a doctor who specializes in bioidentical hormone replacement, then you must find one who does. A gynecologist is no more equipped to handle your hormones than a plumber if they have not gone out of their way to learn and study outside of medical school. Medical school gives approximately four hours of instruction in prescribing hormones, and this includes gynecologists. What doctors *are* taught about menopause and perimenopause is to give synthetic drug hormones like Premarin and Prempro and Provera. Studies have shown the danger of these pharmaceuticals. They do not replicate nature, they are not an exact fit, they are drugs and not natural.

BIOIDENTICAL VERSUS SYNTHETIC HORMONES

The word "bioidentical" means biologically identical to the hormone, an exact replica of what we make or have made ourselves in our own bodies—because of this, these hormones are a perfect fit. Bioidentical hormones are made from soy, plant, and yam extracts and are synthesized in a lab to exactly replicate human hormones. They are natural, made from things found in nature, unlike drugs, which are made from things that are not found in nature.

Hormones such as Premarin, Prempro, and Provera are synthetic—they do not occur in nature. The molecular structure is different from that of a hormone produced in our own bodies.

Premarin is made from equillin, which is pregnant mare's urine. A female horse has thirty-four different estrogens. A female human has three classical estrogens: estradiol (heart protective), estrone (takes away symptoms), and estriol (breast cancer protective). But we also have about thirty other estrogens, some good estrogens and some procarcinogen estrogens, that have been identified, and researchers continue to discover new ones. None of our estrogens is compatible with a horse's estrogens.

On top of all this, the extraction process for the horse is cruel. They put the horse in a stall for life, with a catheter in her bladder to extract the urine, and continually impregnate the horse for fifteen years until she dies. If you are a believer in passed energy, how do you feel about taking a pill every day that comes from such sadness? How good can it be for us to consume a pill made from a horse that is possibly eating poor-quality food and is locked up in a stall all day. And it doesn't even replace our missing estrogen!

The potential side effects of Premarin are devastating. The most pertinent is Premarin's power to raise C-reactive protein, the one absolute marker for heart attack. As a result, cardiologists who routinely check this marker in women on Premarin find it high and then offer a statin such as Lipitor instead of bioidentical estrogen. Check out chapter 21 for how harmful statins can be. Bioidentical estrogen (17 beta-estradiol) never raises C-reactive protein, plus it keeps arteries clear, eliminating the two risk factors for heart disease and Alzheimer's. Yet doctors continue to write prescriptions for synthetic hormones—it boggles the mind!

Hopefully, you will find a qualified doctor at the back of this book who knows about bioidentical hormone replacement therapy. If not, it's worth a trip to the one nearest you. You only have to go the first time; after that, monitoring is done through blood tests, twenty-four-hour urine tests, and other lab work.

Young people today in their late thirties and early forties are very hip to realize that the way of their parents is not the way they want to go. Too many of them have seen their parents' marriages fall apart because Mom got too emotional and Dad could no longer stand it. Too many of them have seen their mothers lose themselves, and their fathers fade away.

Young people know there is a better way and bioidentical hormone replacement is the answer. I sound like an old fart when I say this, but "I wish I knew at their age what I know now." It thrills me to pass this on to younger people. You don't have to suffer. All this misery that women have been going through is unnecessary. Women no longer need to be embarrassed of breaking out in a sweat in front of everybody when it's not hot, or watch their bellies grow larger (when they are *not* pregnant), their arms get bigger, their beautiful lustrous hair turn stringy, and their skin wrinkle, and then experience the diseases that accompany hormonal loss.

The information now available on extending life and health is like a golden key. If people understood that they can now live life in their fifties, sixties, and older with the same quality as when they were in their twenties and thirties, everybody would want it. But we are constantly fighting an establishment that knows if everyone figures out that replacement of hormones keeps us so healthy and happy that we won't need their drugs, it will then affect the bottom line of big business and it will pull the rug out from under all the rest of the doctors who are unwilling or unable to embrace this change.

—Dr. Candice Lane, Westlake Village, California

No, no, no . . . not for the young people, and good for them. They are not stuck. They are not afraid to go against their doctor. This new generation knows their doctor is not God. They want quality of life, and they need it because they are going to live longer than we will and with better quality of life because of this knowledge. Bioidentical hormone replacement is life changing, and the sooner you start, the less internal damage you will have and the better quality of life you will obtain.

MENOPAUSE

If your hormones are surging during perimenopause, in menopause they are bottoming out. The surge and loss of hormones during perimenopause turns into the abrupt absence of hormones as we head into menopause, which can happen from our forties into our fifties. Hormones are crucial to every single function of the human body, yet we are expected to live without them for more than half our lives. Imagine, from your forties on you will most likely feel awful, as if your essence is gone, while techno-logical advancements will keep you alive into your nineties and over one hundred!

Breakthrough doctors understand the vital importance of hormones. As Dr. Thierry Hertoghe says: "Hormones put you to sleep at night and they wake you up in the morning. They control your blood pressure; they build up bone, maintain muscle tone, and lubricate joints. Hormones govern growth; they even make the body produce energy and heat. Hormones burn fat. Hormones govern the menstrual cycle and allow pregnancy (and birth) to occur. They fight stress, prevent fatigue, calm anxiety, and relieve depression. Hormones make and keep memories. Hormones maintain the correct level of sugar in the blood and tissues. They resist allergic reactions and infections. They soothe pain. Hormones control your sex drive, viril-ity, and fertility. They stimulate your brain and your immune system."

So, if hormones do all this, why would you be content to be without them? Frankly, without hormones quality of life takes a big downturn. In my previous books, I have called the horrible symptoms the "Seven Dwarfs of Menopause": Itchy, Bitchy, Sleepy, Sweaty, Bloated, Forgetful, and All Dried Up! If you are in, or have been going through, menopause, you know exactly what I am talking about.

Each one of these symptoms is your body talking. Itching, bad moods, depression, bloating, hot flashes, sleeplessness, and no libido are all the ways your body is trying to communicate with you to let you know that you haven't found the right "hormonal cocktail," individualized just for you. Every woman is different and every woman has different hormonal needs; that is why a "one pill fits all," the standard of care for most doctors, could never work unless you got lucky and that pill happened to be exactly what you need (but that would be rare). Talk with your doctor as often as you must until you have no more symptoms. Symptoms are not about you complaining; a body that is in imbalance is a setup for cancer or heart disease or some other breakdown. Think about it. When you were young you didn't have these symptoms because you were making a full complement of hormones. It's only since your hormones have begun to decline that you are experiencing this discomfort.

Sometimes people are in denial about how bad they really feel. So many people around my age say to me that they "don't have any symptoms," and then I find out that they sleep in separate beds or bedrooms, never sleep more than five hours a night, are battling weight and losing memories and thoughts, have headaches, watery eyes, and "forget about sex, that's been gone forever". . . and this is just for starters.

No one has to live this way. Menopause does not have to be a horrible passage. Nothing will restore your youthful energy and bring back good health like bioidentical hormone replacement therapy.

I bless the day I found bioidenticals; before that, I was a mess and couldn't get rid of those Seven Dwarfs. I couldn't sleep, I woke up every fifteen minutes sweating like I was in a sauna, I completely lost my libido, was depressed from not sleeping, was gaining weight for no reason, had body itches that were driving me crazy, felt pissed off most of the time and didn't know why, and pretty much wanted to pack it in because this was no way to live.

Bioidenticals changed everything, and I have been singing their praises since *before* I published *The Sexy Years* in 2004. Because of that, I get a lot of questions about how they work and where people can get them. Recently I was being interviewed by a TV reporter who took me aside afterward to ask, "Where can I get this? I love my wife so much, but it's as if the essence has gone out of her." He looked sad, like he was helpless, like she was slipping away from him and there was nothing he could do about it. I can't tell you how often I hear this.

After that, she went to one of my qualified doctors and within a few months I happened to run into them again, and I smiled as they both gushed about how great their lives had become again. They were happy and relaxed and the pheromones were definitely present.

It is amazing to me that people like this couple have to search out bioidentical hormone treatment—I can't believe that the medical establishment is so resistant to natural bioidentical hormone replacement. It's not as if they have found the answer to this passage in pharmaceuticals. In fact, the main FDA-approved drugs for menopause have been proven by the Women's Health Initiative to be "dangerous, harmful and even fatal." This particular study suggests that "a woman would be better off taking nothing at all than to take these dangerous drugs."

Then suddenly, like a godsend, a body of doctors (let's call them anti-aging doctors) appears from different parts of this country and the world, Western trained, from all the A-list schools, and they are saying, "Hey, we found the answer, and it's been around for fifty years": If you put back a person's hormones with real bioidentical hormones (biologically identical to the human hormone, an exact replica), then he or she will start to feel great again.

I get what all these wonderful cutting-edge doctors are saying, that "this is the most rewarding work they have ever done." How incredible it must be to make people well and restore quality of life on a daily basis. How wonderful to have satisfied, healthy, happy patients. And that's what is happening . . . every day more and more people are realizing that the answer does not lie in all the prescription drugs people have been taking. When you replace lost hormones with bioidenticals you get your life back. Those in the know understand this. You get to retrieve your optimal prime. You get your health back, your libido returns, the headaches go away, the weight normalizes if you are eating correctly, and you get to feel happy again.

The medical establishment has been trained to have a pharmaceutical drug for every problem or ailment. That is the nature of allopathic medicine. So, instead of replacing a woman's or a man's sex hormones with estrogen, progesterone, and testosterone, and then regulating your cortisol (see page 123) with bioidentical cortisol to "turn off the noise" that keeps you tossing and turning and awake at night, you are given a sleeping pill like Ambien or Lunesta (or how about Prozac for the depression that accompanies lack of sleep?), plus a continuing series of drugs for new ailments to deal with the side effects of the drugs you are presently taking, when in reality all you need is hormones. Enough already! Stop the insanity! There has never been a person who has a Prozac deficiency!

The drugs we are given from middle age on will most likely overtake the bulk of us and require that we end up in a nursing home. Think about that! The cumulative effect of antidepressants, blood pressure medications, diabetes medications, allergy medicine, statins (nasty drugs, see page 288) will eventually leave us so confused and disoriented that our families will have to put us in nursing homes (for our own good). Nice, huh?

If this scenario does not sit well with you, then consider real hormone replacement. I have been on bioidentical hormones for twelve years. These have been the calmest, most satisfying years of my life, and hormones have everything to do with it.

Hormones are the juice of youth, the "plant food," for lack of a better description, that our bodies crave. It's not just me saying this. By reading the interviews in this book, you will see that these breakthrough doctors know that bioidenticals are the answer.

Menopause is easily rectified by going to a doctor who specializes in bioidentical hormone replacement. Qualified doctors understand how to do it and how to work with you to find the "sweet spot," that place where you feel perfect. Do not give up until you get to that place.

How to Replace Hormones

In *Ageless*, I discussed in depth the different ways doctors can prescribe bioidenticals—check it out for a longer explanation. Here are the quick hits:

WHAT YOUR DOCTOR IS TRYING TO DO Your doctor is trying to replicate nature with BHRT. When you were young your body made estrogen every day of the month. Then it made progesterone two weeks of every month, and at the end of that cycle you either had a period or you were pregnant.

CONTINUOUS COMBINED Doctors will replace your estrogen and progesterone with bioidentical equivalents in continuous combined doses, which means both estrogen and progesterone every day. You will not have a period if you take the hormones this way. This would not be my choice, and the doctors I have spoken with all say they have to respect their patients' wishes and that at least they are getting hormones, albeit not the way nature intended. Most doctors prefer to replicate nature and force a period. If we are trying to trick our bodies into thinking we are healthy and reproductive so as to outwit cancer, it makes sense that our bodies should menstruate.

STATIC DOSING Based on your individual needs, determined by a blood test, your doctor will prescribe a static dose of estradiol every day of the month. On days 18 to 28, your doctor adds a static dose of progesterone, based on your lab work. This matches what your body did when you made a full complement of hormones and matches nature.

RHYTHMIC CYCLING This is based on the ancient cycles of nature when women's bodies cycled to the rhythms of the moon, producing estrogen in increments. The first three days were one amount, the next three days another amount, and by the twelfth day the estrogen would peak. As estrogen started to fall, progesterone would rise. Your doctor will prescribe your bioidenticals in accordance with your own rhythms. I take my hormones in a rhythm.

Menopause can be such a pleasurable passage. I know, because I have so enjoyed myself these last twelve years. I even like the way I look, and I think it's because I am happy and healthy and in love. The fact that my husband has embraced male hormone replacement has brought our relationship to new heights. We are in sync and we have such a good time together. If you embrace bioidenticals, then by attraction your husband will want what you have. Read Dr. Thierry Hertoghe's interview (chapter 9) to see what hormone replacement has done for him, and then ask your husband to read it. His story is very inspiring. Dr. Hertoghe started BHRT at age thirty-five. You should see him—Wow, what a hunk!

With bioidenticals it's as though all the pieces have come together at this time in my life. I owe this quality of life to real hormone replacement.

POSTMENOPAUSE

Okay, here's the deal, there is no postmenopause unless you are dead. Menopause never stops. There is no "after"! Once you begin hormonal decline it continues the rest of your life. If you look up death in the dictionary it says "loss of hormones."

So many of my female friends in their seventies say, "Oh, I'm past that." Wrong! You are never past menopause; your body is only past the initial shock of the terrible symptoms of losing your hormones. Your body gets used to feeling awful and you learn to live with symptoms such as sleeplessness or sleep disturbances, no libido, weight gain or weight loss, brittle bones, loss of memory, joint pain, bad knees, bad hips, and a general sense of being "not of the world" anymore. Some women have described it to me as feeling "invisible."

Real hormones give you back your visibility. With real hormones your energy will come back, your sex hormones will charge up again, and even if you no longer have a partner, a woman with "pheromones" puts out a sexiness that people can feel. It makes you feel alive and energetic. The difference between youth and old age is energy. Old people are out of gas. Young people have energy. Now you're probably not going to jog up the Great Wall of China, but there will be a spring in your step.

I have spoken to women in their eighties and nineties in my other books, such as *The Sexy Years*, who are on bioidentical hormones, and they are as young as anyone I know. Read "Eve's" story in *The Sexy Years*. She is inspirational; ninety years young and full of energy with a great-working, sharp brain. She is "of it." She is not on the outside looking in. She isn't the old grandmother the family puts in the corner. Instead, Eve is in the kitchen, working with the young girls of the family.

You can have that, too. None of us has to fade to black with the diseases we have come to expect with aging. Alzheimer's should not be the end point of life, nor should heart disease, nor should cancer. These diseases are so prominent and prevalent with older people because our doctors and medical institutions of higher learning did not anticipate this changing world. Our medical professionals did not see that technology was coming like a Mack truck to prolong our lives. All the wonderful MRIs and CAT scans, PET scans, sophisticated blood tests, and even antibiotics now allow all of us to live longer than humans have ever lived before in history. But they didn't think about the quality of life. Big mistake.

The pharmaceutical companies saw it coming. And they are thrilled. They have a drug for every ailment we experience as we age all the way to the nursing home, and then in the nursing home they supply all the sedation drugs to shut us up until we do indeed fade to black (after we mortgage our houses to pay for the nursing home costs)!

What a sorry way to end a beautiful life. I think often of President Reagan, a man I had the privilege of knowing. He didn't know who he was in the end. He faded to black. I often think, what if he had been with a doctor who realized that his spells of memory loss and fragility during his years in the White House might have occurred because he was so depleted of testosterone (remember, stress blunts hormone production and who in the world would be more stressed than the president of the United States?), and when a man's testosterone plummets he is left with too much estrogen, which leads to Alzheimer's and heart disease. How sad that there was no one knowledgeable around him who could have at least checked. We'll never know.

I'm not going out that way. I want my brain to the very end. I want my energy, I want my rockin' libido to the very end. I want to be laughing on the way out from happiness . . . laughing because I had such a great time. I believe it is possible if I keep my hormones at optimal levels for the rest of my life.

So that is my answer to postmenopausal . . . as long as you keep "filling the tank" with bioidentical hormones in the right ratios for you, you can expect to go out kicking.

ANDROPAUSE

Men experience hormonal drop-off just as women do; it's just not as in your face as the female experience. But make no mistake about it: Men, you must take andropause seriously, or expect to decline in ways you never imagined!

Andropause is male menopause—as hormones decline, men may exhibit the following symptoms:

- fatigue
- tiredness, low energy
- depression
- irritability
- anxiety
- loss of memory or concentration
- relationship problems with partner
- loss of sex drive
- erection problems during sex
- loss of morning erections
- decreased intensity of orgasms
- backache, joint pains, stiffness
- loss of physical fitness
- feelings of being overstressed

Testosterone is a powerful anabolic hormone produced by men and women. In men the adrenal glands produce some testosterone, though most of it is produced in the testicles. To combat andropause, it is important to replace testosterone that has been lost in the aging process. Replacing testosterone can:

- stimulate libido
- improve osteoporosis
- reduce body fat
- improve mood and depression
- improve muscle mass

- improve autoimmune disorders
- fight fatigue
- improve the symptoms of diabetes
- reduce the risk of heart disease
- help in treatment of lupus

Testosterone is necessary in men for erections, ejaculations, and fertility. Testosterone also lowers cholesterol by protecting the heart and arteries, thereby reducing the risk of heart disease.

Moller, a Danish physician, found that 83 percent of patients experienced a significant decline in their cholesterol levels while supplementing with physiologic doses of testosterone. As a benefit these patients felt much better than they would have on a conventional medication (statin), which has debilitating side effects such as nausea, gallbladder disease, diminished libido, liver problems, abdominal pain, muscle wasting, kidney failure, and total transient amnesia.

Testosterone builds muscle and improves muscle tone. It preserves bone mass and reduces fat and cellulite. It also prevents joint and muscle pain, and obesity.

Peak testosterone levels are reached in a man's early to mid-twenties, but as a man ages the Leydig cells that secrete testosterone begin to wear away. Because of this, between the ages of forty and seventy the average man loses nearly 60 percent of the testosterone inside his body. Other lifestyle factors such as overtraining, stress, and alcohol can hasten the deterioration of Leydig cells and cause testosterone levels to decline drastically.

Testosterone stimulates the body's development of muscle, bone, skin, and sex organs, along with masculine physical features such as hair growth. Scientists have recently discovered that testosterone also improves mental power by enhancing visual and perceptual skills. Low levels can disrupt the body's blood sugar metabolism, leading to obesity and heart disease. Its use is popularly associated with enhancing libido, but research indicates that it is a vital factor in the prevention of cardiovascular disease as well as improving energy level, bone density, muscle tone, prostate health, mood, and vitality.

If you are a male and you feel fatigued day and night, if you are losing your self-confidence and feel depressed, anxious, or overly emotional, or if you have constant restless sleeps or disinterest in sex and your memory is suffering, then this is a good indication that your testosterone levels are low.

A qualified doctor is essential in working with you to replace declining testosterone. You must ask your doctor if his specialty is bioidentical testosterone replacement. If the answer is no, he is not the right person to guide you through this passage.

Most conventional doctors give a blood test and announce to the average seventy-year-old male that their testosterone levels are normal. Normal for what? is the question. Normal for a seventy-year-old male is not what you want. A seventy-year-old person is in declining hormones. What you want are hormone levels equal to those of your optimal prime, the period in your life when you were healthiest and strongest. Not only seventy-year-olds can be low in testosterone, it is now happening to men at much younger ages. My son needed to begin testosterone replacement at age thirty-six. Dr. Thierry Hertoghe needed to start replacement at thirty-five. High-powered men with high-powered jobs is a recipe for burning out hormones, and age has little to do with it.

A qualified doctor will understand this and will also know to look not only at your total testosterone levels but also at the free testosterone; in other words, the testosterone that is not bound up. Many males are told that "they have more testosterone than they can use." Males have bragged about this to me and I often wonder how much of that testosterone is useful. If it is not "free" then it is virtually useless and does not do the job.

I cannot tell you the difference testosterone replacement has made in my own husband. Ten years ago he was in serious decline. He was around sixty-one at that time. He couldn't stay awake and he was sleeping and taking naps throughout the day. His energy had drifted away and he really didn't want to do much of anything. He would complain that even though he was working out, his muscles seemed to be shrinking. He was a bit cranky (not his usual self), and his interest in sex had diminished (very unusual for him), but he was so tired he didn't seem to notice. It was like he was beginning to fade away. He wanted to stay in most of the time and his mood changed the energy in our home.

Today, ten years later, he is back and loaded with great energy, great vitality, great health, great libido, and in a great mood all the time. He not only replaced his missing testosterone, but also strengthened his adrenals, replaced his missing DHEA and progesterone, replaced his missing thyroid with bioidentical thyroid, replaced his missing pregnenolone, started a vigorous supplement regimen, makes regular visits to the antiaging doctor to detoxify and build up, and gets eight to nine hours of good sleep a night. He is a new guy.

His friends can't believe how good he looks—well-cut, defined muscles, tan glowing skin. He looks and feels healthy and exudes energy, vitality, sexuality, strength—in other words, he is one sexy guy. And is he happy!

He leaps out of bed in the morning ready to tackle the day with energy and a great outlook. It's been a remarkable turnaround for us, and with both of us on complete hormone replacement our lives have become pretty impressive.

Aging is not an issue for either of us. If this is aging, then bring on more. We both often say that these are the best years of our lives and that we have never been happier and healthier.

Testosterone is a steroid hormone and remains a prescription-only medication. You need to obtain a prescription from your qualified physician that has been individually prepared for you by a compounding pharmacy.

11

DR. JENNIFER BERMAN

It's nice to be alive while you are alive.

—T. S. Wiley

SEX

WHO EVER THOUGHT sex would become a distant memory? All your life, there it was . . . always there, always at the back of your mind, all your life! And then one day . . . Wow, the feeling is gone. What happened? Is it me? Is it him? Is it her? Maybe your partner just doesn't do it for you anymore. But no, that's not it. You want to "feel" but can't. What is wrong?

You guessed it. It's your hormones. It's physiological. It's also emotional because imbalanced hormones create major symptoms. You get depressed, you gain weight, you get allergies, watery eyes, and body itches. You get bloated, hot flashes, angry, tired, fatigued, forgetful, and all the juices in your body dry up. You guessed it, those important juices.

Now sex is no longer pleasant because it is painful . . . it hurts. Lack of natural lubrication is uncomfortable. The vaginal tissue gets thin, so sex hurts on that level. Try as hard as you can, you can't feel anything and orgasm is impossible no matter what you do.

There is good news. It all comes back with hormonal balance. It takes a while until you get the hormonal "song" perfect, but be patient, it will return, and if your experience is like mine, better than ever! I think I have been hormonally imbalanced all my life, from stress, toxins, stress, chemicals, stress, and more stress. When you get your hormones balanced, that "old feeling" will come back. You'll be buying fancy new underwear and lighting candles.

Aging is a fantastic passage as long as you are well, because with age comes wisdom and wisdom is the greatest gift of all. At this age you know something . . . you have a confidence you never had before and a sureness about yourself. Imbalanced hormones rob you of this confidence, but when you find the right doctor for you (see the resources) and get yourself put back together again, your life will go to new great places. Every day will be a good one, and all you have to do to achieve this is restore your endocrine system by replacing every missing hormone.

> Remaking ourselves is the ultimate expression and realization of our humanity.
>
> –Dr. Gregory Stock, *Redesigning Humans* (2002)

This is the second time I have interviewed Dr. Jennifer Berman about the effects of health on one's sexuality. There are so few doctors in the world who have chosen to specialize in this arena. It's almost as though the subject is taboo, yet sex is the one universal human enjoyment that every man and woman experience at some point in their lives. Decrease in libido is becoming commonplace and is very stressful for those who experience it. Lack of desire can be a result of low or missing hormones, toxicity, stress, and/or aging. The good news is that you can rejuvenate your libido, and Dr. Berman is the person to explain how. You will enjoy her candor and openness about such an intimate and vulnerable part of our nature.

SS: Thanks for taking the time with me again. This is our second interview together, and I received so many great comments about you from the last book, *Ageless*. Tell me, is it possible to be sexually healthy if you are not a healthy person?

JB: A lack of sexual feeling is almost always an imbalance within the body. It could be hormonal imbalance, inflammation, stress, nutritional insufficiencies. Not to mention their DNA and own genetic risk factors and/or environmental risk factors they may have been exposed to.

SS: You mean exposure to toxicity, as in preservatives in the food, chemicals in the food, or chemicals in the environment or the house, can affect sex drive?

JB: Yes, absolutely, chemicals affect and blunt hormone production, and hormones are directly connected with our sex drive. Unfortunately, most of my patients think that it's a lack of interest in their mates. They say things like "I'm just not turned on by him anymore."

SS: I think of all the marriages that have ended because of hormonal imbalance—it seems so real when you are going through it, as though you think you really don't have feelings for your mate anymore, when in reality most of the time our hormones have a direct effect on our personality and these feelings very well could be from a hormonal imbalance. I mean, we all remember PMS—that felt real. We all know what it feels like to have hormone "moods": You could punch someone in the face and feel justified when you are in that state. So imagine the toll it takes on a marriage when you are with each other day in and day out and one or both of you have hormones that are "off."

JB: Most of my patients come in wanting testosterone, but I have to educate them: It's more than testosterone: It's a new diet, a new lifestyle; it's taking antioxidants and understanding what they can do for your body; it's vitamins; it's anti-inflammatory products and a reduction of stress. Loss of testosterone and/or DHEA (which comes from the adrenal glands) is a by-product of aging and/or stress. Knowing this, I blood-test to see the adrenal levels. Sometimes we start there.

You see, the concept of looking at only one source of the problem, as in isolating testosterone as the culprit, is no longer relevant. We now know that it is a combination of things. There are changes going on inside the body, in the brain, in the central nervous system and with your neural endocrine system, and they are all happening simultaneously. You might not feel them individually, but collectively they are creating the imbalance. So you have to look at everything and address them in order to effectively treat the symptoms and prevent further decline.

SS: Prevention is the word, isn't it?

JB: Yes, start early. Prevent. Don't wait until you have fallen apart. It makes it so much harder (but not impossible) to treat.

Women in their mid- to late thirties should be addressing their hormones.

SS: Yes, I agree, but there is a big problem, and that is with the doctors. I am constantly hearing from women that their doctors tell them they are too young, or "not to worry," or perimenopause is "nothing," or, worse, that it is all in their heads, or here, "take a sleeping pill" or "take an antidepressant."

JB: Well, that is wrong advice. When a woman is first starting to feel subtle symptoms, or changes in libido, that's when she needs to start with preventative measures. Women in their seventies might not be experiencing hot flashes or night sweats anymore, but they do have sexual function problems; they still have joint pain, and neck pain, and back pain, and rheumatoid arthritis. They might have irritable bowel syndrome. In fact, everything bad or inflammatory gets worse as you age. So these women are telling me all the time that they don't need hormones because they are no longer experiencing the traditional symptoms, but the deep loss of hormones results in cardiovascular disease, bone disease, brain fog or memory problems, aching joints and joints that no longer work, cancer, and Alzheimer's. Replacing lost or low hormones early in life, and the earlier the better, can protect you from ever contracting any of these conditions or diseases. So it's about hormones, and it all ties together.

SS: There is the misconception that hormone loss is just a passage and then it all stops.

JB: The role that hormones play doesn't stop or go away once you've gone through menopause; if anything, that's the time when you need to continue replacement because your ovarian function and adrenals continue to decline even more. Adrenal gland function and adrenal gland hormones support lower cortisol levels, and that is crucial for a person's ability to sleep, among many other important functions. Besides, estrogen is a very potent anti-inflammatory and antioxidant, so it helps with joint pain, back pain, arthritis, and the bones.

SS: Are you leaning more toward natural remedies such as bioidentical hormone replacement as you deal with aging in general?

JB: Yes, but pharmaceuticals have their place when necessary, and as we've discussed in the past, every woman and man needs to be treated individually. Every person metabolizes differently and every person absorbs differently. But aging is linked to inflammation, and when inflammation is present cells die or burst and release more inflammation, which is what damages our adrenal glands and our ovaries, which in turn can cause heart disease.

SS: So it's a never-ending decline and your job is to put the brakes on. It makes sense—the biggest killer of women is heart disease, but in reality what is killing them is hormonal decline.

JB: Right, so my point is that there are things you can do right now to prevent and delay the process and even restore function and health. But most people wait until they are seventy-five and then it's getting a little late, a lot of damage has been done.

SS: So how does all of this translate to sexual decline?

JB: When a woman comes in who no longer has any sexual feelings or sexual drive, I have to look at all the other functions and hormones and glands and organs, and check for inflammation, and talk to her to see where the aches and pains are located in her body. I need to have all that information in order to bring balance back into her body. Without that balance there will be no ability for this woman to rev up her sexuality. The entire body has to be functioning properly for a woman to revive her sex drive, including hormonal balance. It's an entire program. But I can bring them back to life if they are willing to work with me and trust me.

SS: Who are the easiest?

JB: Perimenopausal and menopausal women with low libido are my favorites. They are amenable to medical therapy. I talk with them for five minutes and I get excited because I know I can help them. The most challenging ones are women with orgasmic disorders or primary orgasmic disorders, meaning they have never had an orgasm in their lives. This is not about sexual abuse; these are women who have healthy relationships and for all intents and purposes are normal.

SS: What is the cause?

JB: The orgasm is a learned reflex that you usually discover before puberty. If for whatever reason the brain-genital connections are not made at that time it's like trying to learn Chinese when you're fifty as opposed to five. There's something that goes on at the time of orgasm that is a complex reflex of hormones, neurological, muscular, blood flow, psychological, emotional—it's a symphony. There is a point in time when the frontal cortex of your brain is acutely aware of the moment; it shuts off your primitive brain, and then the LIMBIC SYSTEM takes over. But for people who are nonorgasmic they don't have the capacity to ignite that switch.

SS: So are you able (excuse the pun) to turn them on again?

JB: Yes, but it's with things you wouldn't imagine: meditation, stress reduction, learning how to make themselves vulnerable and let go of control to a degree. Sometimes we resort to oxytocin, which is normally used in labor to cause the uterus to contract. But it has other effects in terms of sexual function.

SS: Yes, I have read about this. In fact, oxytocin is what makes men feel like cuddling after sex, and it enhances erections and orgasms.

JB: Right. And then there are other patients of mine who have secondary ANARAZMIA, which means that after having their baby, or after using oxytocin, or after a hysterectomy or after menopause, they developed orgasmic issues. Those women are easier to treat because they are familiar with the reflex already.

SS: Bringing up hysterectomy, when the uterus is removed, the deep uterine orgasms are gone forever. There is no bringing that back, right?

JB: Yes, the deep pelvic floor uterine types of contractions are no more. Women really need to be counseled when they are contemplating a hysterectomy. Studies say the orgasm doesn't change, but they don't explain that things won't be the same. What they need to make clear is that clitoral orgasms don't change, but deep, vaginal, pelvic-floor-contraction type of orgasms can no longer happen.

SS: Thank you for saying that. I think it is a travesty that one million women a year have hysterectomies and have no idea that this is going to happen to them. I feel cheated that I did not have this information in advance. It would have seriously impacted how I dealt with the bleeding and I would have found another way. I now know that the uterine bleeding most women experience means that they need to take their bioidentical hormones in a rhythm so the estrogen receptor sites open up to receive the progesterone.

If I understand this correctly, the uterus gives us information about ourselves. The uterus bleeds when the hormones are imbalanced. The remedy of removing the uterus to stop the bleeding only takes away the evidence (bleeding) but doesn't address the underlying problem, which is hormone imbalance and the receptor sites not opening. This scenario gives cancer an opportunity to manifest under these conditions; the bleeding is actually a warning system.

JB: Hysterectomy appears to be an easy solution by removing the offending parts, but there are other solutions to uterine bleeding: endometrial ablation, laser and ultrasound, and many others. The uterus should be removed only if there is cancer. Women are getting smarter; especially with books like yours, they are now equipped with questions and knowledge. This generation of baby boomers is not just sitting back and saying okay. They are much more proactive.

SS: But it sure seems like there is a whole lot of sexual dysfunction going on. Is it the stress and chemicals of today's environment?

JB: Yes, but I find people put things off, and it's easy to explain away sexual dysfunction—"We're doing the house" or "After the wedding in Phoenix"—people can minimize or make excuses for these things. By the time they do go to a doctor it's a significant problem. I mean, we don't expect that every day we're going to be bursting, bubbling with libido; it does wax and wane, but if it's chronic and persistent and pervasive and has infiltrated your relationship, then don't put it off.

SS: But it's not just the female. We tend not to look at men as having sexual problems, but they can become hormonally depleted as well.

JB: Right, not only less of a drive, but potency as well—their erectile quality diminishes.

Loss of libido is a sign that your body is not functioning adequately.

Now, if you have low libido, but your testosterone levels are amazing and your IGF levels are off the charts and everything else is in balance and then come to find out that you just can't stand your husband . . . that's another story. But assuming that testing shows that there is an imbalance—and not just a hormonal imbalance but an imbalance in your lifestyle, imbalance in your diet, imbalance in terms of inflammation—then you need to be adjusted and restored and calmed down.

Meditation: I cringe when I say the word because five years ago I would never have stood up in front of my peers and talked about it, but every week the *New England Journal of Medicine* and *JAMA (Journal of the American Medical Association)* have a different article about the positive effects of meditation; it increases chemicals in your brain that are protective and helps to enhance and elevate mood and energy.

SS: So men and women (especially) talk about sex at this age as something that "was," and something they do not miss. But sex keeps us energized and vital and connected to the world. I truly believe it is something we need to treasure and to fix if it's broken.

JB: Men feel intimate and connected as a result of having sex with us. But for whatever reason we withdraw, due to low testosterone levels, or other low hormone levels, or stress. By virtue of who we are we feel less intimate and connected. Women complain to me that their husbands are not as romantic anymore, they are not as thoughtful, they watch too much television, they are not home anymore, which then makes these women less interested in sex, so it can become a vicious cycle.

SS: But if you get their hormones balanced (and providing these two still like each other) it can give a couple a whole new chapter.

JB: Like I said, provided the rest of their health is in check; sick, depleted, unhealthy people are not going to be in the mood no matter how much they like each other. That's why being able to use all the resources and information available helps me create the ideal program for my patients. Then I can individually mold the program to fit each patient. I guess that is what the "art" is, that while my "painting" is unique it is not so much different than the other doctors'. We're all painting the same painting but with a different spin.

My take is that I have a focus of sexual medicine and that is why people come to me. They're not expecting that they are going to be told about their diet when they have a sexual problem. They aren't expecting that all these other things are causing, or affecting, or adding to, or compounding the problem, or that if they don't do this now, things will get worse down the road.

SS: Did you start out with a complete program for sexual health that included hormone replacement?

JB: I started out looking at blood flow to the clitoris. It evolved into hormones, and the role that hormones play in sexual function and response. And then as time went on I started thinking about wellness and how sexual health and sexual problems are a part of general health and wellness. It's not like you have low libido alone. That's when I started to crystallize the relationship between sexual health and general health. But you know, it's not like there is an antiaging atlas or textbook, there is no road map on how to help a person maintain a happy, healthy, sexually fulfilled life. That's where the "art of medicine" comes in again. I pulled pieces from here and there and put it together from antiaging medicine and endocrinology, sexual medicine, sex therapy, obstetrics, gynecology, and neurology, plus the nutritional components, and then I created my program.

SS: And are your patients getting better?

JB: Yes, and they are excited. Their libido is definitely better, but they say things like they have so much more energy and they sleep better and their memory is better, so I now can see that supplementing with all these other components *enhances* the effects of hormones.

SS: Do they get overwhelmed with all the changes you are asking them to make in their lives?

JB: I explain things and make sure they understand and then I write it down and also give them a lot of reading material. I explain how they are supposed to take things and where they are to get them, but, yes, it is a lot to throw at people. It's important that they know the whole program and what kind of results they can expect if they choose to embrace it. It is an evolving process for me also. I am learning every day and it gets better all the time. Right now I am very interested in the brain chemistry and the neuron-endocrine physiology that all play a critical role in treatment. And then there are the anti-inflammatory supplements and antioxidants that offer great protection for the heart and keeping cholesterol under control.

SS: So you're "turned on" by this work?

JB: Oh yes, more than ever. Every day I have happy people leaving my office. It's rewarding to be in a facet of medicine that truly makes people well and vital and happy with their lives.

SS: Thanks, Jennifer.

DR. JENNIFER BERMAN'S
BREAKTHROUGH BREAKOUTS

- A lack of sexual feeling is almost always the symptom of a health problem in the body, such as hormonal imbalance, inflammation, stress, nutritional insufficiencies; genetic and/or environmental risk factors can also affect sex drive.

- Women in their mid-thirties should begin to address the early signs of hormone imbalance to prevent more serious problems developing as they age, including inflammation that can increase the chance of getting heart disease.

- Meditation, stress reduction, and learning how to relax can help women regain their ability to have an orgasm, but doctors can also prescribe oxytocin, which is normally used in labor to cause the uterus to contract.

- When a woman has a hysterectomy, her clitoral orgasms don't change, but the deep, vaginal, pelvic-floor-contraction type of orgasms can no longer happen.

Dear Suzanne,

At forty-five years old, I have been successfully taking bioidentical hormones for the last four years. For the most part, I have had amazing results, but I still could not budge past a certain weight to take off that last five pounds. When I read Ageless, I read the chapter about Human Growth Hormones and wondered if I might be low. My doctor took a blood panel and noted that I was low in HGH. He suggested I begin taking injections.

My doctor, and the doctors you interviewed in your book, explained that they only treat those who are deficient . . . not someone looking to enhance sports performance or look younger.

I can't tell you how much better I feel! It was like the missing piece of the puzzle in my hormone regime as you have said. I have incredible energy. I buzz around all day. I have dropped those last stubborn five pounds. My body looks more toned. My brain is sharper. My skin looks better. I just plain look and feel younger and more vibrant!

My husband was so impressed with my results, he started asking about your book. Now he is taking testosterone and HGH and he's like a new man. He sleeps better. He looks trim and fit. He has the energy to exercise and play with the kids. Thanks to you, we have the "joie de vivre" we didn't even know we were missing!

Thank you, Suzanne.
Eliza and Ben S.

12

STEP 2: AVOID CHEMICALS AND DETOXIFY YOUR BODY

WE ARE UNDERGOING an environmental assault unlike anything humans have ever before experienced. Toxicity is all around us: in our food, the air we breathe, the water we drink, the fabrics of our clothing, household products, car exhaust, cell phones, computers, power lines, pollution, toxic waste. All of this man-made toxic soup spells disaster for us.

These toxins manifest themselves in our bodies in a variety of ways, including decreased immune function, brain damage, hormonal dysfunction, emotional disturbances, and even cancer. Living in this polluted toxic world, we humans now carry in our bodies industrial chemicals, food additives, heavy metals, and anesthetics, plus the residues of pharmaceuticals, legal drugs (alcohol, tobacco, caffeine), and illegal drugs (heroin, cocaine, and marijuana).

We live with over three thousand chemicals added to our food supply, and over ten thousand chemicals in the form of solvents, emulsifiers, and preservatives that are used in food processing and storage, and these chemicals can remain in the body for years.

Recently my blood test results showed I had high levels of cadmium. I asked my doctor (Dr. Michael Galitzer) where I would be getting exposed to cadmium, and he said, "Smoking." When I told him I had never smoked, he said, "What about secondhand smoke?" That's when I remembered my years of performing on Las Vegas stages when audiences were allowed to smoke in the showrooms. I remembered that I used to cough constantly in the mornings, but back then I thought it was because of the dry desert air. I now realize that at that time the air-conditioning in the showroom pushed all the smoke from the audience up to the stage and I, as the star and the singer, was doing the deepest breathing. I never smoked a cigarette in my life, and here I was coughing up secondhand smoke. Now, shockingly, twenty years later, I find I still have residue in my system.

Everyday products like gasoline, paint, household cleansers, cosmetics, pesticides, and dry-cleaning fluids also pose a serious threat because our bodies cannot break them down as we age, or if we suffer from poor nutrition. These changes are occurring faster than the human body can adapt to them. According to Marshall Mandell, M.D., "The current levels of chemicals in the food and water supply and the indoor and outdoor environment has lowered our threshold of resistance to disease and has altered our body's metabolism, causing enzyme dysfunction, nutritional deficiencies, and hormonal imbalances."

> Pesticides and plastics can abnormally increase your estrogen and cause estrogen dominance, which can predispose women to cancer.
>
> **–Dr. Candice Lane, Westlake Village, California**

And you wonder why we are sick?

It's just common sense to understand that we cannot keep on living with this chemical assault and expect to be well. The bad news is that toxicity is not going away, and unfortunately, as the population continues to grow, it will become worse. Breakthrough medicine understands that these toxins put us at peril and that we cannot achieve optimal health until we find ways to counteract the toxins that already exist in our bodies and reduce our exposure to what is in the environment and in the food we eat. We need to detoxify our systems and build up our bodies with nutrition to fight the world we live in. Detoxification is a key component to the 8 Steps to Wellness.

We don't suddenly get sick; it takes a long time for the body to break down. By the time a cancerous tumor was discovered in my breast the doctors had figured, because of its size, that it had been growing for approximately ten years. When you are diagnosed with cancer you try to figure out where it came from, how you gave it to yourself, and I couldn't imagine that I had possibly played any part in this diagnosis. I presumed that my cancer was "genetic."

When I was younger, no one was aware or conscious of chemicals and toxins. Yes, there were always the "health freaks" who looked pasty and ate macrobiotic green-looking stuff and lectured about the dangers of eating red meat, but no one paid much attention to them. Too bad; they truly were onto something. (Initially, all truth is ridiculed!)

I never gave a thought to taking birth control pills for twenty-two years; I figured if my doctor gave them to me they must be safe. No one ever told me that these pills were chemicals and prevented me from fully ovulating, which signaled to my body that I was not a reproductive person (a perfect setup for cancer). I never gave a thought to food additives that were in the groceries I purchased at the supermarket. Luckily I never liked fast foods, so I avoided that bullet, but along with everyone else I was ignorant about chemical-laden foods and toxic household products.

I remember liberally spraying my home with Raid bug and ant spray whenever there was an infestation. I remember rubbing chemical-laden mosquito oil all over my body when we used to go camping; it didn't enter my mind that my skin was transdermal and all these chemicals were going directly into my bloodstream. I remember using full-strength cleaning products and soaking my hands in the solutions.

My father smoked all the time; how much of that secondhand smoke was being taken in by the rest of the family? All the fathers smoked back then, and the women also liked to smoke at night; it looked glamorous, they thought, the movie stars smoked in motion pictures and everyone wanted to look glamorous and cool just like them.

The naive bliss of ignorance—we just didn't know. If we did, surely we would have taken it seriously and made changes. We were ignorant, but we weren't stupid. We trusted and believed.

But now there is good news . . . we know how to rid our bodies of toxins and pollutants, but we must make a firm commitment to ourselves, open our eyes, and accept that poisons are here to stay and if we are to survive in the toxic soup that exists on our planet, big changes have to occur.

Of course, it starts with nutrition. The food we eat has a direct influence on our health. Real food is essential, and label reading is a must. We need to be informed about food additives: terms such as caseinate, autolyzed yeast enzymes, beef or chicken broth, natural flavorings, soy protein, hydrolyzed protein, soy isolates, and soy protein concentrates all indicate a food has harmful glutamates—and humans are twenty times more sensitive to ingested glutamates than monkeys and five times more sensitive than mice. (See Dr. Russell Blaylock's interview, chapter 14, for more on these harmful substances.)

Switching to real food (organic if possible) is a good start to detoxifying your body. By recognizing the devastating effects of chemicals we can now make a new life commitment, a shift in our thinking regarding chemical poisoning. For without taking the food we consume seriously a big crash awaits us down the road.

Here are some other things you can do to detoxify your life:

- If organic food is not available, then washing the poisons off of your food is essential. Stores like Whole Foods sell naturally derived produce washes.
- It is essential to maintain a household free of toxic chemicals. Remove any chemicals and contaminants and toxic household cleansers from your home, or at least limit your exposure to them. Substitute natural cleaning products, such as distilled white vinegar, baking soda, Borax, lemon juice, citrus cleaners, Castile soaps, and safe commercial products. These items can be purchased from health food stores or cutting-edge grocery stores like Whole Foods.
- Pay attention to the air you breathe. The average American spends most of his or her time indoors; the quality of that air becomes crucial. I had not heard of "sick buildings" until I experienced one myself. For fifteen years I stayed at the same hotel in Florida for my once-a-month appearance on HSN. Every time I checked into the hotel my eyes started itching, my sinuses acted up, I started sneezing, I felt headachy. I thought it was *Florida* . . . that I was allergic to something in the air, or the weather. I had not connected my allergic reactions to my hermetically sealed, toxic, mold-filled hotel room. Once I switched to a new hotel with fresh air and windows that could open, the symptoms went away. Tropical climates are especially dangerous in hermetically sealed rooms; mold accumulates and the toxins get trapped. Other toxic substances that are airborne are pollens, dust mites, mold spores, tobacco smoke residues, benzene, chloroform, chemical gases, and the formaldehyde found in the backings of our carpeting.
- Ozone and ionizing air filters are now available for home use. Common household plants can also be used as filters to remove pollution from indoors.
- Filtering your water is essential; unfortunately, our tap water is a major source of toxic chemicals that our livers are required to process. A water filter will help. And reverse osmosis filters are

essential if you have fluoride in your water system. The filter needs to be changed every three months because fluoride will eat through it in that amount of time.

CONSIDER COLONIC THERAPY Now that we've looked at ways to clear toxins from your life, here are some breakthrough treatments for getting rid of them in your body. Colonic irrigation is one of the most effective ways to cleanse the large intestine of accumulated toxins and waste products. Colonics draw toxins from the blood and lymph back into the colon for excretion. Colonic irrigation lasts thirty-five to forty minutes and cleans the entire five feet of the colon, unlike an enema, which cleanses only the lower eight to twelve inches of the bowel.

BUILD YOUR IMMUNE SYSTEM I have had the pleasure of working with my antiaging physician, Dr. Michael Galitzer (see chapter 24), to detoxify my body on a regular basis. I go to him once a month and weekly if I have the time and am in town, not because I am sick, but because I am well and want to stay that way. I travel constantly for my work and get exposed to all kinds of toxins, including electromagnetic radiation from airplanes. Couple that with long work hours, interaction with the public, plus poor air quality during flying, and the result is a weakened system. Knowing this, I go to the doctor not only to detoxify, but also to build up my immune system to stay healthy. It works; I have not been sick in years.

Most often Dr. Galitzer will give me an intravenous vitamin C drip. The relationship between vitamin C and body toxicity is complex. People deficient in vitamin C are more susceptible to environmental pollutants, but exposure to toxins like lead or benzene will deplete a person's vitamin C stores. Evidence also suggests that vitamin C deficiency hampers the body's own detoxification process. Vitamin C also functions as a free-radical scavenger, neutralizing the immunosuppressive toxins produced by infectious diseases. Free radicals are what give us cancer. Antioxidants like vitamin C eat free radicals.

KEEP YOUR LYMPH SYSTEM HEALTHY Keeping your lymph system healthy and moving is essential for detoxifying the body. After radiation treatment for my breast cancer I developed a painful lump under my arm, which was a congested lymph gland, and that's when I took notice of the lymph system. We have three times more lymph fluid in our bodies than blood. This fluid bathes all the cells in the body and carries nutrients from the blood to the cells. The lymphatic system has been called the vacuum-cleaning system of the body, the garbage collector of the body and the immune system.

The lymphatic system is a complicated network of vessels, ducts, and nodes that moves fluid between the cells and tissues and produces and distributes the infection-fighting and -scavenging cells of the body. It feeds literally every tissue and organ. It feeds the blood and is the transportation highway for the immune and repair functions of the body. When the lymph system is functioning properly it effectively cleanses the tissues, aids in cellular repair, and eliminates toxins.

Doctors acknowledge that the lymph system is one of the most important keys to health. It is an essential component of immune function, a network of vessels and lymph nodes that runs throughout the body transporting lymph fluids and eliminating toxins. The lymph system affects every organ in the body and serves as a primary cleansing and filtration system.

When the lymph system becomes congested, it deprives the cells of oxygen and affects the ability of the body to rid itself of its own waste material. Over time, other body systems that rely on the lymphatic system for waste removal will become compromised, setting the stage for pain and disease. A sure sign of lymph congestion is sore or swollen lymph glands, which are most noticeable in the neck, armpits, groin, and intestines. Illnesses as wide-ranging as allergies, fibrocystic disease, and cancer can be related to lymph congestion.

Correct diet, infrared sauna, and manual lymphatic massage can prevent or reverse lymph congestion and will stimulate the flow of lymph. I work with Cynthia Story, a certified lymphatic specialist in Montecito, California. An inexperienced therapist can aggravate a patient's condition by pushing the material to other areas of congestion. Well-trained conscientious therapists can avoid creating such a problem, but only by spending a great deal of time in each session.

Because of the time-consuming aspect of lymph massage, a lot of doctors are turning to a noninvasive handheld instrument known as the light-beam generator (LBG) to restore lymph function and eliminate wastes. This machine penetrates many times deeper than lymphatic massage alone and also increases the effectiveness of manual drainage of the lymph system.

Recently I was the keynote speaker for the A4M (American Academy of Anti-Aging Medicine) Winter 2007 convention in Las Vegas. As many as 25,000 doctors are involved with this group, and I try to attend these sessions on antiaging and alternative medicines as often as possible. There is always enthusiasm and energy around breakthroughs and new advances in natural healing, and it is exciting to be around doctors who have made the leap to change. I have been especially interested in lymphatic relief (selfishly), and I came across yet another marvelous invention called the Ondamed machine. This is a very sophisticated new piece of equipment you need to urge your doctor to purchase. It is a cellular-electrical-biofeedback machine and purports to have miraculous effects for acute-pain management and lymphatic congestion, among other things. This machine has been used successfully since 1993. It is a "spectrum of low-level pulsing magnetic fields that induce the flow of micro-currants within the tissues of the patient." Okay, in English this means it is able to locate underlying dysfunction and provide a treatment for the patient. It can pinpoint the location of the pain, which doesn't necessarily mean where the pain manifests. For instance, your pain may be in your knee, but the Ondamed machine can tell where the pain originated, which might be in your kidney. Safe and noninvasive, it promotes improved circulation, wound healing, bone regrowth, and pain relief, for conditions such as fibromyalgia. These conditions resolve quickly, as though the body simply needs a small signal to jump-start the healing process. (See the resources for more information.)

There are daily routines you can do to keep your lymphs flowing correctly: Dry-skin brushing improves the skin's abilities to remove toxins, oxygenates the tissues, and reduces cellulite. One session of light brisk stimulation of the skin is equivalent to twenty minutes of exercise for encouraging healthy movement of fluid through the lymph vessels.

Another way to keep the lymphs flowing is to jump on a Rebounder, a mini-trampoline. It cleans the system by causing the body's lymph fluid to flow, plus it's fun and inexpensive.

The lymph system, unlike our blood system, has no pump. In order to keep your lymphs moving, exercise and manipulation are essential. If you sit around all day and do nothing, you can bet your lymphs will become congested.

I now use the Ondamed machine and the results have been truly miraculous. In just a short period of time I am no longer experiencing pain, swelling, or tenderness in the breast, and the most exciting part of this treatment is that it requires no pharmaceuticals. What we are doing is healing and unclogging the congestion. Continuous attention has to be paid to the lymphs, as they want to clog up easily. Manual massage, exercise, swimming, aerobic movement, using the Rebounder—any one of these is important for keeping the flow. Then, if your doctor has the Ondamed machine or the light-beam generator, utilize them.

CONSIDER CHELATION THERAPY You can also detox with chelation therapy, which draws lead, mercury, and other heavy metals out of the body. Remember how cadmium from my exposure to secondhand smoke twenty years ago still resides in my system? Think about your mercury fillings and the glass thermometers you used to play with when you were a kid until they dropped and broke so you could conveniently play with the little wiggly ball of mercury. Think about the Ban roll-on deodorant with "aluminum chlorohydrate" you used . . . that was sold to us as a "good thing." Think about the X-ray machines they used to have in shoe stores to measure your feet. How many times did you stand on those, waiting for your mother who was trying on shoes, while you were looking at the skeleton of your foot? All these metals, chemicals, and rads stay in our systems unless we are able to draw them out.

Remember how good a tuna fish sandwich used to be—until we found that tuna was loaded with mercury, as are mackerel and swordfish. Think of all the lead pipes you have inadvertently been exposed to in places of work or in one of your homes.

Chelation refers to a method of binding up toxins such as heavy metals and bodily wastes and removing them from the body, while at the same time increasing blood flow. In chelation therapy a synthetic amino acid called EDTA is administered intravenously and binds to various toxic metals in the blood such as mercury, lead, cadmium, and aluminum. The toxins are then flushed from the body through the kidneys. EDTA is three times less toxic than aspirin and has been tested and used safely for the past thirty years on an estimated half million patients . . . including me.

Dr. Galitzer has me take chelation sessions regularly to remove the heavy metals I have buried in my system as well as new toxins to which I am regularly exposed. This is another safe, nondrug way of keeping healthy and ridding the body of foreign substances.

You must remember that detoxification is ongoing. If we lived in a clean, nontoxic, chemical-free environment, we would have no need to do any of this, but that is not the case. So staying well requires effort, due to the unchangeable effects of pollution.

Other intravenous detoxification drips use ultraviolet light or hydrogen peroxide. Building-up therapies include glutathione, intravenously or with nanotechnology glutathione patches (see more on page 378), the body's natural detoxification substance, which declines with age.

HYPERBARIC OXYGEN Hyperbaric oxygen is another highly effective method of removing toxins. The patient is placed in a sealed chamber that is filled with pure oxygen. Oxygen "burns up" disease-producing microorganisms and toxins in the body. Stroke victims are greatly helped by the treatment, and after chemotherapy some cancer patients successfully use hyperbaric oxygen to detoxify from the chemicals.

(Michael Jackson, the entertainer, was famous for traveling with his hyperbaric oxygen chamber for its beautifying effects. It makes the skin baby smooth and flawless, but it's a rather expensive way to maintain beauty!)

I took one hyperbaric oxygen treatment for this book to see what it was like; personally, I did not enjoy the experience of lying in the glass container. I could see out and watch TV, but I felt claustrophobic. That is just me, but if I were very ill I would not hesitate to take advantage of its tremendous benefits.

INFRARED SAUNA And finally, infrared sauna is a highly effective way to detoxify. It is the only detoxification program that has successfully removed fat-stored toxins. Heat stress removes calcium deposits from the blood vessels and breaks down scar tissue from their walls. Other studies demonstrate that saunas can remove chemicals such as DDE, PCBs, and dioxin from fat cells.

The body uses its own internally generated heat to protect itself from viruses, bacteria, and other harmful substances. A fever is the body's attempt to destroy invading organisms and to sweat out impurities through the skin. Infrared sauna has heat levels that do not go above 180°F but are generally kept around 140°F. The reason is that on lower heat you can stay longer and bring up the internal temperature of the body to do its detoxifying work.

I recently purchased a home unit for $1,900. I realize it's a little pricey, but it saves me a trip to my antiaging doctor to use his. This way I take a forty-minute sauna two or three times a week, and I am always sure to drink lots of water before and after to get maximum benefits. Of course, as with any measure affecting your health, before you try a treatment, consult a doctor or knowledgeable and experienced expert.

DETOXIFICATION is essential in the world we have inherited. Dr. Leon Chaitow in *Alternative Medicine* says, "The need to tackle toxic burdens before they manifest themselves as disease has never been greater. It is clear that the future of health care will have at its very core an absolute requirement for safe and effective detoxification procedures, hopefully instituted before the individual's immune system and vital organs have ceased to operate adequately."

It can't be clearer than that. It's a new world with new health problems, and we can't put our heads in the sand and pretend that toxicity, pollution, and environmental distress are not with us. I feel optimistic that if we embrace this new way to be well, through the 8 Steps to Wellness outlined in this book, we can live a long life with optimal health.

13

STEP 3: TAKE NUTRITION SERIOUSLY

> I was eating bad stuff. Lots of sugar and carbs, junk food all the time, it makes you very irritated.
>
> —singer Avril Lavigne, discussing her angry lyrics

> Food is now nothing more than plastic for people's mouth entertainment.
>
> —Dr. Steve Nelson, Rancho Mirage, California

YOU ARE WHAT YOU EAT, so eat well. Scientists have now proven insights about food made in classical times. What was once called "the Doctrine of Signatures" contends that every whole food has a pattern that resembles a body organ or physiological function and signals the benefit it provides. Here is just a short list of examples of whole food signatures.

A sliced carrot looks like the human eye. The pupil, iris, and radiating lines look just like the human eye . . . and science shows that carrots greatly enhance blood flow to and function of the eyes.

A tomato has four chambers and is red. The heart is red and has four chambers. All of the research shows that tomatoes are indeed pure heart and blood food.

Grapes hang in a cluster that has the shape of the heart. Each grape looks like a blood cell, and all of the research today shows that grapes are also profound heart- and blood-vitalizing food.

A walnut looks like a little brain, a left and right hemisphere, upper cerebrums and lower cerebellums. Even the wrinkles or folds on the nut are just like the neocortex. We now know that walnuts help develop over three dozen neurotransmitters for brain function.

Kidney beans actually heal and help maintain kidney function and, yes, they look exactly like the human kidneys.

Celery, bok choy, rhubarb, and more look just like bones. These foods specifically target bone strength. Bones are 23 percent sodium and these foods are 23 percent sodium. If you don't have enough sodium in your diet the body pulls it from the bones, making them weak. These foods replenish the skeletal needs of the body.

Eggplant, avocados, and pears target the health and function of the womb and cervix of the female—they look just like these organs. Today's research shows that when a woman eats one avocado a week, it balances hormones, sheds unwanted birth weight, and prevents cervical cancers. And how profound is this? . . . It takes exactly nine months to grow an avocado from blossom to ripened fruit. There are over 14,000 photolytic chemical constituents of nutrition in each one of these foods (modern science has only studied and named about 141 of them).

Figs are full of seeds and hang in twos when they grow. Figs increase the motility of male sperm and increase the numbers of sperm as well to overcome male sterility.

Sweet potatoes look like the pancreas and actually balance the glycemic index of diabetics.

Olives assist the health and function of the ovaries.

Grapefruits, oranges, and other citrus fruits look just like the mammary glands of the female, and actually assist the health of the breasts and the movement of lymph in and out of the breasts.

Onions look like body cells. Today's research shows that onions help clear waste materials from all of the body cells; they even produce tears which wash the epithelial layers of the eyes.

THE IMPORTANCE OF UNDERSTANDING NUTRIENTS

The typical Western diet, high in red meats, bad fats, food additives, and carbohydrates is a perfect cancer brew. This brew not only causes cancer but can promote the growth of existing cancers as well.

—Dr. Russell Blaylock

Hormones and diet. Wow! When you get those two issues in balance you are flying high. Bioidentical hormone replacement puts the life force back in you. It gives you *you* back. Your thoughts return, your energy returns, your libido is in tune again. By coupling this with a proper, nutritious, chemical-free diet, you can expect the health that accompanies this one-two punch to be amazing.

We are what we eat. I realize it's a cliché, but that's the bottom line. Good food feeds our cells. Cells make up who we are, and reproduce themselves by the billions each day . . . unless we are in a toxic state. When chemicals and toxins are part of our diet and lifestyle, our cells malfunction and malfunctioning cells are what make us sick and cause disease.

Malfunctioning cells are an umbrella for every disease known to man. You name it: fibromyalgia, lupus, cancer, arthritis, heart disease, toxicity—it really doesn't matter the name given to the disease, *the reason you have the sickness is because your cells are malfunctioning.*

The toxins in your diet make it impossible for your cells to receive the nutrients they need to be healthy and reproduce. Toxins essentially turn your lights out. You fade away, sometimes quickly and sometimes slowly. Toxins wipe out your hormones, and the process of accelerated aging and disease begins. Toxins will kill you, it's just a matter of how soon.

To be healthy you have to take your food seriously. Yet, we rarely give it a thought . . . we are so used to having chemicals all around us. We mindlessly grab that handful of chips, packaged cookies, instant soups, or consume dangerous oils. Trans fats, hydrogenated oils, additives, and irradiated foods are making us sick and killing us. In fact, children now start out handicapped in the womb; pregnant mothers drink diet sodas, thinking they are doing something good for themselves and their growing baby—after all, there's no sugar, right? But the baby is taking in every chemical the mother consumes, and when you read renowned brain scientist Dr. Blaylock's interview that follows, you will see that giving an infant just six tablespoons of diet soda alters his DNA . . . *forever!*

It's so easy to mindlessly consume chemicals. For example, I was sent a gift basket of "healthy treats" by a well-meaning friend. As I picked up the first ingredient, a salami, I looked at the ingredients list. Here's what I found:

- pork
- salt
- corn syrup solids
- wine
- sugar

- dextrose
- natural flavorings (i.e., chemicals)
- sodium ascorbate
- lactic acid starter culture
- sodium nitrate
- sodium nitrate (It was listed twice. Who knows why?)

So . . . is there anything listed here that could be considered nutrients, anything to build healthy cells? Have you ever seen a sodium nitrate plant?

Will this improve my brain?

Will this make me healthy?

Yet all day long, a little of this, a little of that, and the accumulation of chemical-laden foods adds up to a deadly bunch of toxicity. Now that I know this, I can throw out that salami.

Healthy cells; yeah, yeah, yeah, who cares. Right? Think about this: *If all of your cells are healthy you cannot be sick.* If for any reason a cell starts to malfunction it is less able to perform its assigned tasks, which is where the problems begin. When such malfunction occurs in a large enough number of cells that it impairs the body's ability to self-repair and self-regulate, disease occurs.

But, you are thinking, what about diseases that are from bacterial or viral infections? And what role does genetics play in all of this?

I still maintain you most likely can't get sick unless you have a deficiency in your body, and that deficiency would be the lack of enough healthy nutrients (food) your cells need for proper functioning, or it could be the opposite; you get sick in the presence of toxicity.

Most of the time there is both: We don't eat right and we consume chemically laden foods. This combo is a disaster for us. To protect yourself from viruses, infection, or any genetic predisposition, keeping your cells nourished with proper nutrition will keep you healthy in the face of these conditions. Strong, healthy, nourished cells are your edge. This is how you will stay healthy in an unhealthy world.

Toxicity is the biggest deterrent to good health in the world today. Toxicity means that the cells are poisoned by something that inhibits proper function. All chemicals are toxins. According to one of the great scientific minds of this century, Dr. Roger Williams, "Body cells in general die for two reasons: first because they do not get everything they need; second because they get poisoned by something they decidedly do not need." What they need is the right foods, and what they don't need is toxins. It comes down to a choice: take it seriously or face the consequences.

We can live long, healthy lives if we do two things: provide our cells with all the nutrients they need and protect our cells from toxins. With this understanding we can significantly extend the length and quality of our lives. In the world as we know it today it is very difficult to accomplish these two tasks perfectly. As a result, cells suffer, we age, the quality of our life is diminished, and we die. The variable in this sequence is how fast we *allow* it to happen.

Health is everything. There is no quality of life without good health. But health is more than the absence of disease. Health is feeling good, feeling well, without aches and pains and weakness. Health is energy, vitality, happiness, sexuality. Without great health you won't have great sexuality. Sexuality is an inner sense, a glow, radiance, attractiveness. Healthy people are attractive, sexual. They command a room. They look bright and energetic.

With properly functioning cells you have a strong resilience to various kinds of stress—physical, chemical, biological, and emotional. With good lifestyle choices we all have the ability to make daily repairs to our cells, the ability to build healthy new ones, and the ability to efficiently remove pathogenic microorganisms and toxins from our bodies. Health is the state wherein all cells are functioning optimally. Now here's the reality: never do all of our cells function perfectly, so the challenge is to keep cellular malfunction to a minimum.

We produce ten million new cells every second, but how healthy are these cells? This is determined by our choices. Sick cells reproduce sick cells. You're not going to make healthy cells with diet soda. See how it works?

Having a cold or flu is your body screaming at you: "All is not well." Healthy people resist infections and colds and flu. Being sick is not normal. My husband is like that. I have never (in forty years) known him to be sick. It's amazing. All the colds and flus and infections I had in my early years never got him. We would sleep in the same bed while I was hacking and coughing and he never caught anything. The reason is his incredible gravitation to the foods that are good for him.

During the day my husband likes to munch on apples (always organic) or oranges or grapefruits. We are blessed to live in California, where these are so abundant. This is all second nature to him. He does this because he has always done this and his parents did this. Good eating is passed on, just as are poor dietary choices.

In the evening when I am preparing our dinner, he always has a large wooden bowl of fresh nuts in their shells (all different kinds—pecans, walnuts, hazelnuts, almonds), and he will sit there with a nutcracker and eat them for an hour. Then he likes to have some wonderful "peak season" fruit. In papaya and mango season he could sit there all night. For dinner I always prepare lovely vegetables and salads chock-full of great ingredients from my organic garden: fresh fennel, different garden lettuces, vine-ripened or heirloom tomatoes, fresh parsley, shallots, celery, cucumbers; high-quality olive oil; sea salt, fresh thyme, tarragon, or mint. Our main course might be organic chicken legs rubbed with olive oil, turmeric powder, and sea salt. Yum. I'm getting hungry writing about it. This kind of food allows you to eat until you are satisfied because it is so full of flavor. Once you start eating this way and making good choices you won't want to go back to packaged, chemical-laden foods.

So you get the picture: fresh nuts, fresh fruit, fresh vegetables; delicious healthy oils—olive oil, palm oil, flax oil—even butter; organic protein. This is wonderful cell-building food. With ingredients like these, food is exciting and delicious, never flavorless. Every choice you make regarding the food you eat should be made with this thought in mind: Will this food build me up or will this food bring me down?

Everything you eat has an effect. Eat a bag of Doritos (40 percent chemicals!) and you destroy cells in the process from just one serving! Chemicals are not a joke. Our bodies were not meant to ingest chemicals. Wait until you read Dr. Blaylock on diet soda! I doubt you'll ever drink one again.

Dr. Eric Braverman, who wrote *Younger You*, has an impactful interview as well—he talks about the "rainbow diet," which recognizes the effects of the different-colored fruits and vegetables and their benefits. And wait until you read about the value of fresh herbs and how you can turn your already great food choices into "superfood" by adding nature's flavorings. I now grow all my herbs: sage, which is delicious gently sautéed in olive oil and a little sea salt and served with fresh cannellini beans, tarragon, different types of thyme, oregano, marjoram, rosemary, which I use in almost everything I cook, and lots of fresh parsley and cilantro.

My husband and I used to go out to restaurants all the time. When we had blood panels done, they indicated trans fats in our systems. How could that be? I would never have trans fats in our house. But then I thought about our meals out. Restaurants use bad oils—corn oil, vegetable oils, canola oils, soy oil, peanut oil. But aren't these oils supposed to be heart-healthy? Wrong. According to Dr. Blaylock, that's the bill of goods the food manufacturers would have us believe. Dr. Blaylock will explain this in greater depth in his interview, but let me give you a quick indication of why eating these oils can be bad. The first line of defense against disease is the cell membrane. That is the wall that surrounds the cell and carries out many important functions. Healthy membranes, built from appropriate materials, protect cells from harmful invaders, including viruses. Malfunctioning membranes allow bacteria, viruses, toxins, and other harmful substances to damage cells. The presence of poorly constructed cell membranes formed from poor diets is one of the biggest reasons that almost all Americans get sick.

Here's how it connects with the bad oil scenario; these membranes that surround your cells are made of mostly fats and oils. If the membrane is constructed from the wrong oils and fats, the cell can malfunction. Diets with excessive poor-quality oils and saturated fats create rigid cell membranes that lack necessary elasticity. Instead, the surround is more like an eggshell that can crack.

Good oils (essential fatty acids), like olive oil, flax oil, and palm oil, are used to create the phospholipids in cell membranes. These oils are essential because your body is unable to produce them, so you have to bring them in from the outside. When the correct raw materials are lacking, the body makes cell membranes out of whatever raw materials are available, like margarine, vegetable shortening, and other hydrogenated oils. Cell membranes built from these inappropriate fats and oils cause the membrane and the entire cell to malfunction.

So if you build a cell from hydrogenated oil, it impairs the passage of oxygen into the cell and oxygen-deficient cells become *cancerous*. Think about that the next time you reach for one of those supermarket oils.

All the doctors I have interviewed say you should also supplement with essential fatty acids and fish oils to be sure that your cells have enough of the proper membrane-building oils. This membrane is your defense against disease. Remember, if you have healthy cells you can't get sick.

Antioxidants are essential for the reproduction of healthy cells. The cell membranes (outer coating) and the insides of cells can be damaged from oxidation by free radicals. The problems humans experience today from cell malformation are from the onslaught of chemicals: ozone in urban air, chlorine in tap water, fluoride, and many others. All these chemicals cause oxidative damage to our bodies.

Free radicals damage our cells like rust corrodes metal. Free radicals have unpaired electrons. Electrons need to travel in pairs, but an unpaired electron that has had its partner grabbed by a free radical (kidnapped) aggressively tries to find another mate. So it grabs from something else, perhaps a molecule that is performing an important job in one of your cell membranes. Once the electrons have grabbed that molecule, it can no longer perform its job correctly, and to make matters worse that molecule now becomes a free radical itself, aggressively seeking its own electron mate. This chain reaction can result in serious cellular damage commonly associated with aging and disease.

But if the body's tissues are rich with antioxidants they can stop hazardous chain reactions as soon as they begin. Antioxidants are essential and obtained from our nutritious food and by supplementation.

We need more antioxidant protection than ever before because we are exposed to so many more free radicals. We are in crisis because the need for antioxidant nutrients is up while the supplies in our diets are down. We can get it through the food we consume. Also see page 378 on nanotechnology and order the glutathione patches to detoxify your body throughout the day. I wear a patch most days, and follow my good diet to stay healthy.

A diet rich in antioxidant nutrients together with antioxidant supplements is absolutely necessary; eat real, clean food that has not been tainted by pesticides. Stay away from fake foods—foods that have not been grown, picked, plucked, or milked. Avoid chlorinated water—chlorine is in our tap water, shower water, and swimming pools, but it can damage your skin and lungs. Install reverse osmosis filters in your home to protect against chlorine and fluoride and switch your pool water to saline. And try to breathe fresh air.

These changes in your lifestyle are more important than ever before. Your life and the lives of your family depend on it. Think about this when you go to the supermarket. When your kids beg for harmful foods, educate them. Explain to them about free radicals. Draw pictures of cells with happy faces and cells with sad faces. Show them how to eat right. Educate yourself and then educate your children. They will get it. And then they will be able to survive in this sick world.

It's surprising to learn that most Americans are slowly dying of malnutrition. It's not about not having enough food, it's that we consume the wrong kinds of food. In fact, the poorest segments of our population live in areas where fresh food is almost impossible to purchase. These people buy most of their food in a convenience store. There is no real food in a convenience store. The people who shop in convenience stores consume enormous amounts of diet sodas and foods in bags: chips, dips, cookies with bad fats. And as a result, this segment of the population is predominantly overweight and sick.

Chemicals make you fat. They have no nutritional value, so your body keeps urging you to consume more and more to see if one of those bites just might have any usable nutrients. We know of course that isn't possible, but the mechanism is in place, so a person eats and drinks more and more, causing obesity, diabetes, heart disease, cancers, and premature death.

Food is meant to nurture our bodies. I have said this in so many of my Somersize books: Avoid white flour, white rice, sugar, processed oils, and most milk products. Most people are lactose intolerant. Try goat milk and goat cheeses instead. They taste delicious and do not seem to cause havoc in most people's guts. And above all, avoid chemicals.

We cannot create healthy cells if we consume foods from animals that do not have healthy cells. Avoid meat, chicken, and fish that have been fed toxic diets.

Chemicals used during the growing, harvesting, processing, transporting, and storing of produce diminish their nutrients. Food that has undergone these processes cannot support our cell chemistry.

Extended storage of foods in refrigerators or freezers robs them of many of their nutrients. Frenchwomen are healthier than we are—I am sure it has a lot to do with the fact that they buy their food fresh daily. Europeans, in general, live for the most part in small apartments and have small refrigerators, so they cannot store food very well. This seeming disadvantage is actually to their advantage. Our prosperity as a nation allows us to have large freezers, usually more than one. We have large kitchens, so we buy enormous amounts of food and then it sits around, losing its value even if it is organic. Commercial practices that take food from farms to supermarkets can destroy it. They pick produce before it is ripe, and store foods for long periods of time. They subject produce that has been picked prematurely to harmful methods to ripen it or color it artificially for presentation in the "fresh" produce section of the supermarket. In many cases these fruits and vegetables have lost nearly all of their vitamin and mineral content by the time you are in the checkout line.

Think about this. We are trying to achieve the impossible at present if we continue our poor diets and lifestyle habits. We want optimal health, but eating a diet that cannot provide the proper nutrients cannot provide health. You can exercise, which is great, you can take your bioidentical hormones to replace your lost or missing ones, which is great, and you can get plenty of sunshine and think happy thoughts. All of this is great. But if your diet does not provide the proper nutrients, if you are living with toxicity, if you are consuming chemicals, your health goals will fail.

14

DR. RUSSELL BLAYLOCK

For the first time in the history of the world, every human being is now subjected to contact with dangerous chemicals, from the moment of conception until death.

–Rachel Carson, *Silent Spring,* 1962

DR. RUSSELL BLAYLOCK IS EXTREMELY PASSIONATE and knowledgeable about the effects of chemicals on humans. As a brain surgeon, he was able to see firsthand the horrible effects of chemicals on the brain and was profoundly shocked to realize it was happening to younger and younger people.

Dr. Blaylock attended Louisiana State University of Medicine in New Orleans, and completed his internship and neurosurgical residency at the Medical University of South Carolina in Charleston. After twenty-six years of practicing neurosurgery, in addition to having a nutritional practice, he has recently chosen to devote his full attention to nutritional studies and research. Dr. Blaylock has authored three books on nutrition and wellness, including *Excitotoxins: The Taste That Kills, Health and Nutrition Secrets That Can Save Your Life,* and *Natural Strategies for Cancer Patients.*

Dr. Blaylock is devoted to helping us, the patients, understand the devastating effects of chemicals relative to our health. You will never eat the same way after you read his interview.

SS: Thank you for your time, Dr. Blaylock. I know you are a neurosurgeon by profession but you've recently retired. Why?

RB: I decided to devote my time to neuroscience and general nutrition studies. I have a newsletter that I write on all different subjects. For instance, I write about diabetes and hormone problems and anything that has to do with human health. But my primary interests are excitotoxicity, brain function, and nutritional protection of the brain.

SS: I am quite familiar with your newsletter and eagerly wait for it to arrive each month. Explain excitotoxins.

RB: Excitotoxins are a special group of amino acids that are the building blocks of proteins that we call glutamate, aspartate, and cysteine. The food manufacturers add tons of these excitotoxic amino acids to foods of all kinds, including baby foods. The only reason glutamate and similar excitotoxins are added to foods is because they greatly enhance the taste of foods—they make foods taste scrumptious. For instance, MSG (monosodium glutamate) is a dangerous brain-toxic compound that should not be added to baby food, or any food. MSG is not the only taste-enhancing food additive known to cause damage to the nervous system. There is a whole class of chemicals that can produce very similar damage. They all share one important property: When neurons are exposed to these substances, they become very "excited" and fire their impulses very rapidly until they reach a state of extreme exhaustion. Several hours later these neurons suddenly die, as if the cells were "excited" to death. As a result, neuroscientists have dubbed this class of chemicals "excitotoxins."

SS: I believe if the public really understood this they would never consume any food containing these harmful chemicals, yet when you walk through the grocery store, the labels speak. Food-additive chemicals are everywhere.

RB: That's why you and I are speaking. So much negative information had come out initially on MSG that they came up with yet another substance called hydrolyzed vegetable protein that contains three known excitotoxins and, in many cases, also has added MSG. This substance is even more dangerous than MSG. As soon as negative information gets out they always find another way to fool the public; now they are adding even more excitotoxins, but they are called caseinate, autolyzed yeast extract, beef or chicken broth, or natural flavoring.

Ironically, the government regulatory agencies allow food manufacturers to call these excitotoxin additives by any name they choose as long as the glutamate content is less than 99 percent pure.

Now, what if someone told you that a chemical added to food could cause brain damage in your children, and that this chemical could affect how your children's nervous systems formed during development so that in later years they may have learning or emotional difficulties. How would you feel?

SS: I would feel betrayed. Explain the pathway.

RB: Glutamate is one of the many neurotransmitters in the brain—in fact, it is the most common neurotransmitter in the brain. Neurotransmitters function by interacting with receptors on the neurons—sort of like plugging in an appliance into a wall socket. When the glutamate enters the receptor, it turns on the neuron, making it very excited. Because glutamates are so toxic outside the neurons, where they can interact with the receptors, the brain has a very elaborate system to keep these glutamate levels extremely low.

Even slight elevations in glutamate levels outside the neurons can result in widespread brain damage!

Recently they've discovered that virtually every tissue in the body has glutamate receptors and that overactivation of these receptors can cause a wide variety of disorders, including diabetes, heart failure, atherosclerosis, and lung damage—and even make cancers grow faster and spread throughout the body.

SS: I think I need a crash course in glutamate. It's easy to confuse it with glutamine, which is a common supplement many people take.

RB: Yes, they are completely different. Glutamine is made by the body for a number of functions, such as muscle growth, immune function, and function of the cells lining the GI tract. It is converted in the body to *glutamate*, and neurons use the glutamate for a transmitter. Glutamine is only harmful if converted into glutamate in large quantities. Glutamates are not only found in chemicals like MSG but also in hydrolyzed protein, soy protein, soy isolates, soy protein concentrates, or autolyzed yeast extract. When humans consume an excess of these excitatory amino acids, depending on their absorption capacity, you can increase your blood glutamate level from nineteenfold to as much as fiftyfold—which is a huge elevation. Humans have the distinction of being the most sensitive to ingested glutamate additives, being twenty times more sensitive than monkeys and five times more sensitive than mice, the next most sensitive animal. Today, people are exposed to higher concentrations of glutamate additives than at any time in history. So we are at risk, great risk.

SS: Risk for what?

RB: A great number of maladies, including cancers. The link between glutamate in the diet and cancer growth invasion and spread has only recently been discovered. Yet I look at the nutritional recommendations of oncologists and major medical and cancer centers and I am astounded to see two things: one is sugar (and large amounts of sugar are in the recommended diets), and the other is large amounts of glutamates.

Now, sugar is a powerful cancer growth promoter, and we have an impressive amount of scientific literature that clearly demonstrates that glutamates make tumors grow faster and make them invasive, yet doctors encourage their patients to consume more glutamates. Also, glutamates make chemotherapy less effective. In fact, several studies have shown that the prognosis of a number of cancers depends on the number of glutamate receptors found on tumors. Even more exciting, studies are now showing that blocking these glutamate receptors can slow the growth of many cancers and make chemotherapy much more successful, even in lower doses.

SS: It doesn't make sense. If glutamates are so harmful why are they legal?

RB: Because it's a natural amino acid and no one has been able to get the FDA to pay attention. All the way back in 1957, glutamates were found to be toxic to the retina of the eye . . . destroy it. Since that time we've found that it is a very powerful brain toxin and a child is in a very supersensitive state. The infant and child's brain is four times more sensitive to the damaging effects of glutamate than an adult's. In addition, glutamate in excess alters the way the brain forms, because glutamate plays a major role in how neuron pathways develop. Glutamates have a dramatic effect on the neuroendocrine system. In fact, the regulation of all the hormones is profoundly affected by exposure to glutamate, especially in a child because it alters the pathways. Glutamate neurotransmitters are the most important neurotransmitters in the hypothalamus, which regulates the hormones. During the development of a baby, the nerve pathways form in the hypothalamus by controlling this neurotransmitter. If glutamate levels are too high during this critical period of development, when they get older they may have abnormal menstrual periods, premature puberty, and infertility. Physicians are not familiar with the literature explaining the effects of glutamates, so the patient is not getting the proper advice.

SS: What about older people; can glutamates contribute to Alzheimer's?

RB: We are finding that Alzheimer's is much more common in women, particularly women who have low estradiol levels, but the connection seems to be in above normal LH (luteinizing hormone) levels (that is, above 28.5 IU/l for estrogen-free women and 44.6 IU/l for those taking estrogen replacement). During menopause, estrogen levels fall and LH levels rise. In those doomed to get Alzheimer's disease, the LH levels rise very high. Of great importance is the discovery that estrogen is a very powerful *inhibitor* of excitotoxicity, and natural estrogen is protective of the brain. Its effect on protecting the brain occurs mainly in physiological doses, and those are—as you write about, Suzanne—replacement doses.

With men, we know that when testosterone rises above the physiological levels, it becomes extremely toxic to the brain; in fact, it actually magnifies excitotoxicity. So hormone replacement in the right physiologic levels is very protective of the brain and reduces the incidence of Alzheimer's disease, but at doses that are too high, the physiological levels increase the risk of Alzheimer's. So the balance of these hormones, as you emphasize in your books, is what's important.

SS: Just for clarification, we are talking about real bioidentical hormones, right?

RB: Absolutely . . . bioidenticals are certainly more physiologic. I don't think any of the pharmaceutical synthetic hormones should be used. For instance, the commercially available synthetic pharmaceutical hormones break down into a number of brain-toxic substances. This is particularly true for medroxyprogesterone (progestins), which breaks down into a dozen brain-toxic compounds. But when we break down real bioidentical progesterone in the brain, we find two very *protective* compounds are produced. These special brain protectors *are not* produced by pharmaceutical hormones and may explain why tests using these hormones failed to reduce Alzheimer's disease in women.

SS: Let's talk about diet sodas. I know people who drink ten, twelve, fifteen sodas a day. Are they really that thirsty?

RB: Two studies came out recently by one of the biggest cancer research institutes in the world, the Ramazzini Foundation of Oncology and Environmental Sciences in Italy, and they used the largest number of rats ever used to test aspartame. Both studies were very carefully done and they both showed an *increase* in cancer incidence from doses of aspartame equivalent to drinking diet sodas. Previous studies showed that aspartame breaks down into formaldehyde and formic acid, and when they put a radioactive tag on the aspartame to see what happens to it metabolically in the body, they found it not only broke down into formaldehyde, but the formaldehyde also attached to the DNA and caused multiple breaks in the DNA . . . what we call double-strand breaks and those are most associated with cancer induction. We also know that formaldehyde is very difficult for the body to remove from DNA.

We had good evidence before that aspartame most likely produced cancer and now we know it does for sure.

There's more. Both of these studies showed a dramatic increase in leukemia and lymphoma with aspartame exposure, and it was accumulative over time. The second study showed it also increased breast cancer and probably brain cancers. We also know from previous studies that aspartame produces the very same brain damage that MSG does.

SS: So, do you think the high consumption of this product is going to result in a tremendous increase in neurological diseases, particularly Alzheimer's and Parkinson's, and ALS as well as cancer?

RB: We're already seeing that. We are seeing a tremendous increase in one of the brain tumors, the astrocytoma, particularly in young women who consume aspartame. In talking to a lot of these women around the country I find that they are drinking large amounts of diet colas, sometimes as much as a case in one day, because it's addicting.

SS: What is the addictive factor in aspartame?

RB: I knew a nurse I worked with when I was practicing neurosurgery who was so addicted that she would get up at three o'clock in the morning and drink a six-pack of diet soda. She couldn't help it . . . and her immune system was ruined. She was sick all the time.

Recent research indicates that glutamate plays a major role in human addiction. That's because in the brain a nucleus, called the nucleus accumbens, is connected with addictive behavior. This nucleus is activated by glutamate. So when you are eating foods containing glutamate additives or drinking lots of diet colas, your addictive behavior increases.

I had a patient who I told all about the dangers of aspartame and she said, "Well, I agree with you, and I know you are telling me the truth, but I just can't stop drinking them. I'm probably not coming back anymore," and she didn't. She also said, "I'll probably die from this stuff, but I just can't help it. I have to have it." Her addiction to diet soda was as strong as any addiction I have seen to cigarettes and narcotics.

Aspartame is becoming a major addictive substance and the health effects are absolutely profound. It should never have been approved, and it was approved over the objections of some of the major neuroscientists and toxicologists who served on the board of the FDA. They recommended that it not be approved, but it was approved over their objections for monetary reasons.

SS: So, we're going to need twelve-step programs for diet soda addicts?

RB: If they live long enough . . . I've never seen people addicted to anything as much as aspartame, and I believe that many are going to die as a result. It's a terrible addiction.

SS: One of the doctors I interviewed for this book said, "We have to accept that cancer is here. That there's a merging of traditional and alternative medicines to deal with cancer and that we are going to have to learn to live with cancer." Do you agree? Do you agree that cancer is so out of control that it's just going to be a part of everyday life with everyone?

RB: It depends on your lifestyle and eating the proper foods and avoiding the toxins. You have to exercise and get plenty of sleep, take certain supplements, drink pure water, and then your risk will be extremely low. I don't think it's an inevitable thing; rather, people make bad choices for themselves and then put themselves at tremendous risk.

SS: I was surprised to read your negative take on vaccinations. In fact, you have made me realize how blindly I have accepted vaccinations over my lifetime, not only for myself but for my son as well. I mean, when the pediatrician wanted to vaccinate my baby, it never entered my mind (so many years ago) to question. It felt like I was doing the best thing for him, you know, protective. What is wrong with vaccinating?

RB: This obsession with overvaccination is ruining people's immune systems. This is well documented in medical literature, but unfortunately physicians who practice and the general public are totally unaware of this.

Those of us who understand are very concerned that there are so many vaccines being given to people, particularly with mercury contamination that wipes out their immunity. There is a strong connection between overvaccination and excitotoxicity in the brain. This may explain the dramatic rise in autism over the last thirty years.

A number of experiments have shown that vaccinations, especially in excess, can cause chronic inflammation of the brain, which increases brain levels of glutamate, leading to abnormal brain development and function. Studies of autistic children have shown high blood and spinal fluid levels of glutamate. Children are receiving thirty-five vaccines before starting school, and this is playing havoc with their brain function. Some pediatricians are giving as many as nine vaccines during a single office visit—this is unconscionable.

I worry for the children. There's a new study out of *JAMA (Journal of the American Medical Association)* that showed there's a dramatic increase in chronic diseases in children. It's gone from 1.8 percent in 1960, to 7 percent today. That's an almost fivefold increase. Sixty percent of children age five to ten have at least one cardiovascular risk factor and 30 percent have two or more. We have never seen this before.

SS: Is this due to poor diet or toxins?

RB: Mostly diet, but also exposure to an enormous and growing number of toxins and vaccines. People are spraying their yards with Roundup and all kinds of weed control, herbicides, and pesticides. They have no idea of the medical and toxicological literature showing that these toxins from pesticides, even in extremely small doses, are powerful neurotoxins and that they suppress immunity. Some of these chemicals can produce autoimmunity and they are also very powerful carcinogens.

Roundup weed killer is associated with an 800 percent increase in multiple myelomas (bone and blood cancers), which are growing like crazy in this country.

SS: Is there any safe way to use these chemicals?

RB: Wearing gloves and masks around the home when you are using them helps, but think about the children. They are in the yard, the dog is in the yard, then they bring it into the house, and it's on the bottom of their shoes or the animal's paws and they don't realize that just the fumes from this is enough to raise your blood levels of these toxins. What's worse is that all of these compounds are fat soluble so they remain in the body for decades, if not a lifetime. Breast tissue tends to concentrate things like DDT and other pesticides in very high concentrations, higher even than in your blood. The ability of some tissues (like the breast) to concentrate these toxins makes certain organs much more susceptible to carcinogenic effects. We're seeing neurological diseases in much higher concentrations than ever before as well, so prevalent in fact that it's almost an epidemic and it's occurring in younger people with things like Parkinson's and Alzheimer's.

SS: Alzheimer's? That is the domain of old people, right?

RB: *Used to be that the risk of Alzheimer's would go up tremendously after age eighty, but now we are seeing it in people in their forties, fifties, and sixties, which was quite rare.*

SS: What is the reason for this?

RB: Destruction of critical nerve cells in the temporal lobes plays an important role in Alzheimer's. If children are consuming glutamates from an early age, they are destroying nerve cells in the brain, particularly in the temporal lobes of the brain. Also, follow me on this . . . we have forty-five million people in this country who have metabolic syndrome (associated with diabetes and obesity). You can produce metabolic syndrome in experimental animals by feeding them . . . glutamate. Our children are consuming doses of glutamate that exceed what we are using to produce metabolic syndrome in animals. If you expose rats to MSG (monosodium glutamate) as infants, they become grossly obese as adults or adolescents. So we know MSG during the growth period produces grossly obese individuals. There is a strong link between obesity, the metabolic syndrome, and Alzheimer's disease.

SS: So there you have it, chemicals equal obesity and early Alzheimer's. This is terrible. It seems these substances are . . . well . . . evil.

RB: And the government allows them to put on the labels "contains no MSG," yet when I go through a store and look at these labels, I'll find three or four different glutamate toxins added to the food, but they use a disguised name. It will say hydrolyzed protein, or vegetable protein extract, or autolyzed yeast extract, or natural flavor. All of those are disguised names for MSG because the FDA says if it's not 99 percent pure you can label it any way you want. You can even put "contains no MSG" on it. Most of your meats are injected with hydrolyzed protein.

SS: So what you are saying is that virtually every processed food contains glutamates.

RB: Yes, it's very difficult to find a processed food that does not contain it. Let's talk about Doritos chips. Doritos has three powerful excitotoxins in it. Of special concern, it has MSG in high doses and sodium caseinate. But if you look at the labels, you'll see sodium or calcium caseinate on hundreds of items in the supermarket, and these are the things that children are eating the most.

SS: How did it get this way?

RB: It's about selling food. In World War II, the Japanese were putting a lot of MSG in their rations; afterward American scientists analyzed it and found that this was the reason their rations tasted so much better than our GIs' rations and so they shared it with all the manufacturers. They held a conference with the major food processors and concluded that this additive used in processing would make food taste better. So since 1945 they've been adding this to our food. In 1970, 262,000 tons of MSG was added to American foods. Because we send food all over the world, we're beginning to see people from all parts of the globe starting to have a problem with obesity, even in places where they never had obesity before.

Unfortunately, everybody is looking at sugar and exercise and saying kids are playing too many video games, but think about it, when you and I were kids we ate tons of sugar and you rarely saw an obese kid in your class . . . maybe one, maybe two at most.

SS: Yes, and even then we were getting a fair amount of MSG. I remember that our mothers were convinced that Accent, the meat tenderizer (which is MSG), was the only way to marinate a steak, but we didn't have the fast-food places like we have now. What happened to real food? When did we stop eating real food? Did it start with those frozen TV dinners I used to beg my mother to buy?

RB: Yes, not only were you getting glutamate from them in the form of MSG, but also aluminum from heating the TV dinner in the aluminum trays, which is toxic. Here's the problem . . . Americans have gotten used

to the taste of glutamate additives. So it's a dilemma for the food manufacturers. If one of them says, "I don't put MSG in the food," he's not
going to be able to compete with the guy who does, because that guy's
food will taste so much better. This is the dilemma that keeps the food
manufacturers doing it.

SS: I truly believe when people find out about this, they will be willing to forgo this fake taste, get used to the real taste of food again, and
even be willing to pay more for food that is not loaded with MSG and
other harmful glutamates. This information makes me happy that I did
not have much money when my son was a child—I was a teenager and
we only ate real food. Rarely fast food, because it was something I could
not afford. Mothers today are going out of their way to do the right thing
with their children. It seems to me that the doctors need to be educated.
Most doctors are very poorly versed in nutrition. And we operate in an allopathic medical system where every complaint has a drug attached to it.
This is a big problem also. Am I being naive?

RB: You are right, it's about awareness. If people understand just how
toxic this is they will stop. But most people don't understand, most people I speak with say things like "I'm not allergic to MSG" or "I'm not affected, it doesn't bother me."

The first thing you have to understand is that it's not an allergy. It's a
toxic sensitivity and everybody is sensitive to the toxicity. Some more
than others because of different variables like antioxidants and detoxification systems, but everybody is sensitive and it's the silence of toxicity
that's most dangerous. When you give animals doses of MSG, it starts destroying brain cells but the animal appears normal. But when you slice
the brain of this animal, you can see the loss of great numbers of brain
cells, and over time the animal, just like humans, will become demented
or lose its ability to think cognitively.

This obesity epidemic, the diabetes epidemic, this cancer epidemic, endocrine problems . . . all these things can be directly related to the intake
of aspartame and particularly MSG. When you take the two together, it is
frightening, and hundreds of millions of people are doing just that worldwide. In fact, studies have shown that adding aspartame with MSG
greatly magnifies the toxicity and raises blood glutamate levels much
higher than when either is used alone.

SS: Your message is that we need to understand these toxicities.

RB: Yes, people need to understand just how important this is. It's not
just one more thing to scare you. This is real and of major importance. It
exceeds most of the other things that are being talked about.

Look at mercury toxicity. Mercury destroys the brain by triggering excitotoxicity. If you block excitotoxicity you block most of the mercury's toxicity . . . same thing with lead. Pesticides affect our brain, also triggering excitotoxicity.

When you are eating a lot of glutamate, it makes pesticides more neurotoxic, it makes mercury more neurotoxic, so you are magnifying *the toxicity of every environmental toxin by eating these foods. That's what people need to understand.*

I read in your book *Ageless,* Suzanne, that your mother had macular degeneration. Well, macular degeneration is now considered to be an excitotoxic disorder of the retina. These neurons become overexcited and burn themselves out.

SS: Can we detoxify from excitotoxins like glutamate and MSG?

RB: The number one detoxification is to stop exposing yourself. And then you do simple things that stimulate repair. Most important are things like DHA from fish oil. The DHA in the fish oil is the most beneficial for the brain and for everything else, including cancer treatments. DHA helps repair a lot of the damage that has been done—plus a lot of B vitamins, thiamine, B_6, niacinamide, help. They play a big role. Also, B_{12} and folic acid help you repair the damage; selenium is very important because as your immune system repairs itself it helps repair the brain as well. These things help reduce inflammation and, as you know, chronic inflammation is what leads to most of the diseases. If you look at diabetes, arteriosclerosis, cancer, neurodegenerative diseases, they are all associated with chronic inflammation. Chronic inflammation significantly magnifies excitotoxicity, not just in the brain but also in all the tissues in your body, so that interconnection of inflammatory cytokines and excitotoxins causes a great number of disorders.

SS: In my last book I wrote extensively about inflammation and urged all my readers to get the highly sensitive CRP (C-reactive protein) test as the best way to gauge the amount of inflammation. It's so simple . . . it's just a blood test. Strangely though, so many don't want to do the tests because they don't want to know. What they don't know won't hurt them is the thought process. Much of what I am trying to get across in this book is the notion that we now have the available information and tests to catch problems before they take hold.

RB: Yes, and most people don't think about atherosclerosis and the connection to excitotoxins, but a recent study showed that if you fed an animal MSG early in life for about six doses—six doses, that's not much—when they reached adolescence (and the same goes for a human being having the same amounts early in life), these animals were still generating high levels of free radicals in the walls of their arteries at an age equivalent in humans to ages twenty and twenty-five. That's just one short dose of MSG early in life that is still producing free radicals for *two decades*, which is the *cause* of arteriosclerosis, not elevated cholesterol as it was thought to be. *Cholesterol has little to do with it*. In essence, what I am saying is that the high excitotoxin additive intake causes chronic inflammation and this results in most of these diseases. The good news is that an elevated CRP can be lowered by dietary changes and a few special anti-inflammatory supplements. The problem is that people are eating diets that dramatically promote inflammation.

SS: That's kind of overwhelming when you consider the bad diet and lifestyle habits we all have or had until some time ago when some of us woke up. So, help me out here. If the chemicals are still residing inside us, is there any way to get it out of our DNA . . . out of our cells?

RB: It's not a matter of getting it out. It's that the early exposure altered your genetic activation of inflammatory processes. The glutamate is long gone; what's left is that it turned on a free-radical-generating process that lasts for a long period of time. The answer is to do the things nutritionally that we know would do the opposite of that, which is to shut down the free-radical generation and produce anti-inflammatory responses. Flavonoids and carotenoids powerfully inhibit inflammation. That's how you reverse the process, and as we get older we need much higher doses.

FLAVONOIDS AND CAROTENOIDS

Flavonoids provide powerful protection against cancer and other diseases. Flavonoids are plant pigments responsible for the color of flowers, fruits, and sometimes leaves. Researchers believe the flavonoids that plants supply provide the natural anti-inflammatory and antioxidant magic bullet so important for health.

Foods that contain flavonoids:
Onions
Lettuce (whole plant)
Basil (leaf)
Garlic (bulb)
Cabbage (leaf)

Kale (leaf)
Brussels sprouts
Kohlrabi (shoot)
Spinach (leaf)
Asparagus (root)
Fennel (fruit)
Soy (seed)
Scarlet runner plant (whole plant)
Lima bean (leaf)
Kidney bean (fruit)
Garden pea (shoot)
Adzuki (seed)

Herbs that contain flavonoids:
Dill (seed)
Tea (whole plant)
Basil (leaf)
Thyme (whole plant)
Cayenne
Coriander
Peppermint
Chamomile
Anise

Carotenoids are natural fat-soluble pigments found in certain plants and fruits. Carotenoids provide the bright red, orange, or yellow coloration of vegetables; they serve as antioxidants and are a good source of vitamin A.

RB: People don't realize how much you increase DNA damage from free-radical generation as you get older. Your DNA oxidative damage at age seventy is about fifteen times higher than at age twenty-five. That means you have to resupply the antioxidant network, not just a few antioxidants. The best defense a person can have is to massively improve their antioxidants and to understand that antioxidants always act as a network, not individually. This is where the medical profession goes wrong when they do a study and they say, we'll give them vitamin E and see what happens. If you have diabetes and you're producing enormous numbers of free radicals and you're given just vitamin E or vitamin C, what happens is that the single vitamin becomes oxidized itself and it then becomes a free radical!

That's why you need the whole network: vitamin C, vitamin E, all the flavonoids and B vitamins and zinc, selenium . . . then that network of antioxidants will neutralize all the different types of free radicals, because there is not just one free radical, there are dozens and dozens of types of free radicals. Each antioxidant neutralizes a specific group of these free radicals and that's why they work as a network. Plus your body has inborn antioxidant enzymes and these enzymes decrease in activity as you get older. Then if you develop disease, these enzymes decrease further and the toxins significantly decrease their activity. But you can change that.

SS: How do we do that?

RB: Well, for instance, melatonin dramatically increases these antioxidants in the brain as well as in the rest of the body. Some of these other antioxidants, like flavonoids, white tea extract, and white tea itself, dramatically improve these antioxidant enzymes. The level of glutathione, which is in every cell, is very important. Very low magnesium levels dramatically lower your glutathione levels and increase inflammation and excitotoxicity. So magnesium in your diet, along with supplementation, has a multiple effect of reducing inflammation and reducing excitotoxicity, while dramatically increasing your cellular glutathione, which gives you tremendous resistance against environmental toxins as well as diseases.

SS: What do you recommend as an average melatonin dose per person? I take 20 milligrams nightly. I sleep like a baby . . . usually nine, sometimes even ten hours. I also wear a nanotechnology sleep patch on my foot, which I explain in chapter 31, "The Future Is Now." To me, sleep is vital to health. Combine that with my balanced hormones and life is very sweet.

RB: Sleep is a huge component of health. People should start on the lowest dose of melatonin and then work up. Anything that is a hormone or a neurohormone should be taken at a range where it is effective.

SS: You mean when you find that sweet spot, where you don't have any symptoms of hormone loss?

RB: Yes. For instance, DHEA is a very powerful protector against excitotoxicity and it promotes plasticity (that is, regrowth of brain connections), but if the dose is too high, it inhibits . . . the same thing with melatonin.

Here's something else: MSG has been shown to block the enzyme in the pineal gland that has to do with the production of melatonin, so if you're consuming a lot of MSG you are reducing your melatonin production, which makes your brain more vulnerable to free radicals.

SS: And it would produce insomnia.

RB: Correct. One of the most common complaints I hear is people saying, "I can't sleep at night." They stay up all night with what we call "forced thinking," and then we discover they had MSG in a significant dose. There's a lot of MSG in hot dogs, and I keep telling the mothers, "Your child is all dosed up on MSG, no wonder he can't sleep."

SS: I take my diet seriously. I eat amazing food at home and it's all fresh and organic, I grow it myself. But I travel a lot and have to eat in restaurants. I recently had a blood test that showed I have trans fats in my system.

RB: Well, we'd all like to live a perfect existence, but sometimes we are forced to eat in airports or restaurants and it has a major impact. When you get back, increase your antioxidants and return to eating right, and take your supplements. Then what you are doing is stimulating your reparative processes.

Curcumin (turmeric) has the ability to stimulate wound healing. Curcumin is also one of the most powerful anti-inflammatories—it equals steroids as an anti-inflammatory. It's also one of the most powerful anticancer agents. It does so by affecting the cell-signaling apparatus, among a great number of other anticancer mechanisms. Curcumin supplementation is going to be one of the leaders, along with quercetin and ellagic acid. These are very powerful in protecting your brain against degeneration and they are the most powerful antioxidants against cancer.

SS: What is ellagic acid?

RB: Ellagic acid is the substance that is beneficial in pomegranate juice and walnuts. When they tested animals with horrible arteriosclerosis, ellagic acid produced over a 1,000 percent *decrease* in arteriosclerotic lesions. This far exceeds anything any statin drug could do.

SS: Ah yes, statin drugs. Lipitor and the gang; what is your feeling about them?

RB: I think statin drugs should be outlawed. They are one of the most harmful drugs ever created and have no more benefit than taking an aspirin a day as far as heart attacks. It's a scam. Number one, cholesterol is NOT the cause of arteriosclerosis. These conditions are due to oxidation of every lipid in the vessel wall. All of the lipids are oxidized, not just cholesterol, and it is oxidation of these lipids that results in the atherosclerotic crud (plaque) we see in coronary arteries and blood vessels to the brain. If you look at an arteriosclerosis lesion, the number one cause is overconsumption of dietary omega-6 fatty acids, and no one is telling the public.

SS: Why are people getting excess amounts of fatty acids?

RB: Because food sources high in omega-6 fatty acids are oils such as corn oil, safflower oil, sunflower oil, soybean oil, canola oil, cottonseed oil, and several other related oils. The very oils they are telling everybody they should eat because they're heart-healthy, yet they contribute significantly to atherosclerosis! Canola oil is a mixture of omega-3 and omega-6 but has been shown to promote cancer and, because it is easily oxidized, could promote atherosclerosis. So I do not endorse its use.

SS: Why are these oils bad for us and why do they cause atherosclerosis?

RB: Because they oxidize very easily and this leads to inflammation that damages the arterial wall, which is considered the major mechanism for formation of atherosclerotic plaques and eventual blockage of the vessel by blood clots. This has been shown in a number of experiments. The most abundant oxidized oil in the wall of atherosclerotic blood vessels is omega-6 oil and NOT CHOLESTEROL!

SS: What about olive oil?

RB: That's fine; it is a monounsaturated fat and it does just the opposite. It contains a substance called "lignans" and a lot of other antioxidants that dramatically reduce arteriosclerosis.

SS: I must say I'm relieved. I would have a hard time without my olive oil.

RB: I mix mine with turmeric because turmeric contains curcumin, which is a powerful flavonoid antioxidant and it protects the oil so it won't oxidize, plus you get the beneficial flavor in your food from the turmeric. You can use other spices as well; many of them, like rosemary and others, are very powerful antioxidants. They are also antiviral. If you already have a disease, you're producing a lot more free radicals than normal, so for instance, you could take bilberry extract because it's much more concentrated than eating bilberries, or the same thing with grapes. If you concentrate the part of the grape with resveratrol, then you get a much more concentrated effect than from eating grapes.

SS: How about wheelbarrows full of red wine?

RB: [laughs] Well, the power of red wine . . .

SS: Please say it's good for me, doctor . . .

RB: Red wine has resveratrol, which is a powerful antioxidant, but sorry to say, California wine has fluoride in very high levels. They use cryolite as a pesticide. Cryolite contains both aluminum and fluoride.

SS: Is that why you get a headache?

RB: The headache comes from the sulfite in the wine. It can also cause wheezing and other problems. On the other hand, the fluoride and aluminum are powerful neurotoxins. Most California wines have very high fluoride and aluminum levels. The sulfites spontaneously break down in the body into an extremely powerful excitotoxin that's ten times more potent than glutamate. Sulfites can produce significant exci-totoxic damage. There is evidence that the fluoride and aluminum, when combined, can greatly magnify the damage caused by the sulfite.

SS: I must say that there are several wineries in California that are going organic. I know in Malibu, California, they are producing some ex-cellent organic wines; also, there are Napa wineries producing organic, as well as a couple of wineries in Oregon. I see it as a trend. If people de-mand it, they will answer the demand, and we here in California are so proud of the wine that is produced in this state.

RB: Well, organic wine would most certainly be better. European wines have much lower levels of fluoride than American wines, particularly Italian, French, and some German.

SS: It seems to go against the grain . . . to put pesticides in wine. Wine is this natural beautiful thing . . .

RB: It's because they use the cryolite as the pesticide and spray it on the grapes, and it is then absorbed into the grapes. Once fluoride enters a food it is impossible to remove. Fluoride is a very reactive substance and it binds to the plant so you can't remove it. This is the problem with some teas, like black tea, which has an enormously high fluoride level. Green tea has far less and white tea has the least, plus it has the highest antioxidants of any tea. I wrote about it in my newsletter.

SS: As I said, I always look forward to your newsletter. Please tell my readers how to order it.

RB: Go to www.russellblaylockmd.com.

SS: The whole fluoride thing astounds me. In Los Angeles County we were "treated" to fluoride since last November and there is nothing we can do about it.

RB: You have to understand it's all a payoff system. Fluoride is a waste product. Communities keep trying to refuse it and they come back every year and try again. They offer the city contracts, government contracts, and dangle the possibility that they are going to do a big project if this community agrees to fluoridate the water supply. One of the biggest chapters in my *Health and Nutrition Secrets* book is about fluoride. We now know beyond any doubt that fluoride does not reduce cavities; in fact, it *increases* cavities, so there is no justification for putting fluoride in the water. Even the ADA (American Dental Association) admits it, be-cause the studies were so overwhelming that there was no benefit what-soever from drinking fluoridated water. The ADA has been lying to dentists and the public all these years.

Fluoride is one of the most poisonous substances on earth. It tends to accumulate, particularly in the bones and the thyroid gland, and in the brain. It lowers IQ. It's associated with Down syndrome and it triggers excitotoxicity. But the people who are promoting it, primarily the government and the ADA, have so much influence through the media that you really can't get the truth out. People are just not aware how enormously toxic fluoride is, particularly when combined with aluminum. When you mix them together, which they do in drinking water, where they combine chemically, they form a substance that acts as a false transmitter for what is called G-protein receptors in brain cells as well as other cells and wreaks all kinds of havoc. We also find that tumors, like breast tumors, also have these G-type receptors, some of which are glutamate receptors, and that fluoride activates them. So this connects to the finding that fluoride increases cancer growth and cancer mortality.

SS: Well, I grew up in San Bruno, California, and I remember when the city proudly announced that our water was "fluoridated." (I later had breast cancer, by the way, a large tumor, and so did my sister. There was no prior history of breast cancer on either side of our family.) So as a child I was exposed and now today as an adult I am exposed again. It's very maddening.

RB: When you fluoridate whole communities, you are just assuring a lot of cancer patients that their cancer is going to recur or it's going to be more difficult to control because of the fluoride. As you fluoridate the water, you fluoridate the plants. We're seeing a bioaccumulation of fluoride all over the United States, and the National Research Council said the average American is taking in about two to three parts per million fluoride whether they want to or not. The ADA has stipulated that everybody needs one part per million of fluoride (who knows why), but you are already getting three times that amount. Because people drink a lot of water, especially in the hot summer months, their intake of fluoride is much higher. This is especially so for babies and small children because of their low body weight and high fluid intake. Incredibly, aluminum is also added to drinking water to clarify the water.

SS: Well, the first thing I am doing is searching the house for any leftover tubes of fluoridated toothpaste. But let me ask you, if we have a filtration system in our homes doesn't that help?

RB: Well, that depends. There are only two ways to remove fluoride. One is a reverse osmosis filter. With reverse osmosis, the fluoride burns the filter, so it's important to replace the filter pretty near every three months. The other way to remove fluoride is to use a distiller, which distills the water, removing most of the contaminants. The better distillers have a built-in carbon filter to remove volatile chemicals as well.

SS: It's amazing that we are all still walking around.

RB: Well, as we're looking at this accumulation of toxins and the widespread use of pesticides and herbicides, particularly around homes and yards and inside houses, when we see the vaccination program with all of its aluminum and mercury and overvaccination effect, when we look at the food adulteration and food additives, we're just going to see a lot more serious disease in younger people and a severe drop-off in the number of people who are able to reach their seventies and eighties. *The New England Journal of Medicine* had an article explaining how we may have seen the peak of our improved life span, and that now we are going to start seeing a decrease of life span because of all of the above. The more they look at diseases, the more they are concluding that environmental pollution is playing a major role. We're just exposed to so many environmental toxins and our ability to resist is so attenuated by our diets.

Detoxification is important, and detoxification of the human body is purely based on nutrition, and yet the medical profession is totally unaware of that. Most doctors today have no conception of the effectiveness, the dramatic effectiveness, of certain nutrients to enhance the body's ability to detoxify these environmental toxins.

You ask the average physician about detoxification and he says it's what happens in the liver. He doesn't even realize that detoxification takes place in every cell in the body. You have these same enzymes in each cell of the body. In addition, the GI tract has a lot of them because that's where the first assault occurs . . . the food you eat. When things are working right, when the food is nutritious, it is detoxified before it even gets in the body. Doctors also don't realize that, and they don't have any idea that nutrition plays such a vital connection to keeping that detoxification at a peak level.

If we look at people with chronic disease, most are affected by poor detoxification systems and, as I stated, it's nutritional. If you boost people's detoxification ability they do a lot better, particularly cancer patients undergoing chemo and radiation. The toxicity of chemo kills cells, which are then released, and internal toxins in the body can cause the detoxification systems to become overwhelmed. That's why there is such a high mortality in patients who have chemo and radiation. I would wager that the death rate from traditional cancer treatments is infinitely higher than they're reporting, which is already high enough. These treatments are causing a lot of patients not only to die earlier but they're also converting curable patients into incurable patients.

SS: I have to say, when I saw the last appearance of Tammy Faye Bakker on *Larry King Live*, I thought to myself, was it necessary to poison her and degrade her health so dramatically? Or could she have just let it take its course, without all the poison, and die naturally?

RB: You're exactly right. You see, this is how they deceive cancer patients. They tell them this tumor responds very well to this agent, but what you need to understand is the word "responds." They never say the word "cure." What they are really telling you is that the tumor will, in most cases, temporarily shrink and then it will start growing again like wildfire. That's because when tumors respond to chemotherapy, the cancer cells respond by producing what we call a multidrug resistance, which means that they become resistant to all other chemotherapeutic agents. Then the cancer just grows as if you'd put fertilizer on it. That's why these patients die so quickly afterward.

SS: And die so horribly.

RB: Yeah. And, you know, in studies forty years ago they posed the question "Why do cancer patients die?" and they found out most of them die because they starve to death. The cancer steals all the nutrition; that is, it selectively steals the nutrition for itself. If you looked at Tammy Faye Bakker, the poor woman starved to death. Forty or fifty years ago they were afraid to feed cancer patients because they were afraid they would feed the cancer at the same time, so they would purposely restrict their nutrition. Then one bold oncologist said, "Let's try feeding them," and they did a lot better and their cancer did not grow any faster.

SS: What about radiation?

RB: In some cases it's beneficial, but it's used too much. For instance, a mammogram is the craziest thing I've ever heard of in my life. Radiation is the only known carcinogen for the human breast. Yet, we're telling women to go every year and have their breasts irradiated, and if you have a family history of breast cancer, do it every six months. The reason one has a family history is because one has defective DNA-repair enzymes. We have special enzymes that will fix damage to DNA. Radiation damages DNA, and if they already have a defective ability to fix the DNA and then you're irradiating them every six months, you are going to increase the incidence of breast cancer.

Studies show this: Mammograms increase the incidence of breast cancer from 1 percent to 3 percent, and one radiation oncologist said it's actually higher than that—it may be as high as 10 percent a year.

SS: Wow. I'm sure a lot of women will feel as I do right now. I believed them and I faithfully had mammograms for ten years before I was diagnosed with cancer. This is wrong. This is the information that has to get out, but business is in the way. Radiation and chemo and mammograms are big business, and not many women can afford MRIs.

RB: And that is a tragedy. But what rational woman would say, "I have normal breasts, but I'm going to go out of my way to increase my risk of developing breast cancer by 30 percent over the next ten years by having my breasts irradiated"? That doesn't make rational sense. At least, if you're going to do it, take curcumin because curcumin has been shown to prevent radiation-induced breast cancer.

SS: What about for someone like me for whom it has already been done? Is it too late?

RB: Curcumin will help because it continues to reduce inflammation. In Hiroshima and Nagasaki, people exposed to radiation continued to produce huge amounts of free radicals for decades afterward. The reason the Japanese who were exposed had a lower cancer rate than expected is because they have the highest flavonoid intake in the world, the largest omega-3 intake, and the lowest omega-6 intake. (Omega-6 increases cancer risk.) So the Japanese had the best diet in the world to be exposed to this massive radiation dose.

Americans have the worst diets, so they are far more sensitive to radiation side effects. The average woman who is getting mammograms and eating Doritos and junk food and frozen foods and has a high intake of omega-6 fatty acids has breast tissue so sensitive that when she is irradiated she's going to produce a far greater number of breaks in her DNA than the Japanese experienced and it's going to lead to cancer. Add in things people use daily in this country like NutraSweet (which is composed of 40 percent of the excitotoxin aspartame) and the rest of the other chemicals people are eating and then you have brain toxicity and neuron damage as well.

SS: Okay, I've got to ask again . . . why don't we know this, why aren't we mad as hell?

RB: I was warned when I submitted my book *Excitotoxins* to my publisher to be prepared for a backlash from the food industry, and especially the glutamate manufacturers. These two industries have joined together to fight anyone who would dare criticize the use of flavor enhancers. In fact, they have formed a special group, called the International Glutamate Technical Committee, and it is made up of representatives of major U.S. food manufacturers and the Ajinomoto Company, based in Japan, which by the way is the chief manufacturer of MSG and hydrolyzed protein. I'm sorry, but I felt the message was too important to be left alone. The FDA has failed in its stated purpose of protecting the public from harmful substances being added to the food supply. Millions of lives are at stake, including those of future generations. People must be warned.

SS: What do you see for the future? Are we going to "get it"? Are we going to realize we are on a path of no return and change the ways we are living our lives?

RB: The only thing that's going to save us is for people to become aware of the enormity of the problem. Then they need to become aware of the solution to the problem. Most important, they need to be dedicated to following that solution.

Unfortunately, I predict disaster in the next twenty years. Today's children are so widely and intensely affected now that when they reach thirty and forty they are going to be sick and dying . . . in much greater numbers than today. A lot of them are going to end up in total care and we're going to have to build facilities all over the country just to take care of the demented and seriously ill thirty- and forty-year-olds. And it's going to bankrupt the nation. So I pray that people start paying attention. If this scenario develops as I predict, they will pay attention. I spend a lot of my time talking with young people who are having these health problems, and when I explain that the cause is nutritional and environmental, they listen. In fact, the young people I speak with are listening much more than the middle-aged people who are set in their ways.

Suzanne, you have a perfect opportunity with the popularity of your books to really make an impact. Let people know this is not some silliness, this is deadly serious, and we are going to pay a huge price if people don't listen. As I look over the horizon to the next twenty years, I am saddened to contemplate the amount of death and disability we will see in very young people.

SS: I can see it coming. My friends are starting to die and be sick.

RB: I've lost quite a few friends, and then you hear about all these young athletes dying of sudden cardiac death; well, that's due to magnesium deficiencies in the face of high glutamate intake. You know how kids eat. We are going to see more and more of this. It's awful; I've never seen so many people stricken with multiple sclerosis or fibromyalgia or lupus. And the fact that 1 in 150 children and 1 in 65 male children born now are autistic is terrifying. **We are witnessing the destruction of a whole generation and it's just the beginning. And the answer is so simple!**

SS: Thank you for your courage. Thank you for your passion and intelligence. Thank you for your time. I will do my best to see that your message is heard.

DR. RUSSELL BLAYLOCK'S
BREAKTHROUGH BREAKOUTS

- Food manufacturers add harmful excitotoxic amino acids such as MSG (monosodium glutamate) to all kinds of foods to enhance taste. The government regulatory agencies allow food manufacturers to call these additives by any name they choose—such as caseinate, autolyzed yeast enzymes, beef or chicken broth, natural flavoring, hydrolyzed vegetable protein, soy protein concentrates, soy proteins, soy isolates, and autolyzed yeast extract. All of these names are disguised names for glutamates, but as long as the glutamate content is less than 99 percent pure it is legally allowed by the FDA. All of these substances can and do cause brain damage. Learning how to read packaging for these tricks will keep excitotoxins out of your diet and will save your life.

- Diet soda is not only addictive, but just one diet soda can kill the neurons in your brain within six to eight hours. These chemicals literally "excite" the neurons to death, which is why they call them "excitotoxins." Their regular consumption can cause brain damage and cancer, as aspartame increases your cancer risk.

- Get a highly sensitive CRP test to check for inflammation. Chronic inflammation significantly magnifies excitotoxicity not just in the brain, but also in the tissues in your body.

- To diminish free-radical damage, take a full course of antioxidants.

- Avoid omega-6 so-called heart-healthy oils such as corn oil, safflower oil, canola oil, peanut oil, soybean oil. Dr. Blaylock and other doctors in this book believe they are the primary source of arteriosclerosis.

- Canola oil contains both omega-6 and omega-3 fatty acids but has been shown to promote cancer.

- The right balance of real hormones, or bioidentical hormones, is protective of the brain and reduces the incidence of Alzheimer's disease.

- DHA from essential fatty acids such as fish oil, plus B vitamins, thiamine, B_6, niacinamide, B_{12}, selenium, and folic acid *are essential antioxidants* and help your body repair the damage done by toxins.

- Reduce your risk of cancer by exercising, getting plenty of sleep, taking cancer-fighting anti-inflammatory supplements such as curcumin and other antioxidants, and drinking pure water. If you have fluoride in your water supply, install a reverse osmosis system and change your filter every three months.

- Shut down free-radical generation and produce anti-inflammatory responses by eating foods that contain flavonoids and carotenoids, which powerfully inhibit the inflammation that can lead to disease.

- Curcumin as a supplement is necessary to prevent radiation-induced breast cancer. Curcumin reduces inflammation.

15

DR. ERIC BRAVERMAN

If people are educated, we can save them.

–Dr. Eric Braverman

DR. ERIC BRAVERMAN IS A RARE DOCTOR of great vision and insight. He teaches that brain health can be both monitored and measured, and that this analysis is the key to unlocking every individual's health. Dr. Braverman is a leading expert in antiaging medicine and has skillfully combined conventional wisdom with his unique knowledge of the workings of the brain to unravel the mystery of what makes us age and how disease in one area affects the entire body. Through his unique creation of what he calls AgePrint, he identifies the parts of your body that are aging most rapidly and in doing so can turn back time. He is passionate in his devotion to finding the problems before they can harm you. He is the director of the Place for Achieving Total Health (PATH) Medical Centers in New York City and Philadelphia. He has written two books, *Younger You* and *The Edge Effect*. My hours spent with him were an education for which I am incredibly grateful. Your understanding of your brain and its connection to your health will be demystified when you read this interview.

SS: I took your AgePrint this morning. I'm happy to say I'm in pretty good shape.

EB: Well, we're only as young as our oldest part.

SS: You make that point. Your approach is so different; explain your protocol. What is your strength?

EB: My strength is the brain, the mind, hormones, the entire body, the treatment of all chronic degenerative neuropsychiatric, neurodegenerative diseases, excluding end-stage cancer and surgery. It's a giant field, in that you can literally rescue a person and turn his health around.

SS: Tell me what is wrong with the approach of conventional medicine?

EB: What's wrong is that it misses the brain. It misses in particular a woman's brain, and misses the importance of memory and attention. It misses the entire idea of checking out the brain while doing EKGs of the brain, it misses the importance of hormones affecting the brain's twenty-one bioidenticals, it misses the importance of nutrition and lifestyle on the brain. And it misses the role of aging in everybody's life; how we all age and lose hormones and that every disease that presents is also presenting with multiple aged human parts, so that a person who has lupus also has estrogen problems and pregnenolone problems and metabolic syndrome, so it misses the idea of people as whole human beings.

It misses the important role of imaging, of lifestyle. Traditional medicine saves imaging until a part is broken. For instance, in traditional medicine they will run a CT scan of the lung on someone once he has lung cancer, but not do the same thing for a smoker (who should have it done every year) to find lung cancer at an early stage. Traditional medicine misses the fact that a physical exam with the finger in the rectum and the vagina is simply . . . a joke.

SS: A joke, why?

EB: Because it's inferior to a computer in every way, because now you can image a person's body with computers. You see, traditional medicine has become a death industry, where the hospitals are addicted to government money, so basically what we're doing is making expensive deaths. Hospitals have also gotten addicted to the drug industry (and this applies not only to hospitals but also to the patients) and the idea that the drug solves every problem. We have become a country that has lost faith and is unable to cope with death, so medicine has taken over the role of religion and medicine has taken over the process of dying. All of this is because as a society we can't cope with death anymore because we have no faith. As a result we have decided to spend all our money on dying rather than on improving our lives.

SS: What about vaccinations?

EB: More people are vaccinated now than are baptized or circumcised. It's crazy, and we are ruining people's immune systems with over-vaccinations.

SS: We live in an era of specialization, so the diabetes doctor only looks at the diabetes, neglecting the rest of the body. There seems to be no thought given to the side effects of the drugs prescribed for diabetes that in turn will have a deleterious effect on the rest of the body.

EB: Right, and the majority of diabetic patients have memory problems, attention problems, and hormonal problems—men deficient in testosterone, pregnenolone, and DHEA, and women with estrogen and thyroid problems. It turns out that diabetes always exists with a brain, mind, sleep, mood disorder component in addition to a hormonal component.

We describe in *Life Extension* magazine our ability to reverse blood sugars of 500 with a nutritional regimen, and completely change people's lives with hemoglobin A1Cs of 14 to normal. The conventional wisdom is that drugs only take off 2 points of 14.6 or 13.5, so that is 7 or 8 points, but we can do four times better than drugs alone by using drugs plus hormones, nutrients, and brain health measures. And by the way, I believe that's true with every disease. So I'm saying, drugs are one component, hormones another, nutrients another, lifestyle another, and when you put them all together you've got four times better medicine than drugs alone.

SS: Is diabetes ever reversible?

EB: Type 2 is almost always reversible by weight loss, mood change, sleep improvement, diet—meaning fiber, and using our *Younger You* rainbow diet with all its vegetables, fruits, and spices. A big component to our diet is that we have people average three spices per meal. Meaning we have them put cayenne pepper on their brown rice, we have them put turmeric on their eggs, cinnamon in their yogurt. We train people to get more out of their food by improving the density. Spices improve the density of nutritional foods. The more nutritious the food is, the more nutrients in it, the better. Every time you put three or four spices in a meal you have just upgraded your food. You have made it a superfood.

SS: How much is enough? I mean, how much turmeric could you put on your eggs to make it mean something?

EB: Well, I certainly have patients who average a teaspoon of cinnamon in yogurt. When you make a chicken soup you can put a lot of sage in it. You can cook with raw basil; many of my patients make their eggs in the morning with basil instead of spinach. Right now you can buy twenty spices in the raw at Whole Foods and cook with them. I tell people to go out and buy $50 worth of spices and $50 worth of herbal teas. There are over four thousand flavonoids that have been discovered in teas that are all anti-inflammatory.

SS: So you put pesto on your omelet and you've done something not only tasty but also good for yourself—it's kind of like eating delicious medicine. What foods have these nutritional values?

EB: Here's your basic rule of aging: You burn up, you dry up, you swell up, and you turn to stone, so calcium comes out of your bones. With age comes inflammation, but there are anti-inflammatories all over the place: oranges, carrots, nutrients, teas. I have my patients drinking four or five cups of herbal tea a day. I ask them to aim for a goal of consuming fifteen to twenty spices a day. Green tea is a cornerstone, but so is turmeric, or cumin, all the spices, they're all good. This is a breakthrough in dieting.

SS: That's exciting. Essentially you are turning good food into delicious medicine. I love cooking with herbs and spices, especially turmeric. I make a roast chicken with olive oil and ground turmeric rubbed all over it. Absolutely delicious. What about chemicals? Is that at the top of the list as far as what to eliminate?

EB: Yes, chemicals are killing people. I tell my patients to buy fresh fruits and vegetables, get whole grains, spices, and buy organic protein.

SS: I've heard that a doctor is taught to determine what is going on with a patient through observation in the first five minutes of an office visit. Can you tell just by looking at people?

EB: Well, I'm not Superman with X-ray vision, but I'm pretty good at picking out problems. There are a lot of tips; people with a bad waistline and those who are fat or are getting fat, and then you know they are also getting heart disease. We know that people with ear creases have a lot more heart disease; bald men have a lot more prostate problems. Blond women with blue eyes tend to get hunchbacks more often, as well as osteoporosis.

SS: Hmm . . . you've piqued my interest . . . what would you tell a blue-eyed, blond-haired woman to do?

EB: Get an osteoporosis check at twenty-five. Women do it automatically with their vaginas with yearly checkups; doctors are trained to focus on the vagina and breasts. But those are not the only organs that need preventative medicine. Early detection is key. Women have a lot of osteoporosis and that feeds depression. In New York, the typical East Side woman misses (regarding early detection) her hormones, misses her osteoporosis, ends up with a sleep disorder, mood disorder, ends up in the hands of a shrink, divorced, and ineffective as a parent when she gets older. That's America . . . spending galore on Gucci and placenta creams and face-lifts.

SS: So you're saying mixed-up priorities. What did birth control pills do to us?

EB: Well, they raised sex hormone–binding globulin, created a lot of emotionality in women, a lot of depression and anxiety, blood clots, heart disease, and liability. Women kind of came out the loser.

SS: I love what you call "internal plastic surgery." Please explain what that means.

EB: We scan people and then rank each body part.

SS: Geez, that sounds like the way it used to be with the boys in high school!

EB: This is the impression you gave to me when I saw you speak at the ACAM conference in Las Vegas. Your mind is young, and so is your face and your whole creativity is fantastic. You would "rank" as a thirty-year-old woman externally. But in my office we would scan you internally with PET scans and ultrasound, and then we may find that you've got gallstones or kidney stones or cysts or lumps or bumps and whatever those things are that are going to hurt you later on. We find the problems now so we can treat them before they become a problem.

SS: Proactive medicine.

EB: Yes, we would want to reconfigure your program to treat your oldest part. No one today should be surprised by any disease. In the future, there will be no need for tragic situations like the premature deaths of Tim Russert, Peter Jennings, John Ritter, or Dana Reeves (Christopher Reeves's wife). There will be no more Jim Fixx, no more aneurysms, and no more people who make $10 million a year and are dying because they didn't have a $500 ultrasound. It's ridiculous. When I watched Senator Tim Johnson from South Dakota coming home from the hospital, recovering from his brain aneurysm, and he was slurring his speech, I thought to myself . . . so unnecessary. Why doesn't everyone have transcranial ultrasounds as we do in my office as part of our physical? In doing so, I find these aneurysms all the time. Why aren't these being done routinely?

SS: I'm sure the answer is insurance . . . which I am beginning to believe doesn't really give us any insurance on *health*; rather, we get insurance on *disease*. Insurance will pay for us when we are sick, but will not pay to prevent us from getting sick, which doesn't make sense. It's a plan without vision. We have all these incredible preventive tests, but not everyone has the luxury to afford them . . . or the good sense.

EB: I see it all the time. I have patients who spend a hundred grand on designer watches, but don't want to spend anything on health care. This is the individual's mistake. The government cannot possibly cover discretionary health care.

SS: So this is money you just have to put aside.

EB: Are we so afraid of death that we choose not to see it coming? The only time we watch death is on TV, but we're so afraid to know what's going on inside of us, we'd rather die than know the truth.

SS: I believe the way we are practicing traditional medicine in this country is a direct route to the nursing home.

EB: There's no question. There's a lot of dementia and frailty and all of that is preventable today. We have parathyroid injections and growth hormones. We have so much available that is preventative. I believe you can end human frailty, meaning the person who is shriveled up, shrunken, dried out, and skinny. You've seen it, the completely demented soul.

SS: When you say parathyroid injections and growth hormones, do you mean replacing all the low or missing hormones to reverse the inevitable ravages of aging? And, do you use real bioidentical hormones?

EB: Yes. For instance, Forteo (a bioidentical parathyroid injection) and growth hormones are key to the frame. Forteo gives you bone strength and growth hormone gives you muscle strength, and human frailty is dependent on muscle more than human bone. All the hormones are important.

SS: Why is zinc so important?

EB: Because it cleans out your body. There are a hundred different enzymes in the body that use zinc. It's a very prevalent trace mineral.

SS: How do you decode the aging process?

EB: Section by section. The same way people decode anything in their lives: you know, the way they do the gutters, or the floors, or the kitchen. Instead I decode the brain and I keep decoding and segmenting it . . . the brain, mind, muscle, bone, immune system. I deal with each one and I rank order and then we have genetic coding.

We all hope and pray genomics and stem cells march on, and I believe eventually they will, but even then, let's say the life span is 200, people will still be getting breast cancer at age 103 and dying and it will be considered premature. I know it sounds crazy, but that's the future. If we adopt my method of catching disease before it manifests, we have a real opportunity to live and die healthy.

SS: That is certainly a noble goal. That's my goal . . . to die healthy at whatever age.

EB: If people are educated, we can save them. Everyone has got to understand that they have to have their brain checked. The brain is the most important organ of human beings. You *are* only as young as your oldest part. We have great healing uses for all the different body parts using the East-West Paradigm. You need to scan and find out what's old before it finds you . . . because it'll find you, and then it will kill you.

SS: Besides scanning and taking advantage of that technology, what else can we do to keep our brains young?

EB: You have to understand that the main chemicals in the brain are the dopamines for energy and the acetylcholines to keep the brain well fed with good blood, a good oxygen supply, GABA for relaxation, and serotonin, which is serenity, which I call the Zen zone, nirvana. And, of course, you need a healthy body.

These are the four major components for the healthy brain; we want to be intense but calm; we want to be aware but happy. Good health requires that for any given body function, all four neurotransmitters must be processed in a specific order and in precise amounts. Small electrical imbalances turn into bigger health problems. The slightest deviation in the brain's activity can be felt in the body, and small electrical imbalances can become amplified into bigger health problems. If your brain chemistry becomes imbalanced, your brain will be unable to process electrical cues correctly, which will lead to one or more of the neurotransmitters becoming deficient.

SS: What would be the effect of that?

EB: These deficiencies will lead directly to decreased physical and mental health. Research scientists are always looking to understand why the body fails. As a doctor, I'm looking first to heal, then to prevent illness, and ultimately to create abundant health over a long life span. Biochemical deficiencies in the brain lead to poor health. But a balanced brain maintains good health and is essential to maintaining a sound mind and body over the long haul. If you enhance your brain chemistry you can reach new personal heights, a state of physical and emotional bliss where you can achieve the balance of a peaceful mind, a power zone in your body, and a spiritual pinnacle for your soul.

SS: In other words, a balanced brain produces sharpness.

EB: Yes, not only that, but a balanced brain enables us to love others, remain calm, and effectively put our intelligence to its best possible use.

SS: Most women experience memory problems once they are in menopause. It happens to men also, but it seems to happen faster to women. It's extremely stressful and a vulnerable time.

EB: Yes, and they should take it seriously. One measure for memory and attention is the speed at which the brain processes information. This is influenced by all four neurotransmitters, but especially *acetylcholine*. A normal brain processes a thought at the speed of roughly one-third of a second. Each of the four primary neurotransmitters has a characteristic hormone associated with it. When a particular biochemical becomes deficient, this hormone comes in to take its place. For example, the body naturally increases production of *cortisol* when there is a dopamine imbalance. Cortisol is the backup adrenaline hormone, so when you are under stress, your cortisol levels increase. Your pulse quickens, you become red-faced, and your blood pressure goes up.

SS: So, when a woman is having memory problems in menopause, she has to determine which of the four major components are deficient?

EB: Right. In my book *The Edge Effect*, you can take a test to determine which of the four components is your type. But acetylcholine deficiency can cause conditions such as memory lapses, trouble walking, and lethargy.

SS: Isn't there an estrogen connection to the brain?

EB: Yes, estrogen raises acetylcholine and dopamine. That's another reason why women have such poor attention in menopause.

SS: What do you see as the effects of the chemicals we are all living with either knowingly or unknowingly?

EB: Just terrible. The average American has four plastics, six pesticides, and nine heavy metals in their blood, and we've got a demon called industry. As a country we need an internal baptism. Chelation is one technique to detoxify, zinc is another, and there are many other techniques of detoxifying. All modern scientists know that the cancer epidemic is fed by the toxic chemicals in society.

SS: Personally, to combat the environment, I take intravenous treatments of vitamin C, glutathione, chelation. I'll do hydrogen peroxide, ultraviolet light, and several others . . . not all the time but whenever it is necessary. I believe in building up to combat the environment. But it's a pretty hard sell to the average consumer, right?

EB: Yes. But if you see from your lab work that you need to detoxify, then you need to do intravenous treatments, or you can use zinc or selenium, which gets rid of a lot of heavy metals. Antioxidants get rid of many organic chemicals. I find that the average American is willing to take three or four vitamins to detoxify, and most adults realize the importance of antioxidants to deal with the assault.

SS: Have you ever experienced someone who had bone loss who rebuilt bone with bioidentical hormones?

EB: Yes, I have reversed twenty years of bone loss with Forteo, growth hormone, and vitamin D on a regular basis. We can reverse all the pauses.

SS: So you're saying no one is hopeless?

EB: Well, if you're dead more than three years you shouldn't come to my office [laughs].

SS: I guess that would be too late.

EB: This is what is so exciting. The antiaging miracle can take today's middle-aged American and expand his middle age by fifteen to twenty years; for example, eighty will be sixty-five, fifty-five will be forty. You, Suzanne, are a living example of that. You may be sixty chronologically, but your sixty is really thirty. You are living the middle-age breakthrough.

It's much more difficult to achieve with an eighty-year-old. I have patients who bring in their eighty-five-year-old grandmothers and want me to give her growth hormones. Unfortunately, her tissues are not that responsive anymore.

This is not where the power of this medicine is. I mean, it's good, and it shouldn't be neglected. It will help. But the power of this protocol right now is to the economy, the country, and to people in general to give them fifteen to twenty more *productive* years. It's ridiculous that women are pushed out of the workforce at age sixty as a general rule because of menopause. Menopause is like a boulder dropped in a lake in which wave after wave keeps hitting you. Then the woman lying on the shore asks, "God, where are these waves coming from?" They don't get that it's correctable, and that is why women in general are doing so badly from middle age on.

SS: With all due respect, there's another component to the misery of middle-aged women, and men for that matter. I think it's the doctors who don't get it. Most doctors have been caught unprepared. It's a real tragedy for women. We have been left adrift with little choice but to choose drugs to control this passage, this condition, leaving us a shell of our former selves, fat, and lethargic on sleeping pills and antidepressants. It's a cruel passage, and yet you and I know there is a simple solution: replacing the lost hormones with bioidentical hormones.

EB: A woman came to me, sixty years old, her vagina was as dry as the Sahara, her skin was dry, her memory and attention were impaired, her hair was falling out, and she kept insisting she was past menopause, that it was ten years ago. I couldn't reach her. She kept saying, "No, my ovaries are dead and they've been dead for ten years." She was miserable. The problem is that it doesn't get better. It doesn't level out; the impact of it gets worse and worse. Women don't seem to understand that they don't have to feel like this.

SS: I do find with the seventy-year-olds and older that they think they are past menopause. It's hard to convince them that hormone loss never stops; that it keeps draining out until you are left like a pile of Jell-O on the floor.

EB: Suzanne, you've got to understand that you are writing for the next generation of forty-year-old women.

SS: Forty-year-olds do want to jump on this fast-moving train, but I don't give up on the older women. They need this so badly. I keep trying to make them understand that without replacing lost hormones they are likely (most likely) to end up in a nursing home.

EB: Even the forty-year-olds are slow to get it. You know, a clock should go off: thirty-five, get ready. Get yourself together. Balance your hormones, fix your bone density. Don't get sold by the miracle creams. It's not about this branding superficiality. They need to be told, "Get into you as a person."

There's a beautiful article in *Science News*, "Aging as the Cause of Cancer," not hormone decline. Even *Science News* doesn't get it. I mean, seeing that hormones decline with age and that's when we get our cancers, the whole hypothesis becomes null.

SS: Tell me for this book, for the sake of my readers, do you think lack of hormones causes cancer?

EB: There's no question. It's obvious; most of the cancers begin when we are in hormonal decline. It's the hormonal loss and the genetic change they create that cause cancer, and this has been well documented in many studies. That's why we should be treating hormonal decline in the thirties, forties, and fifties.

SS: Tell my readers why they shouldn't take synthetic hormones.

EB: They should only take bioidentical hormones because the body recognizes them. They are bioidentical . . . biologically identical to the human hormone. We've had trouble with every existing synthetic hormone. Bioidenticals work and make my patients feel good again.

SS: Everyone I talk to has GI problems: IBS, carb addiction, acid reflux, bloating, and more. What triggers trouble in the gut? Why are everyone's guts so screwed up?

EB: Because our brains are imbalanced.

SS: Back to the brain again.

EB: Yes, the brain and the gut connection. Remember the four components, the four types of personalities; when any of these individual types becomes imbalanced, there is a reaction.

So IBS is anxiety, and serotonin is used to calm and treat it. Then there's the dopamine type. You get a lot of dopamine when your brain is running on too much energy, and it drives your acid high; caffeine drives your acid high, as does sugar. A lot of people have trouble with constipation and that's an acetylcholine imbalance. Sphincters wear out with age, just like your esophagus can wear out and be a little too wide open so you get acid reflux. There is anatomical wear and tear, just like when a knee wears out. Then there are the GABA types who are often plagued by irritable bowel syndrome. So it's important to find out your type and treat the deficiency.

SS: How do you do that?

EB: Take my AgePrint test. It's in both of my books, *The Edge Effect* and *Younger You*. You can treat irritable bowel with serotonin agents, and you can cut your acid by becoming calmer. You can improve your GI tract through sleep, more enzymes, fruits, vegetables, becoming aware of your food intolerances, and getting desensitized to certain foods.

SS: I think a lot of the obesity comes from chemicals and food intolerances. What do you think?

EB: I tend to view things from a brain perspective. Obesity is a disorder in a society that has brains damaged from watching murders on TV, and by being bombarded by chemicals, salt, sugar, and junk food. We are a society that has lost its taste for spices, herbs, and vegetables, and in doing so we have continuing damage to the brain. Once people get into carbs and salt, there's no stopping them. It's like alcohol addiction. I recently worked on a panel for a conference of the National Institute on Drug Abuse where it was concluded that obesity should be classified as a brain chemical disorder.

Obesity is a neuropsychiatric disorder where a person gets addicted and food intolerant because of a brain chemical disorder, which then triggers the wrong choices, and then the wrong choices trigger a whole cycle of intolerance, allergy, and illness.

SS: So when you get the brain back in balance . . .

EB: Everyone's brain chemistry is in imbalance when they are eating wrong; anxiety, depression or the blues, salt cravings, sugar cravings, carb cravings, fat cravings, and want of portion control are the results. Each one of those cravings correlates to brain imbalance—dopamine being sugar cravings, acetylcholine being fat cravings, GABA being protein cravings and portion control, you know, loss of boundaries, and serotonin is salt cravings. These cravings come from brain chemical imbalances, and they become addictive and compulsive. People know they shouldn't be doing it, but they're still bingeing on popcorn at midnight and buying hot dogs on the street and eating at restaurants that in New York charge $150 for a dinner that is nothing more than salt and fat. That's addiction.

Then there's the spice/tea component. Tea chemicals cut the appetite and a host of spice chemicals cut appetite by giving you antioxidant nutrient density.

The third component that's missed is that obese people have medical illnesses that are usually undiagnosed such as hormonal imbalances—which you know about, Suzanne—liver disease, gallbladder disease, lung disease, immune disease, thyroid disease, and more. When you are that sick, even if it is undiagnosed, there's no way to successfully diet.

The number one enemy in America right now is obesity. Fifty percent of the population is overweight. We have a catastrophe in this country.

SS: How do you feel about diet soda?

EB: How do you feel about urine?

SS: [Laughter]

EB: I mean, we try to stay away from drinking it, don't we? We have to break the addiction. We are able to do it with nicotine. A lot of people smoke, but we are able to break the addiction with the same chemicals that nicotine hits: acetylcholine and dopamine. With that we are able to kill people's appetite for junk food and that includes diet soda.

SS: For the readers' sake (and mine), explain the pathways.

EB: Well, there are dopamine circuits in the brain that we've identified. There are studies that show that a dopamine gene controls what we call reward circuits. I mean, how come people are puffing cigarettes and downing salty, greasy garbage and being satisfied by it? What triggers the reward in their brain?

SS: Because we have gotten used to this taste, that we've developed a taste for chemicals, that we've developed a craving for cigarettes because it makes most people feel better? I think what we have to ask is why are people needing to satisfy themselves, what is missing in their lives? What are we medicating? Is it stress?

EB: Well, it becomes an irresistible drug . . . the same way men chase women at eighteen. This is enhanced reward. It's called impaired inhibitory control, so people are no longer able to inhibit in the prefrontal cortex of the brain, they can't inhibit the food intake once they start. All of a sudden it feels good, like a heroin addict. Areas of the brain are triggered: the hypothalamus, a section of the brain called the nucleus, and another section in the ventral part called the parietal lobe.

SS: What does this do?

EB: These sections of the brain get conditioned to the stuff that is raising the pressure. I mean, why are people eating things that are destroying the liver, fattening the liver, setting them up for cancer? These things clog the brain, and then the dorsal stratum of the brain triggers these people to feel that it's actually doing good. They want more.

SS: Can hormones be addictive?

EB: Yes, they change brain chemistry in a way that a person may want more than is good for them. For instance, I have seen men take too much testosterone and growth hormone because they think big is better.

SS: I think the only time a woman would take too much human growth hormone is if she thought it would make her thinner.

EB: But, of course, it usually doesn't. Too much GH in a woman causes bloating if they are not on the correct amounts of estrogen. There has to be the correct ratio in all hormone replacement.

SS: I always say not too much, not too little . . . has to be just right.

What do you think about chemotherapy and radiation? Do you think they have a place?

EB: Yes, but one has to choose carefully. I've had Hodgkin's lymphoma patients who have lived a long time, and breast cancer patients who have lived a long time. My strength is knowing we need to find cancer early. That's what we do in my office. Find it before it's a problem. The colon, the anus, the prostate, the breasts, and the vagina are not the only five organs to get cancer. To focus only on those five parts for early detection is scandalous.

SS: You said earlier you treat the brain, the mind, hormones, really the entire body, and focus on the treatment of all chronic degenerative neuropsychiatric or neurodegenerative diseases, excluding end-stage cancer and surgery. So, if a cancer patient came to you, would you send him to another doctor?

EB: With cancer you have a spreading, infectious, often terminal, illness. That's a whole other field. But we can provide them with the brain component. Cancer patients don't sleep very well and we get them sleeping seven to eight hours a night. We help them get rid of their depression; we help them with their anxiety. We give them nutrients, intravenous drips to build them up, to strengthen them. We also send them to alternative cancer doctors.

SS: Why is fibromyalgia so prevalent?

EB: Because people want to avoid the scandalous viewpoint that they have depression. They won't treat it, so they live with a whole body that aches to hell until they are willing to accept that they have a chemical depression. Most people view psychiatry from a perspective of guilt.

SS: That's interesting; so you're saying fibromyalgia is an emotional disease. Of course, a lot of emotional diseases are due to hormonal loss, so the depression that relates to, say, estrogen loss could contribute to the depression that leads to fibromyalgia, right?

EB: Well, I'm talking about the brain connection. Fibromyalgia is a brain chemical imbalance that responds to serotonin. We work with patients who come in having been in bed for seven years with fibromyalgia and chronic fatigue; now they are living like they were never ill.

You see, the brain is the most important organ. We use medications, nutrients, and, yes, hormones to change a person's memory, attention, and brain well-being. But sometimes fibromyalgia is actually due to cancer. It's called Lamberg-Eaton syndrome, where you get muscle aches and fatigue, and there are other cancer syndromes that will give you chronic fatigue. The hormonal component is important to every patient, and chronic disease responds to BHRT and gives the patient a sense of well-being and energy.

SS: When is an antidepressant necessary?

EB: Sometimes I have patients who are so severely depressed only Adderall will bail them out. But in a perfect world, it would be my hope that these patients would get to me sooner, so I wouldn't have to resort to such strong drugs. There is a role for strong drugs. There is a role for morphine. I'd rather go home and die on morphine than spend $200,000 in a hospital dying.

It's crazy, we have children down the block here in New York City who can't afford vaccines or vegetables, and we spend these ridiculous amounts of money on dying. Our priorities are skewed. . . . America's child knows more about Viagra than vegetables, and the average American adult will buy Viagra sooner than he buys vegetables. We have a society that has a value-structure problem. We need to reconstruct health care. We have to tackle faith, mistrained doctors, the environment, the role of the pharmaceutical industry, the failure of education, the addiction industry's role, the lifestyle role, the hospital's role, the food industry's role, the insurance industry's role, and the clergy's failure to make an impact on anyone.

SS: You'll get no argument here. What do you tell your patients about sleep?

EB: The average American is stressed out, so they start running on their own high cortisol. You can tell by looking at the typical New Yorkers who take the subway every morning, with their swollen red faces. I tell my patients they have to have a minimum of seven hours of sleep every night if they want to be well. That is the best way to lower cortisol and then everything starts working better.

SS: What do you see for the future?

EB: *The future of medicine will be a new society. We will all live in new nontoxic homes in a new culture. The future doctor will make the brain and the mind and our emotional well-being number one. Doctors will have a new mind-set. The reason they are not doing hormones correctly and the reason they are not implementing new ideas is that they are not finding and do not know how to find disease soon enough! The present physical exam is useless to the patient. All the new imaging techniques need to be put into a modern physical exam, a kind of "Star Trek Physical." So it's a new home, a new culture, a new brain, a new hormonal-based medicine.*

It's all missed now. A patient has twenty signs of aging and they treat that with a Band-Aid. What you are touching with your Ageless movement, Suzanne, is the failure of the physician to recognize that all diseases are in the context of aging.

SS: Thank you, it's my privilege. I'm just a messenger; it's doctors like you who are leading the way. What drives you?

EB: I'm driven by wanting to see the world reach a new era, a new age of longevity, a golden age for human beings and God. I get driven a lot by a vision of what the world can be and how my family can share in those benefits when all of us are living longer, better, safer, healthier, more loving, caring, moral lives connected to a higher power spiritually. That's what keeps me going.

DR. ERIC BRAVERMAN'S
BREAKTHROUGH BREAKOUTS

- Adding an average of three spices per meal can transform your foods into superfoods. Spices improve the density of nutritional foods. It will be like eating delicious medicine. Natural substances in spices and teas also cut your appetite.

- Practice proactive medicine by finding potential health issues before they become problems. Get PET scans, ultrasounds, and (for women) an osteoporosis check at twenty-five. Take advantage of the technology.

- Forteo, growth hormone, and vitamin D taken on a regular basis can reverse bone loss.

- Treating hormonal decline in our thirties, forties, and fifties with bioidentical hormones can reduce the risk of cancer.

- Sleep seven hours a night to lower your cortisol levels, which will reduce stress and make the body run better.

- The brain ages just like the rest of the body. Finding your brain type, and then testing to see if there are deficiencies, can circumvent many diseases and give you a better quality of life.

16

DR. STEVE NELSON

A low sex drive is an indicator that a person is sick.
  –Dr. Steve Nelson

ONE EVENING I was watching TV and Dr. Steve Nelson was being interviewed. He was discussing new cutting-edge treatments and said to the interviewer, "Aren't you tired of giving in to modern medicine's 'drug for every ailment' approach?" He was focused on prevention and natural cures, and I realized I wanted to get to know more about him.

Dr. Nelson is a vibrant and exciting healer. His focus is on wellness. He is the founder and director of the Synergy Wellness Clinic in Palm Desert, California. Every Wednesday night at 7:00 Pacific Time he offers a telephone conference call free of charge, where he will answer your questions. The number is 616-712-8000, and the passcode is 890255#. Enjoy. He is not only full of information but also a lot of fun.

SS: Good evening, and thank you for spending this time with me. Explain the Synergy Wellness Clinic that you founded, and what is unique about what you are doing?

SN: At our center we have adapted to the problems of today's world. We recognize there is an environmental assault, we know the toxicity of today's world is affecting people, and we work with this understanding, knowing that pollution and toxicity are making people sick. We build up the body to counteract the onslaught of environmental poison. We detoxify the body and we use unique new testing like hair samples to analyze deep toxicity within the DNA, and we also work with cell renewal.

SS: What do you mean by deep toxicity and cell renewal?

SN: Hair samples are very accurate and can show toxicities that people carry over their lifetime in the DNA of their hair . . . deep toxicity.

I'll give you an example. A forty-year-old patient of mine in Whitby, Ontario, Canada, who had been on insulin since she was twenty-eight, was labeled a juvenile diabetic. I knew that couldn't be true because juvenile diabetes is diagnosed between the ages of eight and twelve, but she persisted to have sugar problems and was spilling ketones into her urine. But her blood sugar wasn't elevated nor was it that low. So this is not a true diabetic.

We took a hair sample; we ran the scan and found that she had a subacute virus in her liver, but the primary problem was that she had been poisoned by paraquat and DDT. We started detoxifying her with nutritional IVs, gave her homeopathic drops, and today she no longer needs to be on insulin.

SS: She is lucky. . . . She was misdiagnosed, then she was put on the wrong medications, and as a result the problem continued to degenerate. Had she not found your kind of medicine, she would still be getting progressively worse because they were treating a disease she did not have. This must be happening all the time.

SN: We are encountering strange conditions never before seen, a lot of neurotransmitter disorders, sleep disorder; either people can't go to sleep or they can't stay asleep. A lot of fear reactions, rage reactions, what we call discongruent neurotransmitters; either too much serotonin or too much dopamine, but we are able to order neurotransmitter panels for that and find the problem. Chemicals can cause anything because they affect all the nerve pathways.

SS: Are the chemicals coming from plasticizers and plastic bottles?

SN: There is a fallacy about bottled water and plastic bottles. If people are going to buy water they need to buy it in glass bottles.

SS: I would think especially in the desert where the plastic bottles sit around in the car in that intense heat.

SN: Yes. You get what they call a direct petrochemical evaporation coefficient from plastic bottles. In other words, you get higher evaporation of the petrochemical in the water at higher temperatures. My recommendation is you keep a cooler in your car with a little ice in it. Newer cars actually have bottle coolers.

SS: Women e-mail me almost every day about their inability to sleep. It's about hormonal loss and high cortisol, right?

SN: Yes, to an extent. . . . You have to detoxify and replace hormones simultaneously to get the maximum benefit. We also give people 7-keto

DHEA, which is manufactured by Biotics Research, which does not get shunted to cortisol (which would prevent sleep) by the adrenal cortex, the medulla, or the liver. You never want to shunt cortisol or you will have defeated the purpose. DHEA is very central to antiaging, as is balancing all the hormones, but you also have to detoxify.

SS: What is the procedure at your clinic?

SN: We take a history, but it will be a unique approach. I want to know where you've traveled, toxic exposures, medications you've been taking, particularly antibiotics within the last year. I ask about your dental history, I talk about dental meridians, shocked teeth, amalgam fillings. I ask about radiation exposure they might have had (everybody is exposed to radiation every day). I ask about sex drive, because it is a known fact that people with low sex drives are sick. If you are hormonally balanced and detoxified your sex drive should be at least an 8 out of 10.

SS: I had not thought about lack of libido as an indicator of poor health, but of course it would signal that all is not well.

SN: When I see patients I want to know about their energy levels at different times of the day. You want your adrenal cortex levels highest in the morning and lowest at 10:00 at night; if not, we have an adrenal/cortisol problem.

I ask my patients if they've ever remembered being food-poisoned. I ask about their bowel habits. You should be having a bowel movement twice a day if you are eating properly.

Then I do muscle testing, thyroid testing, figuring out deep frequencies and shallow frequencies. We'll get blood chemistry if their budget allows it, and then we offer to do a neurotransmitter panel to see what is going on in the brain.

SS: That's a wide variety of treatments. . . . I would be excited as a patient to encounter this kind of new, cutting-edge health care.

SN: I'm excited, too. Lymphatics are another area, and we treat with energy units, called SR attenuates. We can eliminate a lymphatic blockage on someone in about ten minutes.

We deal with headaches, gallstones, kidney stones, and we give medicinal mudpacks to patients to take home to reinitiate energy where they had surgeries and scar areas, like C-sections and episiotomies.

SS: What could dental history tell you?

SN: First of all, each tooth in the mouth corresponds to an organ system, so dental history will tell me a lot, especially if you have had a lot of fillings and they have pulled them out. Amalgam leakage is one thing and mercury is dangerous, but we are finding other metals affecting these meridians: palladium, beryllium, and a lot of other metals used in alloys. Just because you have a crown doesn't mean that tooth is healthy. The other problem is if a tooth is cracked, it will cause problems with the meridian related to it. For instance, if it were a first or second molar, these are correlated with heart meridians.

I've had patients with cardiac issues and once these teeth are fixed, the cardiac issue goes away. The other thing is malocclusion, as in not balancing the bite. If the bite isn't balanced that patient is going to be sick; they will have TMJ problems, headaches, visual trouble. In fact, I have a patient right now who was losing her hearing in her right ear, and it turns out that the tooth right below her right ear was decayed. We got her tooth fixed and now her hearing is coming back.

SS: Why is it still legal to use mercury and amalgam fillings?

SN: Good question. I can tell you this: If you lived in Germany or France and your dentist were to put any form of mercury in your mouth, you could report him and it would be immediate loss of license. We're just not that conscious here.

SS: Well, also amalgam is easy to handle and it's cheap.

SN: You don't have to be a great technician to use it: You press it in, scrape it off, press down, and you're done.

SS: I never realized the connection between dental and body health. You tend to think of body parts as individual, as in on their own, but as with the hormonal system it's all interconnected, so of course the teeth are a part of the "dance."

Let's talk about the effects of radiation.

SN: Where do I start? . . . Inflammation, dehydration, and practically every symptom you can think of: nervousness, depression, dry skin, lack of appetite, constipation, diarrhea, just for starters.

SS: Why are they still using radiation?

SN: [Laughs]

SS: I get it, business.

SN: And the system we're in. There are other methods of achieving the same results without the trauma to the body: ultrasounds, thermography.

SS: What about MRIs?

SN: They have their place, but MRI sets up an electrical field. It's no different than having a cell phone to your ear all the time. It has a drying effect on the system and dries out the cells.

SS: And of course hydration is what cells need, so dehydration works against cell replication. If a person used ultrasound and thermogram and it's very clear there is a tumor, say, in a woman's breast, what would you recommend?

SN: Our first recommendation is to do the Asyra scan so we can find out where the deep toxicities are located. (To find out more go to Asyra.com.) Then we look at the deep functionalities and take a very good look at hormone levels, because I have *never* seen a woman with a female cancer who does not have high estrogen. Not one.

SS: What about diet?

SN: Absolutely. We would start cutting out junk food in the diet and usually eliminate dairy, wheat, soy, pork, and corn; those are enemies to everybody. We would follow this individual, and if it became an invasive ductal cell then, of course, there has to be some surgery. But if the woman does not desire surgery we have other approaches: high doses of digestive enzymes, eliminating coffee and stimulants. We use iodine topically. Iodine is a nutrient. It's antiviral, antiparasitic, antifungal, and we have these women rub it right on the breast three or four times a day—that way it gets right into the skin. Then we would use mudpacks to start drawing toxins out. Another thing I have noticed is that all these women have yeast. And excessive yeast is a huge issue; there is now a surgeon in Italy (Simancini) who has been able to place a catheter directly into a tumor, infuse high doses of sodium bicarbonate in it, and shrink it.

SS: Are we doing this in our country?

SN: Unfortunately, hospitals in this country will not let doctors place catheters in some tumors, so if I had a patient who found this treatment desirable I would send her to Italy.

SS: Why can't a doctor in this country treat cancer creatively such as with this method? Why is the only method—standard of care—surgery, radiation, chemotherapy, and after-care drugs? What is this about?

SN: Politics. If a doctor is going to put a catheter in, why not put in a drug? It's frustrating, and it is so simple to infuse bicarb. I put any woman who has cancer on a teaspoon of bicarb twice a day.

SS: You're excited by your work, aren't you?

SN: It brings tears to my eyes. You have no idea how many people we are helping. All I can say is why aren't we thinking preventatively instead of getting our foot stuck in a bucket? Why aren't we thinking about prevention? Why are we not bombarding the country with good information about nutrition and detoxification and therapies to build up people's bodies? Why? Because these nondrug therapies cannot make money for the drug companies and they have such a stronghold.

So you don't discount anything that is going on in a person's life; if they are in a negative relationship, something has to be done because it will make them sick. If they are contributing to a negative relationship it needs to be addressed. When people come to our clinic we advise them that the mind-body connection is important. Happiness is important. People today aren't happy, and it has to do with the pace of society, and environmental toxins are evoking this. Research tells us that 70 percent of kids in this country are ADD by the time they are six years old. Now that is an epidemic and it's not being addressed.

SS: What is the cause of this?

SN: Toxicity, but not only that. Their mothers were toxic when they were carrying them. There's nothing in food anymore. Food is now nothing more than plastic for people's mouth entertainment. If people don't supplement and apply homeopathic therapies and pay attention to their bodies, they are going to continue to get sick.

SS: Let's talk about the lymph system, which I believe is not only misunderstood but, frankly, not understood at all.

SN: You've got that right. It's 100 percent of your body. There are millions and millions of miles of lymphs. Without keeping that lymph clean and moving, you will be forever sick. Lymph is made of salt water, and if you don't consume at least a teaspoon of sea salt every day and drink enough water, your lymphs are going to jam up. If you don't exercise (for example, walk a half a mile a day), your lymph system will get clogged. The lymph system is paramount to your health.

SS: From my understanding we do not have a natural pump in our bodies for the lymph system. For instance, the blood pumps through our bodies without our even thinking about it, but the lymph cannot move unless we move.

SN: You are right. Movement (as in exercise) and water plus sea salt are the only ways to keep the lymph system healthy. People say to me, "Well, I drink iced tea, that has water in it," or "I drink beer, that has water in it." Water is water. If you drink a cup of coffee, you have to counteract that with that much water. If the average male is 180 pounds, he needs to drink 90 ounces of water each day. You take your weight, divide it in half, and drink that in ounces, and then consume one teaspoon of sea salt every day. You are made of salt water. You are 70 percent sea water, and if you don't replace it you will shrivel up. How many women do you see walking around with wrinkled skin? They're not drinking water.

SS: But we go to the doctor and we are told to stop eating salt.

SN: *Doctors equate salt with sodium chloride, which is table salt. But sea salt is 97 percent minerals. There is very little sodium in sea salt. I have actually lowered patients' blood pressure with sea salt and water.*

SS: This is fantastic news. I have always preferred sea salt to table salt. I use Celtic sea salt or Himalayan pink sea salt.

SN: When a physician puts a patient on a salt-restricted diet, what they mean is a sodium-restricted diet. With sea salt, we're not giving them sodium, we are giving them minerals, necessary minerals.

Table salt is very dangerous. It's high in sodium, has very little potassium, and the anticaking agent in table salt is aluminum. We do not need to add aluminum to our systems. Celtic sea salt and pink salt are the best, just like you are using.

SS: And the best-tasting. I'm a cook, so salt is very important, and sea salt brings food to another level. I am so glad to know it is good for me.

SN: The average person doesn't know this and it's very important to get this information out.

SS: Back to the lymphs—how do you break up a blockage?

SN: There is an instrument called an SRT unit, and only one hundred of us have them in this country. It was designed by Dr. William Tiller at Stanford, a genius in energy dynamics. It takes the frequency of the cell and renormalizes it. When the cell wall gets normal frequency it starts to expel the toxins and the lymph starts to move and drain. It's fabulous. We use lymphatic drainage formulas and certain nutrients to get the lymph moving.

SS: I have been plagued with a lymph blockage under my arm from my radiation treatments. There are so many side effects from radiation— I wish the doctor would have been straight with me. He kept saying that radiation is "a walk in the park." I got frightened into radiation by all my doctors at the time, but my side effects were six weeks of incredible nausea; it burned the inside of my upper stomach and left internal scar tissue, caused acid reflux for life, ruined the skin on my chest, and clogged my lymph system. I work with a lymph specialist to unblock, which relieves it, and I also jump on the trampoline for five minutes daily, but your SRT machine sounds rather miraculous. There is also the Ondamed machine, which unclogs the lymphs.

SN: We have had incredible success with ours. People have been amazed with their results.

SS: The sex drive is a big one. It's amazing to realize that people from age thirty-five on are not feeling like having sex. I believe chemicals, toxins, and the overuse of pharmaceutical drugs has a lot to do with it, especially statins. What's your take?

SN: Overuse of drugs is definitely a detriment to libido, particularly drugs like Lipitor or any of the other statins, and we also have to look at the hormonal pathways. Imbalances of hormones are a detriment, then there's prescription medicine, particularly antidepressants, which have to be addressed.

But sex drive is not a simple issue. It's emotional, it's physical, and there is a toxicity component. It could be the makeup they are wearing or the hair color they are using, which could affect the thyroid or the pituitary; or it could be adrenal; or it could be the sex hormones—any of these things could be affecting the neurotransmitter field. So it's a number of things and they all have to be addressed.

I believe in bioidentical hormones, but if you replace the missing hormones and the person is still toxic, you're not going to hit the home run. You might get to second base, but you're not going to get all the way home.

A big factor in sex drive, believe it or not, is fatty acids: We need to have raw oils in our diet. There is a major connection between having sufficient good oils in our diets and the sex drive.

SS: I'm trying to understand. So good oils are crucial to cell reproduction, healthy cells give us our energy, and energy and good health are what drives the sexual part of us?

SN: Yes, it all works together. So, yes, lack of a sex drive is about declining hormones, poor diet, toxicity, prescription drugs (like statins, antidepressants, and sleeping pills) and their side effects; put it all together and you have a recipe for sexual dysfunction, among many other things.

SS: How important is it for men to keep their testosterone levels at optimum?

SN: Optimal levels are important as long as the man is not converting to DHT. If you are overconverting to DHT (dihydrotestosterone) in the presence of any type of prostatic insufficiency, that needs to be examined. DHT is a marker for prostate cancer. The prostate stores DHT. If the DHT is low, you are well and good.

SS: If it is not low, how do you lower it?

SN: We use natural therapies like saw palmetto, selenium, iodine, phosphorus, even rubidium and other trace minerals, and fatty acids.

SS: It seems to me that men start having prostate problems when they decline in testosterone.

SN: You are right. The testosterone levels have to be kept at optimum,

but you have to be sure that the metabolism of testosterone does not produce a lot of DHT.

SS: Right, but what raises the DHT?

SN: The prostate has a metabolism. When you get toxins like petro-
chemicals, parasites, yeast, bacteria, or viruses, all of these things will disrupt the metabolism of DHT whether in the prostate or the liver, and
that will cause the DHT to build up. So there it is again, toxicity is the
culprit.

SS: What do you say to your patients who are diet soda addicts?

SN: Dangerous stuff, toxic and dangerous. There are actually cases of
reported liver damage from diet soda. But how do we replace the urge?
Believe it or not, we have our patients eat dark chocolate and that will
pick up some of the neurotransmitters—the darker the chocolate, the
better. Diet sodas are dangerous, no question about it.

SS: Do all people carry viruses in their bodies?

SN: Yes, viruses, parasites, bacteria in yeast, and they all need to be
detoxified from the body.

SS: How?

SN: If parasites are suspected I put my patients on a twelve- to fifteen-
week parasite program of botanicals; then we reset the digestive fields, test
for pH balance, and then I have to convince my patients to stop putting
garbage in their bodies. Nothing actually kills viruses, we all have them
and will until the day we die, but we can control them with various nutrients like garlic, garlic products, green tea. The Chinese are way ahead of us
in this arena; they consume garlic and green tea every day.

SS: How come everyone is so constipated?

SN: No one is drinking enough water, and then there's a lack of sea
salt and fatty acids, a lack of exercise, and poor diets . . . and there you
have it—constipation! But most people would rather take enormous
amounts of laxatives that only relieve things temporarily than the permanent solution, which is water, sea salt, good oils, and exercise. Do this and
you should have two bowel movements a day.

SS: That sounds heavenly.

SN: It's heavenly if you know what you are doing. You also have to
have fiber to keep the gut running smoothly—fiber supplements are essential (usually they're in powder form), along with eating lots of fruits
and vegetables. Then we must recolonize with probiotics, because we are
all exposed to chemicals and toxic metals: heavy metals like mercury and
aluminum and cadmium, and then there is toxicity from old lead pipes.

We all encounter toxins on a daily basis . . . all these things wipe out the gut flora.

SS: Where is the thyroid in the constipation scenario?

SN: Low thyroid means you are usually constipated, but you may not have a true measure. The thyroid will absorb any toxin to it, and I find a lot of times when I detoxify a patient, they no longer need thyroid replacement. Heavy metals can disrupt the thyroid; viruses can disrupt the thyroid because of malabsorption of the proper amount of amino acids.

SS: Older women complain to me that they are eating less, exercising more, and yet they are *gaining* weight. What's that about?

SN: It could be a thyroid problem—in energy medicine, the thyroid is the backup to the stomach, so I would check the thyroid and also the digestive fields. If you're not digesting your food by producing enough acids, then you are going to gain weight because you are not absorbing the energy force, therefore not breaking it down. When this happens you get a putrefaction mechanism in the bowels, plus undigested foods.

SS: Ewwwww! Do most adults need to supplement the hydrochloric acid in their gut?

SN: About 70 percent of my patients require it. The best form of hydrochloric acid is betaine, because it causes methylation in the stomach, which is what you want. With most adults, they have two things going on: stomach fields that are shut off and a gallbladder that is jammed up, because the gallbladder is backed up by the stomach. If the stomach is not doing its job, the gallbladder tries to take over. If you have nausea, headaches, feeling full all the time, bloating and gas after meals, your gallbladder is probably overworked and damaged.

If your stool is clay colored, there is not enough bile getting into the bowel, which means that your gallbladder is not doing its job. Stools should be mahogany colored. The most common cause of headaches in people is backed-up gallbladders.

SS: It could also be low estrogen.

SN: Yes, low estrogen will cause headaches, but I've found if you get the liver metabolism going properly, the estrogen level will probably come back. Headaches that are right-sided stem from the gallbladder; band headaches that are around the head are usually adrenal in origin, and mean you need to start taking a look at blood sugar levels.

But then you need to ask the patient about head injuries, or surgeries to the head, and even X-rays because all of these things can knock out the energy fields. We treat this with mudpacks on the head every other day for a month, and it will repair the broken chi energy field. Lastly, constipation can cause headaches.

SS: So when a patient complains of headaches, you have to be like a detective . . . eliminating each possibility until you stumble on to the precise reason for the headache.

SN: That is what I do. I peel away and peel away until I find it. It's part of the reason I love this work so much—when we do find the answer, it's very exciting not only for the patient but also for myself.

SS: Do you believe in intravenous treatments?

SN: Absolutely. I give a lot of intravenous nutrients, never intravenous drugs. I give IVs for energy and sex drive, memory, detoxification, vitamin C, glutathione. Some people don't like to take pills, so they come in twice a week and they joke that it's like getting an oil change, but they leave my office feeling great.

SS: Let me be devil's advocate . . . why would we need to supplement with IV treatments? It seems rather extreme.

SN: We supplement with IV treatments because people are not absorbing or digesting or utilizing the nutrients in their food. When you eat you should feel energy. If you don't, there is something wrong, and 80 percent of this is due to the environment, poor diets, and lifestyle habits. Emotional issues are also a factor.

SS: So we're dealing with two worlds here: the pharmaceutical approach that has a drug for every condition and disease, and then the nondrug, "build up" approach that you and the other doctors in this book follow. Are these two worlds ever going to cross over?

SN: That's a very good question. . . . I do think it will merge at one point. The drug companies would like the nutrient companies not to exist, but they are not going away, and there are too many patients starting to cross over to the natural approach. They aren't getting better on the drugs, so they want to try something different.

SS: Hey, the drug companies would like me not to exist!

SN: That's true—you are a high-profile lady, and I'm in your corner— but there is either going to be a merger or there will be a separate set of practitioners, and that is what is evolving right now. At my wellness center we are not only practicing nondrug therapies, but there is also a psychological aspect. You cannot separate the mind from the body; we know this and our approach is about treating the mind, body, and spirit. We get to the root cause whether it's physical, spiritual, or emotional.

It's not simply slapping on a Band-Aid and then forgetting about it. People need to understand that this is a naturopathic program. We teach them that this approach takes some patience, that they didn't get this way overnight, so we can't heal overnight—but in the end we are about healing, not abating. If the patient is willing to hang in there, we can change the quality of their lives and they will get better.

SS: Where do you find the joy in the work you are doing?

SN: I find the joy when I get a call from a patient who tells me how great they are feeling. That's why doctors go into medicine—we get joy from making patients well. I feel joy when I make a child better; I never had any children of my own, so if the child is ADD or ADHD, and as a result of our treatments they start to speak normally and interact with other children normally . . . this is very rewarding. I get joy when I am able to save a man from losing his prostate, and avoiding the prostate drugs that would have changed the quality of his life. I love what I do, and I love being able to restore and repair and help people truly get better.

SS: And we love you for it.

DR. STEVE NELSON'S BREAKTHROUGH BREAKOUTS

- You should be having a bowel movement twice a day if you are eating properly, and stools should be mahogany colored. The permanent solution to constipation is water, sea salt, good oils, and exercise.

- Consume at least a teaspoon of sea salt every day and drink enough water. This combined with exercise will keep your lymph system from clogging up, and the lymph system is paramount to your health. Don't be afraid of sea salt—there is very little sodium, and it is 97 percent minerals. Celtic sea salt and pink salt are the best.

- Natural therapies like saw palmetto, selenium, iodine, phosphorus, even rubidium and other trace minerals, plus fatty acids can lower the amount of DHT stored in a man's prostate. DHT is a marker for prostate cancer.

- Eat dark chocolate in moderation—the darker the better—to help substitute for your addiction to dangerous and toxic diet soda until the cravings subside.

- Fiber keeps the gut running smoothly—fiber supplements are essential (usually they're in powder form), along with eating lots of fruits and vegetables. Hydrochloric acid in the form of betaine helps you digest and break down foods and also helps with acid reflux.

17

STEP 4: CREATE A HEALTHY GI TRACT

Chew your liquids and chew your solids until they are liquid.
  –Dr. Paul C. Bragg

There is no such thing as "junk food," only "junk diets"!
  –Dr. Helen A. Guthrie

SO MANY OF THE DOCTORS in this book talk about having a healthy gut—they know that the path to wellness lies in our GI tract. There is no good day when you don't feel right in your gut.

Brenda Watson, R.N., president and founder of Renew Life Formulas, is a person who understands the journey of food from the first bite all the way to the last stop, the anus. It's quite a journey. Understanding what is involved in order to digest properly helps to have better respect for the GI tract. When all is well, it is a smooth journey, but when things get "off," you can suffer greatly.

In this chapter I'll write about the GI tract, informed greatly by what I learned from Brenda. If you want more information, you can order her video/book program and be wowed by what she has to say. Google Brenda Watson and order her book *The H.O.P.E. Formula* for optimal digestive care.

Initially I never gave my gut a thought. If there were a grade I would have gotten a D. I'm sure most of us are this way. We eat, we go to the bathroom, we eat some more, and the cycle continues. We don't connect what we eat with how we feel.

It all starts with our food, and right now our food supply is out of gas. The food nature gave to each of our cells to allow them to replicate perfectly over and over has been degraded from pollution in the air and soil and by toxic chemicals such as pesticides and herbicides. Food needs to be rethought and understood as an absolute necessity to live this long and healthy life. Food is our life force, food is our health, food is the fuel our bodies need to work efficiently, to replicate healthy cells, and to stay healthy.

Before I truly understood the importance of the digestive system and the part I played in it, I unknowingly abused my GI tract on a continuous basis. I would skip meals, eat too fast, was thoughtless about chemicals, and didn't think too much about getting the right amounts of the right foods on a daily basis. I didn't understand fiber or the importance of vegetables, and sugar was my friend. For every infection I would run to the doctor for an antibiotic, never realizing that by not recolonizing with probiotics and digestive enzymes, I was creating havoc in my gut. Like so many, I would grab a salad and eat it in the car while going through e-mail on my Treo. I would gobble it down, hardly noticing how good it tasted, just shoveling it in. In fact, I could have worn a feed bag for all the enjoyment I got out of it. I didn't read labels. I didn't understand the importance of eating the highest-quality food I could afford. I didn't appreciate the fact that a healthy gut was a gift and essential to living a healthy, comfortable life.

It's the same everywhere, and every day I hear the consequences of our inattention to our GI tract. Someone is always complaining to me about their gut. "Oh, I'm so bloated"—I hear constantly—"I'm constipated," "I have acid reflux," "I have irritable bowel syndrome," "I have indigestion," "I have this cough," "I have phlegm."

It is estimated that as much as 40 percent of the population suffers from some form of digestive stress. By the time a person finally goes to see a doctor he is usually well into a chronic disease state requiring lots of pharmaceutical drugs and/or surgery. In so many cases these drastic measures could have been avoided with a proper understanding of nutrition, digestion, elimination, and stress management.

Your gut begins at your mouth, includes fifteen feet of hollow tubing, and ends at your anus. It is pretty much a person's entire being. It's the center of things. Without a healthy gut you cannot have health. Most people think of the GI tract as something that allows us to eat. But it has now been proven that this vital passageway plays a major role in many aspects of human health. For example, the GI tract is the largest component of the immune system.

The GI tract is one of the more complicated systems in the body and has, in fact, been referred to as the second brain. This is because it contains an extensive network of nerves, neurotransmitters, and nerve receptors that allows it to operate largely independent of the brain.

The only control we have when swallowing is placing the food or drink into our mouth and pushing it back into the esophagus. At that point the nerve networks embedded in the esophagus grab the food and move it downward toward the stomach using a wave of muscle contractions called peristalsis. It's all done automatically. In fact, according to Dr. Russell Blaylock, if you wanted to you could swallow water while standing on your head.

Once you understand how the gut works you will have a new and profound respect for the center of your being. At that point (most likely), a shift in your habits will occur. When I finally got it, my habits changed. There was no way I could continue to eat chemicals or gobble down my food the way I used to. Once I comprehended the devastating effects of poor nutrition, stress, and my nasty bad habit of eating on the run, I realized that gut health was essential to my quality of life and longevity.

Gut health feels great: no bloating, no gas, no burning, no coughing, no acid reflux, no indigestion, no stuffed feeling. I now know if you want to eat on the run, then be prepared to live with "the runs," and/or constipation and sickness.

We all live stressful lives regardless of where we reside. Recently I was working in one of our largest cities and was overwhelmed by the noise, the craziness, and so many people. It exhausted me, and I felt stress but couldn't pinpoint why. I didn't connect my feelings with the noise pollution. Brenda Watson says:

> We breathe toxic air, drink polluted water, and generally pass bacteria and viruses around so often it's amazing we survive at all. The fact that we do survive for decades in relatively good health is, in part, a testament to the strength of our digestive system.
>
> We were never meant to drink fluoridated water or swim in chlorinated water. Milk was never meant to be homogenized. And who thought of irradiating our food? Who decided it was a good idea to put preservatives in our food? How is it that our government has "safe" recommendations for pesticides and chemicals; what makes them think any chemical or pesticide is safe for human absorption or consumption?
>
> In spite of all this toxicity and trauma to our bodies our digestive system functions for years doing its best to break down foods and liquids into the few nutrients that are available. Our digestive system is crucial and vital to our health and well-being, and yet we put it to the extreme test every day by taxing its abilities to operate optimally. The

digestive system also has to (in its spare time) filter and eliminate tox-ins, parasites, fungi, bacteria, and viruses.

Great health comes from the body's ability to digest nutrients and eliminate waste. That's what the digestive system does: Its purpose is to be sure that you digest your foods completely and eliminate wastes natu-rally. We are what we eat, but equally important is that we are what we digest. According to Brenda Watson, "It is essential we break down (di-gest), take into the bloodstream (absorb), and take into the cells (assimi-late). The problem is that not all the food we consume is properly utilized. Even assuming that we eat the highest quality food available (and most people do not) we cannot achieve optimal health unless our digestive systems are functioning at their peak."

Aging, poor-quality food, faulty preparation methods, and external toxins or parasites can lead to a premature decline of our digestive sys-tems and long-term chronic diseases. These diseases include arthritis, dia-betes, fibromyalgia, chronic fatigue, Alzheimer's, irritable bowel syndrome, macular degeneration—it all starts in the GUT!

When our digestive system doesn't function correctly we are not able to reap the full benefits of the food we eat. Aside from digestion, our sys-tem must be able to eliminate wastes and toxins quickly and efficiently. Elimination of toxins is particularly problematic. In today's world we are constantly exposed to so many toxins in our air, food, and water, as well as in the workplace and at home, plus we generate toxins in our own bodies. These toxins produce irritation and inflammation, adding to the burden of our digestive system, and when the digestive system becomes overwhelmed, it is no longer able to adequately perform detoxification functions. That creates "toxic overload."

There is a solution. You can keep your body operating at optimal levels through proper nutrients and keeping the digestive system clean and well maintained. In order to do that you have to understand what happens to your food from the time it enters the mouth until it leaves the body. You also have to learn what can go wrong in the process and why. And most important you need to learn how to avoid, as well as correct and reverse, problems with digestion and elimination.

HOW IT WORKS

Information is power. Understanding the mechanism of digestion will help you to connect the dots to your personal problems. Thank you again to

Brenda Watson and her terrific book; I've paraphrased here some of the information she explains. Follow this closely.

Let's say you just took a bite of food. Here's what happens to it . . .

The DIGESTIVE SYSTEM begins in the mouth where the teeth chew food into smaller particles. Then saliva coats and softens those food particles with enzymes that break down carbohydrates. Saliva also contains enzymes that attack bacteria and their protein coats directly. This is the body's first line of defense against parasites and foreign invaders. Once chewing is completed, and sometimes even when it is not, food is swallowed and transferred down the esophagus to the stomach.

Now your food has hit the ESOPHAGUS.

We all have an esophagus, which is a wonderful ten-inch-long muscular tube lined with mucus-producing cells that lubricates the food so that it passes through with ease. Mucus in this case is a good thing. The esophagus transports food to the stomach through the action of its wavelike muscular contractions (peristalsis).

The muscular valve at the bottom of the esophagus is known as the lower esophageal sphincter. This valve remains tightly closed when food is not being eaten so that stomach acid cannot back into the esophagus and cause heartburn. It opens and closes quickly to allow food to pass into the stomach.

Now we move on to the STOMACH.

Very little absorption actually occurs in the stomach because it is essentially a holding and mixing tank for food. The stomach's main functions are storage and preliminary digestion. It works like a big blender, churning and liquefying food.

The properly functioning stomach secretes five important substances:

1. *mucus*
2. *hydrochloric acid (HCl)*
3. a digesting enzyme called *pepsin*
4. *gastrin*, a hormone that regulates acid production
5. gastric *lipase*, which assists in the digestion of fat

Here's why you need to understand this mechanism. A mucus lining coats the cells of the stomach to protect them from the HCl and enzymes that must be present for proper digestion. This alkaline mucus lining can be damaged by dehydration, overconsumption of food or aspirin, or by the bacterium *Helicobacter pylori (H. pylori)*. (If you eat at restaurants frequently, you are most likely exposed to *H. pylori* through chicken.) This damage can often lead to gastritis (irritation of the stomach lining) or to a stomach ulcer.

Here's something interesting—most people with heartburn produce *too little* hydrochloric acid. Yet the usual remedy is to take an antacid, which removes acid, exactly the opposite of what your stomach wants. It actually needs *more* hydrochloric acid. Without enough HCl, you may not be able to sufficiently break down proteins. This can lead to bloating, gas, and heartburn. Low HCl production can also result in problems with bacterial infections or parasites. HCl is available in tablet form. I often supplement with three betaine HCl during mealtimes (it should be taken with food) and it has eliminated my bloating and discomfort.

HCl is produced by parietal cells (tiny pumps) in the lining of the stomach. This acid is needed to ensure the proper functioning of the stomach. HCl has two primary functions: It provides the acidic environment necessary for the enzyme pepsin to break down proteins, and it helps prevent infection by destroying most parasites and bacteria.

At the end of the stomach is the pyloric sphincter, which controls the opening between the end of the stomach and the duodenum, which is the first section of the small intestine.

We're still on the journey. Remember, this all starts with that bite of food you took in the mouth.

Now we're in the DUODENUM.

When your food leaves your stomach, it enters the first section of the small intestine known as the duodenum. The food is now called "chyme," a mixture of food, HCl, and mucus, which should be a liquid consistency by now. If you took the time to chew your food initially, you will be in good shape at this point. Everything should be running smoothly. But if you didn't chew properly, the whole system is working doubly hard to break down this large clump of food. As the duodenum fills, hormones are released from the duodenal lining and

- delay gastric emptying
- promote bile flow from the liver and gallbladder
- promote secretion of water, bicarbonate, and potent digestive enzymes from the pancreas

The surface of the duodenum is smooth for the first few inches, but quickly changes to a surface with many folds and small fingerlike projections called villi or microvilli. These projections serve to increase the surface area and absorption capabilities of the duodenum. Properly functioning accessory organs (liver, gallbladder, and pancreas) are crucial during this first stage of digestion.

Now we're in the PANCREAS.

The pancreas is vital to digestion. Because of excessive chemicals entering our bodies, pancreatic cancer is on the rise. You want to avoid this life-or-death scenario.

The pancreas is a six-inch-long accessory organ that has three main functions important to digestion. It

1. neutralizes stomach acid
2. regulates blood sugar levels
3. produces digestive enzymes

Digestive enzymes digest proteins, carbohydrates, and fats, and these are only activated once they reach the duodenum. These secretions (pancreatic enzymes and bicarbonates) are delivered directly into the duodenum, the upper portion of the small intestine. The pancreas also secretes hormones—insulin (sugar lowering) and glucagon (sugar raising)—directly into the bloodstream, which help manage blood sugar levels.

We're getting there. . . .

The LIVER is now involved.

You probably didn't realize that the liver performs important functions relative to digestion. Remember, the gut extends from the mouth to the anus. The liver produces about 85 percent of the body's cholesterol (only about 15 percent comes from food). About 80 percent of the cholesterol produced by the liver is used to make bile. Bile is composed of bile salts, hormones (including cholesterol), and toxins. It acts to emulsify and distribute fat, cholesterol, and fat-soluble vitamins throughout the intestines. Bile is an alkaline substance that neutralizes stomach acid. Between meals, it is stored in the gallbladder, a pear-shaped organ located just below the liver. When food (chyme) enters the duodenum, a signal is sent to the gallbladder to contract, thereby releasing bile into the small intestine.

We've only got four more steps of explanation: the small intestine, the large intestine, the rectum, and the anus.

Ninety percent of all nutrients are absorbed in the SMALL INTESTINE, which is twenty to twenty-five feet long. This is where the food is completely digested and absorbed. It has three sections:

- The duodenum is the first foot of the small intestine and primarily absorbs minerals.
- The jejunum absorbs water-soluble vitamins, carbohydrates, and proteins.
- The ileum absorbs fat-soluble vitamins, fat, cholesterol, and bile salts.

The walls of the small intestine secrete alkaline digestive enzymes, which continue the separation of food: proteins into amino acids and fats into fatty acids, and glycerin and carbohydrates into simple sugars.

The LARGE INTESTINE (or COLON) is the last organ through which food residue passes. It has three major segments: ascending (right side of the body), transverse (connects right side to left side), descending (left side).

Chyme enters the ascending colon through the ILEOCECAL VALVE. This is a one-way valve that connects the small and large intestines and regulates the flow of chyme entering the large intestine. Now, think about that bite of food. If you did not chew it long enough to break it down, large clumps of food have been trying to work their way through this maze called the gut, making everything more difficult. You are going to be feeling indigestion and have acid reflux, gas, and bloating, to name a few. When it reaches the ileocecal valve (which is a small passageway), big clumps of food that you didn't properly chew will get stuck and back up all the rest of the food you have eaten after that. The ileocecal valve (ICV) is designed to let waste pass through and prevent it from backing into the small intestine. Have you ever felt the area of the ileocecal (right-hand side, around the ovaries in women) and it's been sore to the touch? That's trouble. Now for sure you're going to be constipated, but this constant trauma can result in appendicitis and other gut-related and uncomfortable symptoms and disease.

After food reaches the ileocecal valve it leaves the small intestine and begins its journey into the large intestine. The chyme passes through the ICV and into the very lowest portion of the ascending colon called the CECUM. At this point the food is in a liquid state. Food waste travels up the ascending colon, across the transverse, and down the ascending portion of the organ. As it moves across the transverse colon, liquid is extracted. It is the job of the colon to absorb water and nutrients from the chyme and to form feces.

The lowest portion of the descending colon is the sigmoid, which empties into the RECTUM. Fecal matter passes into the rectum, creating the urge to defecate.

The ANUS is the opening at the far end of the digestive (GI) tract. The anus allows fecal matter to pass out of the body. The anal sphincters keep the anus closed. Read Brenda Watson's book to understand this in greater depth.

There you have it—the GI tract from mouth to anus. The core of "who we are" physically.

When any part of the GI tract is not functioning well, it creates discomfort and can become diseased. This should be incentive enough for the one simple act of *chewing your food slowly*! It makes the whole GI process work.

It's unfortunate that most of us wait until we have a problem or are already in a disease state before we decide to take charge of our health. The deterioration of the digestive system can occur silently for some years, producing no symptoms or only minor ones, like headaches, low energy, and lowered resistance to infections, gas, bloating, constipation, and indigestion. These symptoms are your body talking to you. They can be a prelude to chronic degenerative disease, which begins by the toxicity produced by digestive dysfunction.

If allowed, and the GI tract continues to deteriorate, you may experience more serious problems—allergies; cancer; autoimmune diseases like rheumatoid arthritis, scleroderma, and lupus; chronic problems like irritable bowel syndrome, Crohn's disease, and ulcerative colitis; and skin diseases like psoriasis and eczema. Surprisingly, macular degeneration has its origins in the GI tract . . . recently discovered as a result of low hydrochloric acid (for more on this see Dr. Jonathan Wright's interview, chapter 2). In fact, virtually any chronic disease can have its roots in poor digestion from poor absorption of nutrients, increased intestinal permeability and dysbiosis, all being the hallmarks of digestive dysfunction.

Now that you've seen what can happen if you don't take care of your gut, follow these simple steps to keep your GI tract healthy:

- Take the time to eat clean food (organic being the best).
- Learn to chew your food thoroughly and slowly.
- Eat probiotics like acidophilus and bifidobacteria.
- Take digestive enzymes.
- Eat some raw foods daily.
- Consume optimum amounts of fiber and essential fatty acids.
- Replace lost stomach acid with hydrochloric acid.

Dear Suzanne,

I am a Wall Street guy. I eat right and do all the other things you suggest in your books. At your suggestion, I started on bioidentical hormones about two years ago. I thought I felt good before hormones. . . . But now I feel incredible. I feel better than I felt in my thirties.

Then I had a problem. My libido soared as my wife's diminished. These days we have hallway sex (you know that old joke). We pass in the hallway and she says screw you and I say screw you too! (Just kidding!)

But seriously she has become real bitchy (not usual). When I feel her in bed she is soaking wet. One minute she turns on the heat and then kicks off the blankets and then she turns the AC at 60 degrees. Up and down like a goddamn toilet seat.

My wife's doctor told her she has all the hormones she needs and why would she listen to that Suzanne Somers anyway?

I love my wife, truly love her, but don't know how much more of this I can take. I seem to be the object of all her unhappiness. It is really tough when she lashes out.

I begged her, begged her to go to one of your doctors.

Well, she finally did, and wow . . . we are getting things back on track. It's not perfect yet but I know she will get there.

I am sure it's usually the wives who get the husbands to go to these doctors, but I see this as our opportunity to live happily ever after.

I love you, Suzanne Somers, because my wife trusts you. When a woman looks at you she wants to feel like you look. I'll keep you posted but I know we are going to make it.

All we both do is rub a little cream on our body parts each day. Simple and makes a world of difference in our lives.

Thank you very much,
John

18

DR. HOWARD LIEBOWITZ

To fight disease after it has occurred is like trying to dig a well
when one is thirsty or forging a weapon once a war has begun.

—*The Yellow Emperor's Classic of Internal Medicine*

Dr. Howard Liebowitz is another ER doc—they're the fearless ones, and
not afraid to speak up. He works with women and men, but men flock to
him because of the way he looks (who wouldn't want what he has?)
and also because he is passionate about this changing medium of medicine.
When you see him you realize he walks the talk—vital, strong-looking,
and glowing with health. It's inspirational. He is the medical director of
the Hall Center and excels in bioidentical hormone replacement for
women and men. He is a weight management specialist, bringing the entire spectrum of integrated health to his center. And as a functional medicine practitioner, he is an expert at lowering cholesterol naturally,
managing blood pressure naturally, and treating the root cause of digestive
problems. He is passionate, concerned, and at the top of his game.

SS: I've been looking forward to this interview. I have seen the major
impact you have on so many lives. But you spent fifteen years working
the ER at Cedars Sinai and then made this switch to practicing antiaging
medicine. Why did you make that transition?

HL: I've always had a passionate interest in prevention. I also worked
at the Pritikin Center in Santa Monica, California, and I was medical director at the Centinela Hospital Fitness Institute. I've worked a lot with
sports medicine, and that requires a healthy outlook on wellness and all

things natural, so functional medicine and preventative medicine seemed a logical extension to me.

SS: A lot of ER doctors tend to be very cutting-edge.

HL: That's true. When emergency medicine started in the seventies it was a very new and challenging profession and no one felt it was going anywhere, but it became a huge specialty. I think the type of doctors who went into emergency medicine had to be very forward-thinking, plus willing to take the risks that sometimes go against the conventional medical grain. It's just the personality of ER doctors.

SS: What is the fear of trying new alternatives in conventional medicine?

HL: There are a few reasons. One of the main fears is litigation. Lawyers and malpractice threats have put a damper on doctors, as in if you follow the flock you won't get in trouble. If a doctor is out there on his or her own and you step outside conventional thinking, no one is going to come to your aid. Unfortunately, this fear has poisoned a lot of the medical care in the United States. So many decisions by today's doctors are made to cover their butts. By necessity, a lot of money is spent on documentation to back yourself up in case you end up in court.

Another problem in medicine today is that a lot of the medical education is handled by drug companies. Doctors go to conferences where they have organized lunch meetings, which are most always sponsored by drug companies, so the information they hear is what the drug companies want them to hear. It's a very forward-thinking doctor who goes to an ACAM (American Academy for the Advancement of Medicine) convention to hear about unusual advances in medicine.

With this new medicine you have to use your own instincts and judgment, and then you try to do what you think is best for the patient. There are not always long-term double-blind studies on nonpatentable medicine like bioidentical hormones. But all of us in this field of medicine are seeing the profound results with our patients; when a patient improves this dramatically without drugs it's pretty encouraging.

SS: Well, nonpatentable medicine is of no interest to the pharmaceutical companies.

HL: But our patients are getting better. The difference between conventional doctors and a functional medicine doctor, such as me and my wife, Dr. Prudence Hall, is that conventional doctors treat an *illness*. If there is no disease they don't have a lot of options. With functional medicine we're able to work with people who don't have a *disease* but do have chronic pain or chronic malaise or exhaustion, or they've been diagnosed with fibromyalgia or chronic fatigue syndrome. As we work with them we often find that they actually have hormone imbalances and conditions that other doctors didn't recognize or feel were significant. We get these patients balanced and put them on good diets and work on restoring their adrenal glands and get them resting and sleeping, plus we take all the toxic substances out of their diets, and amazingly they start to get better. It's incredibly rewarding because this type of medicine really works.

SS: And I haven't heard you mention a single pharmaceutical.

HL: It's like turning a huge ocean liner around in the middle of the ocean—it just takes lots and lots of repeated information to come down the pike before you are able to convert a new patient and get them to feel comfortable doing it. This new medicine allows doctors to think again and use our brains; we see it working day in and day out, but there is definitely a force working against us.

For instance, recently I went to a conference where a very prominent physician presented several papers talking about hormone balancing. Ten papers were in favor of hormone balancing and the next ten slides were saying exactly the opposite. On any subject you can find another very good paper discounting it. So basically you have to use your own judgment and do what you think is best for the patient.

SS: I know a woman who has been enmeshed in conventional medicine. She has had lung cancer and quadruple bypass surgery, has no energy, sagging skin, missing eyebrows, dead eyes, stringy hair, is totally hormonal and on synthetics, hot, cold, her knees are giving out, her hips are giving out . . . you know this type of person.

HL: Is she alive?

SS: Hardly—at least not what I call living. But where do you start?

HL: Well, we often start with a hormone profile. Patients who have become this degraded medically are going to come in with a lot of medical records, so it's not necessary for us to do these big workups. They've already had all the medical evaluations and, medically speaking, they are all labeled up. Because of this we're really not looking at their labels, but it is important that we keep their information in the back of our minds because sometimes we find they have been misdiagnosed. In my years of experience I am constantly picking up on things that other doctors have not deemed significant. Most of these patients are on heart medicine, blood pressure medicine, and diabetes medications, but what really hasn't been addressed is their hormone status. What is their adrenal status? As antiaging doctors we look at the thyroid differently, and we do a tremendous amount of work impressing on the patient the life-altering benefits of nutrition and detoxification.

If it's a man, we get his testosterone levels and look at his DHT (a type of testosterone that is three times more potent than regular testosterone— it is derived from testosterone and can contribute to male pattern baldness and prostate enlargement), we look at his PSA (prostatic specific antigen) and see if he is aromatizing—aromatization is an enzyme pathway in the body that converts testosterone into estrogen. We look to see if he is creating estrogens, which can make him feel pretty lousy.

SS: What about the digestive tract?

HL: Absolutely. We put a lot of importance on that. If people have thyroid problems, a lot of times it stems from digestive disorders like leaky gut.

SS: Ah yes, back in "my other life" I had that diagnosis, but it was never connected to thyroid.

HL: Leaky gut is a syndrome where the cells that line the digestive tract are kind of like the bathroom tiles on the wall, and the grout between the bathroom tiles are like the spaces between the cells. When there is inflammation in the digestive tract (GI tract), the cells swell up, and when they swell up, they get puffy and tend to pull away from each other. When the spaces between the cells open up, then microscopic particles (proteins, usually) leak out from the inside of the digestive tract and get into the bloodstream, where they're not supposed to be because they haven't been completely processed. That's leaky gut syndrome. When these proteins leak out, they are free to go anywhere and they end up lodging into all sorts of tissues. The thyroid is very susceptible because it is so engorged with blood and so much circulation goes through that thyroid. The thyroid doesn't have a filtering mechanism, so these proteins get lodged into the thyroid.

SS: What does that do?

HL: These proteins are foreign and not supposed to be where they are in the blood; they get attacked by the immune system of the body, and that's how you end up with autoimmune phenomena. Plus the thyroid gets damaged and the patient ends up with a nonfunctioning or low-functioning gland.

SS: So this is how so many people end up with fibromyalgia and lupus. Who would have thought fibromyalgia and other autoimmune diseases start in the gut. How do you treat this condition? How do you treat fibromyalgia and lupus?

HL: We work on detoxification, balancing hormones, cleaning up the gut, IV vitamins, and energetic body work through combinations of yoga, breath work, acupuncture, and body mechanics.

SS: But most people have terrible diets, which works against what you are trying to do.

HL: Yes. Bad foods, chemicals, too much sugar, high amounts of toxic substances in the food, antacids, all this weakens the digestive system, so their digestive enzymes are decreasing and the foods aren't being properly broken down as they go through the digestive tract. Even something as simple as not chewing your food well affects the GI tract.

SS: Chewing your food is so crucial. I have tried in this book to show the pathway from the time a piece of food enters your mouth until it is eliminated, so that my readers can grasp this concept.

HL: If you don't chew your food properly (twenty or thirty times), it goes through the GI tract in a state that it is not supposed to (large pieces), and chronically over time the digestive tract becomes inflamed by being barraged with these poorly processed foods.

The other things that happen to many people are food intolerances or food allergies. If you continue to eat food to which you're intolerant, over a long period of time it causes inflammation. A lot of people can't tolerate wheat or dairy. Raw dairy is often the better choice, because the pasteurization denatures the protein in the dairy that we might have tolerated when it was in its raw form.

SS: Is that being lactose intolerant?

HL: Lactose intolerance is a different phenomenon. Lactose is a type of sugar, milk sugar. Some people don't have the ability to break it down over time.

SS: Even if it's raw?

HL: Yes. There are other things we look for, Candida and bacterial imbalances, because the digestive tract is loaded with bacteria. Almost two-thirds of the volume of the stool is bacteria and it's completely essential to our digestion. These bacteria make vitamins that we absorb; they help break down our foods. We also look for parasites, in other words, the protozoa in the digestive tract that we pick up easily in the food chain and also through water, and certainly from traveling. With so many people traveling all over the world today, they come home with parasites and don't realize that any of these things in the GI tract can cause inflammation. However, if you have a healthy GI tract and the immune system is functioning well, you can actually fight these things off and they don't become a problem. Just because you are exposed to an organism doesn't mean it's going to end up causing an inflammation. You have to understand that the digestive tract makes up 75 percent of our immune system; it has lots of lymph nodes, it houses the spleen, the liver, and all of these organs are immune-functioning organs.

SS: So you are saying that if anything negative is coming through the digestive tract, the healthy person's immune system immediately goes on a heightened response, and it can kick off a ripple effect through the rest of the body if that insult is too great?

HL: Right. The digestive tract tends to be our greatest interaction in humans between the inner environment and the external world, and it's completely controlled by what we put in our mouth. This interaction is an important function in the body and to our health in general. We are impacted not only by *what* we are eating but *how* we are eating it.

SS: When you say what we are eating, you mean real food?

HL: Absolutely. Quality, real, good food, not laden with hormones, antibiotics, insecticides, or pesticides. We have to try to eat organic as much as possible, especially vegetables and fruits, and you have to wash them really well, and make sure to have a balanced diet where you are eating good-quality protein with every meal. The biggest problem facing the Western world nutritionally is sugar and carbohydrates; instead, we should be eating more protein and complex carbohydrates like vegetables.

SS: It's quite a job educating the public about eating.

HL: The number of diabetics in this country is mind-boggling and it's getting worse. It's an uphill battle we face here at the Hall Center all day long. Part of the educational process we put our patients through comes down to making healthy food choices, lifestyle choices, getting enough sleep, getting enough rest, and exercise. All of these things are incredibly important.

SS: Okay, two words: diet soda!

HL: I consider diet soda a poison. There is nothing nutritionally sound in it. It's got artificial flavoring, artificial sweetener, artificial coloring. It's completely nonnutritious and it stresses the body, especially if you are consuming large volumes, because you are overwhelming your body's detoxification mechanism to get all these toxins out of your body. Eventually it's just going to burn out your adrenal glands and your immune system. Then there's the caffeine in diet sodas; people who are burned out (adrenals) use the caffeine in diet soda and regular Coke as a stimulant. I had a patient, a welder, who was having aches and pains everywhere, plus headaches, and he just couldn't lose weight. He was having trouble doing his job, and I found after talking to him that he kept a refrigerator in his welding shop and the only thing in it was Coca-Cola. He was drinking it all day long . . . for years. There's nine teaspoons of sugar in a can of Coca-Cola. Do you ever put nine teaspoons of sugar in anything?

SS: No. Never!

HL: Diet soda doesn't have sugar but it has the caffeine. People with burned-out adrenals go to sugar and caffeine to get them through the day. I don't think you could do anything worse for yourself than drinking diet soda and Coke all day long.

SS: I got your message. How about IBS (irritable bowel syndrome)? Everybody is complaining about that one, too. How do we get that?

HL: IBS is an extenuation of leaky gut. It's due to a complex presentation of food intolerances and decreased digestive enzymes. People take antacids, which decrease their stomach acid, and then they eat foods that irritate the digestive tract. When I have a patient with IBS I put them on a gut-healing smoothie. It has medical food in it and it's called Ultra-Inflamax by Metagenics. We mix it together with MSM (methyl sulfonyl methane, a natural source of sulfur), a very powerful anti-inflammatory, and then we also add glutamine, which is a nutrient that enhances the function of the cells that line the digestive tract. They drink this once or twice a day, and my patients will come back in a week or two telling me their GI tract feels better. Then, of course, we take them off the very highly reactive foods like dairy and wheat. In Paleolithic times there were no breads and bakery products. We were not genetically designed to consume wheat.

SS: Well, I know when you took my husband, Alan, off of wheat his health turned around. He feels well all the time, where before he was bloated, uncomfortable, and tired.

HL: The other thing I see are people drinking coffee all day long, and it's very irritating and stimulating (not in a good way) to the digestive tract. Also when our stress hormones go up, which can be exacerbated by stimulants (caffeine, chemicals), we produce a lot of adrenaline and cortisol. When these hormones go into high gear they are very disruptive to the digestive tract.

SS: Yes, they call the GI tract the second brain because of the neurons and neurotransmitters. These neurons would respond to stress and affect the gut. What about bloating? That's a biggie. I don't know a woman who isn't bloated.

HL: It's so prevalent. A lot of women who come here for bioidentical hormones complain about bloating after we've started them on their regimen because the HPA axis has been distorted.

SS: Let me see if I can remember what the HPA axis is. The hypothalamus, pituitary, and adrenal glands act in concert to read cues in the woman's environment or lifestyle. For instance, if she has been out of whack, as in hormonally symptomatic (not sleeping, poor diet, stress), this HPA axis is "off."

HL: And because they have been imbalanced for so long, the HPA axis has been distorted, and the glands don't have the normal or natural neurotransmitter levels they need for normal digestive processes. So when we change a patient's hormone levels, it can exacerbate the problems and symptoms, and this is all due to stress: stressful living, stressful eating, eating foods that are stressful to the digestive system and that are hard to digest, too much sugar, too much caffeine, and too much alcohol. This is when we make adjustments hormonally, but also lifestyle adjustments. The patient needs to work with us in order for this to work.

SS: And not sleeping is another big complaint.

HL: That, too, is disregulation in the HPA axis. That's when I suggest melatonin. As we age, melatonin is produced in the pineal gland. It comes out when we sleep in very dark, dark environments; jet-setting around, long hours, working on the computer until all hours of the night, all of this depletes your melatonin supplies. Then you get in a vicious cycle where you can't sleep because you are not making enough melatonin.

SS: So those computer lights and TV lights are a bad thing.

HL: Really bad. Even streetlights are enough to disrupt the sleep pattern; if your room isn't very dark then you need to sleep with eye shields.

SS: But most everyone of middle age is taking sleeping pills like Ambien or Lunesta. That little butterfly in the commercial that comes and sits softly on your shoulder . . . ahh, sleep. What's that going to do in the long term?

HL: Well, these are toxic substances in your system. Your liver is your primary detox organ, and it is going to have to deal with this toxic load. Ambien is not a natural substance, so basically you are just drugging yourself to sleep, which becomes a vicious cycle and it's hard to break.

Patients come to me with years of unhealthy and bad lifestyles that have led them to this situation. They now find themselves overweight, unhappy, and unable to sleep. We work on their diets, we detoxify them, we put them on melatonin, and they'll come back in two or three weeks and say it isn't working. I try to explain to them that it took years and years to get this unhealthy, and it is going to take a while to restore them. But for a lot of people they lose patience if it doesn't work immediately and they lose interest in it.

SS: How does that make you feel?

HL: I've learned over the years in medicine that things in nature and things in the human body actually change very slowly when we are trying to change major systems like circadian rhythm or bioidentical hormone rhythms or dietary rhythms. The digestive tract has its own rhythm of when things are secreted. All these functions take a long time to find their rhythms, especially when the rhythms have been out of line for so long. So, yes, it's frustrating when patients doesn't have the patience, but of course I encourage them to keep going. I know their health will turn around if it is given the time.

SS: It's difficult to connect the dots. Pharmaceuticals work fast. If they stop working a person can get something stronger and so on. It's rare for a person to be able to see down the road to the long-term consequences of constant pharmaceuticals. It's a direct and sure route to the nursing home, but none of us ever believe that that could actually happen to us. But *you* know and I know that it's more a probability than not.

HL: That's one of the reasons allopathic medicine is favored. Patients want something that is going to work right now. They want to go home, take the pill, and be done with it.

SS: How do you motivate people to stay with it and get well permanently without drugs that do not heal?

HL: I am like a health coach. I tell them what to do, but they are the ones who have to go down on the playing field and play the game. I can't play for them.

SS: Yes, but they are the ones who are going to get the gold medal at the end.

HL: I empower them to take their health in their own hands and take control of it and make themselves healthier. I'll be there to teach them and coach them. I bring all the knowledge I have and all the experience that I can impart to them on the path to greater health. I have never given up on anyone. I figure if they are here in my office they must be trying to change their lives. It's that cruise liner in the middle of the ocean; some people are just turning around slower. You never know when you're gonna click with something you do with them, and all of a sudden they are going to have a breakthrough.

SS: What are you excited about these days in the medical arena?

HL: Stem cells! The possibilities are thrilling. The people involved with stem cell banking talk about the possibility of reversing diabetes, or if your heart were failing they could regenerate your heart, if your lungs were failing they could regenerate your lungs; a huge benefit would be kidney regeneration for all those people on dialysis. People with cystic fibrosis could grow new lungs. How about new teeth, and new eyes? The future of it is mind-boggling.

SS: And now there is really no controversy; they are taking stem cells from your own adult body, and they have located fetal cells in the bone marrow of the adult body. That is exciting. That eliminates the controversy.

HL: We are so excited about this we are offering this service at the Hall Center with the NeoStem Company.

SS: Yes. And I am very excited at having banked my own stem cells with NeoStem. If I ever need to, for whatever reason, I will be able to regrow parts of myself from my own stem cells. It's truly exciting and it is so easy to do.

Let me ask you this: When is it too late for someone? If you are overweight, feeble, and not thinking well, on a lot of medication, and can't sleep—have you reached the point of no return?

HL: It really depends on how much end organ damage there is. If a person is already in dementia, it would be very hard to reverse that. If one has a really bad heart and it's weak and barely pumping, that would be difficult to reverse, but if the organs are basically sound we can work with that.

SS: It shows you the importance of building up the organs and glands that have become weakened. So many of the doctors in this book are also involved in energy medicine, which strengthens the weakest organs and glands.

HL: I think another amazing hormone that hasn't been fully addressed is growth hormone. I see HGH as truly regenerative, and in my practice I see many people who need it and who have very low levels; you can actually spot them across the room. People on growth hormones look dramatically different from those not on it. I wish it were not so expensive—so many of my patients just can't afford it.

SS: That is disappointing. I have a GH deficiency and have been on HGH for two years, along with my other complete hormone regimen. The difference in my metabolism is spectacular. My body responds to exercise as it once did when I was young, I feel a spring in my step, and there is an internal feeling that the "song" is complete.

HL: I understand what you mean by the "song." Hormones are like a symphony orchestra, and you have to have all the different hormones playing well together. Imagine if each hormone was a different section of that orchestra and one hormone system is "off"; that orchestra won't sound very good no matter how great the other systems are. If you have beautifully balanced hormones but one system is weak, like the adrenals (and some people live such stressful lives that their adrenals get pooped out and they never quite come back to normal), and then you add growth hormone, it's not going to be able to carry the load. Growth hormone is a very powerful metabolic hormone, and if your adrenals or any other hormones are low, then you don't get the benefits of growth hormone. Growth hormone is added when all the other systems are in balance. Growth hormone is the final touch, but pretty much ineffective and a waste of money if you haven't balanced the rest of the systems.

SS: Well, for those who have burned out their adrenals (and I bet that is more the norm than we realize), does that mean they will never get the "song" correct? How do you strengthen the adrenals?

HL: To strengthen the adrenals you have to rid the body of everything that is stressing the adrenals in the first place. You have to be on an optimal diet, you have to get enough rest and sleep. These things are paramount to adrenal healing.

SS: Well, that must fall on deaf ears. We laypeople are told this so often by our doctors that we don't hear it anymore. You know, yeah, yeah, yeah . . . sleep and rest and diet. But I've been burned out; I flatlined my adrenals four times in my career. That's when I started "hearing." Burned-out adrenals feel like death. It feels like the end of the road: inability to sleep, depression, weight gain, irregular periods, no energy, no ability to think, racing heart, sadness. Just awful. In fact, my last bout of burnout was the real "come to Jesus" moment for me. My doctor told me that I was on my way to a heart attack. I was forty-five years old. I had no plaque in my heart or arteries. The child of an alcoholic in me had almost worked me to death.

HL: Yes, it's that serious. Skin rashes, irritability, high blood pressure, the list goes on.

There are supplements we use: high doses of vitamins B, B_5, B_6, vitamin C, biotin, Co-Q_{10}, sometimes carnosine. These are all nutritional supports. Sometimes we use acupuncture and other modalities that de-stress, like meditation, calming exercises, stretching exercises, and yoga. A lot of these things help to calm the mind and the body. I try to impress upon my patients to get into some sort of spiritual pursuit and take the time to be introspective. These things can help quite a bit, and of course if a person is not sleeping that presents a huge challenge because sleep is key to healing the adrenals.

But there's also more to it. You have to avoid toxic substances. I call them SNAC: sugar, nicotine, alcohol, caffeine. These are the common substances that many, many people are using and they are highly toxic to the body. If you are using these substances and you are not sleeping and you are running around, it's going to be very hard to heal the adrenal glands. The adrenals are critical to everything, they are absolutely paramount, and cortisol is the one hormone we can't live without. We can live without a lot of the other hormones (and not feel so well, but we could live), but without cortisol (made in the adrenal glands) and healthy adrenals you are pretty much done. The adrenals are critical.

SS: What's going to happen to us as a society? Most people are overworking, like I used to. Most people pride themselves on sleeping as little as possible, as I used to do. I would brag about getting three hours of sleep. Now I would be embarrassed, because I know the damage that's done by missing even one night's sleep.

HL: It is a prevalent and dangerous trend. So many people come to me feeling awful. I put them on bioidentical cortisol, called Cortef, or hydrocortisone, which is bioidentical and made by a compounding pharmacy, and it's like a miracle supplement or hormone. People will feel dramatically better in days. I use low physiologic doses that have been proposed by Dr. William Jeffries in his book *The Safe Uses of Cortisol*. Replacing cortisol allows the adrenal glands to recover, which will give the body enough cortisol so that the rest of the hormone systems will work, and the body will function closer to a normal physiologic basis, and the person will feel much better. Then I can work on resetting the hypothalamic-pituitary axis (HPA axis) so I can get circadian rhythms back on track. This way I can make some headway on healing and it won't suppress normal adrenal function. If I can move a person in this direction, the adrenal glands have a chance for recovery.

SS: What if, like me, because of a lack of understanding, a person has burned out repeatedly (I will never, ever do it again; I would quit my job before I would ever do that again), could you stay on bioidentical cortisol for life?

HL: Yes. You just have to know that if something very stressful happens in your life, for instance, like your house burning down, Suzanne, or a serious illness, you might need a little more cortisol during those very stressful periods. When the stress decreases, then you taper down slowly to your individualized physiologic dose. Some people like you will probably need to replace cortisol for life, just like all the other hormones that need replacing for life.

So often when patients come in and they are in bad shape, I would like to give them everything they need right away. But if I did that I know they would be overwhelmed, so I proceed in little baby steps, hoping they will stay with it so I can get the body running perfectly once again. There are very few who are willing to take it all on immediately, so I usually start with what is the worst thing going on. For a menopausal woman it is usually going to be her estrogen and progesterone; by starting there and replacing those hormones she's going to feel human again, and then I start working on the diet and other hormone systems. After that, I work on the gut; I love to get women into detoxification as soon as I can.

SS: Let's talk about detoxification. What does that mean?

HL: We start off with a fundamental nutritional detox for two or three weeks. First, we take the patient off animal protein and put them on lots of vegetables. This alkalinizes the body and helps enhance the function of the hormone systems and enzyme systems. This takes a lot of stress off the body. Second, we take them off sugar. It's radical, but I ask them to do these things for two weeks at a time; then no starches, no carbs, no alcohol, no caffeine. This leaves them with a pure environment of vegetables, and of course I ask them to drink lots of water. The third thing we do is colon therapy. The colon is the primary organ for reabsorption of nutrients and fluids in the body, and often the colon can have bacterial overgrowth and *Candida*, so cleansing the colon enhances reabsorption of nutrients and fluids. Fourth, we give them intravenous vitamins during this period and this supports immune function. We give high-dose vitamin C to rid the body of viruses and to stimulate the immune system. Fifth, we use acupuncture to do the same thing and promote energy. And sixth, Far infrared sauna treatments to promote sweating and detoxification. Infrared sauna is different from regular sauna because regular sauna is going to heat your skin and get you very hot because it has a very hot ambient temperature, and you'll start sweating but you can't stay in very long. Infrared sauna is a low-temperature sauna, so you can sit in there for a long time and it raises your core temperature. By keeping your core temperature up it allows for your metabolism to stay high. So sitting in an infrared sauna for thirty or forty minutes a day has the same effect on your metabolism that you would get from exercising. It's a great thing to add to your exercise regimen, and for people with a disability it stimulates their metabolism just as exercise would do.

SS: Wow. That will sell Far infrared saunas right there.

HL: Yes, you can sit in there for an hour and you'll be sweating profusely, but you don't feel that hot. I exercise a lot, so my body core temperature actually stays up pretty high. I don't have any problem detoxifying because I sweat a lot, and sweating is actually a sign of good health. Far infrared sauna does this for you.

A lot of people don't sweat usually, due to an iodine deficiency—which is very important for mineral health. The Japanese have the highest amount of iodine in their diets of any population and they also have the lowest incidence of cancer.

In fact, iodine deficiency is being related to stomach, breast, ovarian, and uterine cancers, and especially thyroid cancer. But this doesn't replace exercise. You have to keep the body moving or it will stiffen up.

SS: What do you do on a daily basis?

HL: I've always exercised every day. I rarely miss. Even if I only have a few minutes, I'll do something: yoga, rowing. I've done the Ironman Triathlon in Hawaii three times. So daily I take testosterone, thyroid on an empty stomach, DHEA, then I go downstairs and whip up a smoothie that I've been on for years for my gut. I put in a lot of fiber—psyllium, flax—MSM, and glutamine. I put some frozen berries in the smoothie and that's my breakfast. I brew up a huge pot of rooibos tea; it's organic, from South Africa, and it has the highest amount of antioxidants of any plant on the planet. It's free of caffeine and contains no tannic acid, so you can leave it brewing all day and it just gets stronger in its antioxidant content. I drink it in the morning, and when I come home from work at the end of the day I drink it as iced tea. I drink about five or six cups a day.

SS: What about supplements?

HL: Absolutely. Besides hormones, I take melatonin at bedtime; and in terms of my supplements I take high-dose B, C, and taurine, which is an amino acid that regulates heart rhythms to keep my heart beating regularly. I take Co-Q$_{10}$, saw palmetto, 5-alpha-reductase inhibitor, which blocks the production of DHT (dihydrotestosterone) from testosterone, which keeps the prostate from enlarging. Melatonin is a hormone and an aromatase inhibitor that blocks the production of estrogen from testosterone, which is a good thing for men. As men get older they convert more testosterone into estrogen, especially if they are putting on weight because the conversion takes place in fat. Then I take antioxidants—krill oil, which is a very highly concentrated omega-3 oil. I like it because it is free of toxic mercury, and fish oil treats cholesterol problems.

SS: You take your health seriously. Most men prefer to be given a pharmaceutical prescription. It's just easier.

HL: Yes. But they won't get better that way. They won't build up. They won't be able to take advantage of antiaging by using pharmaceuticals. Most of the men in my office are brought here by women. For the most part men don't direct themselves toward their health, because they are driven in terms of business and achieving, and excelling and competing. You would think they would have the same kind of drive when it comes to their own bodies. Men just seem to accept the fact that they are going to get older and lose their vitality. It's strange to me, because you would think they would want to be able to function physically. I was speaking with your son, Bruce, who is also a cyclist, and he was in agreement with me that if he misses his fifty-mile bike ride on Sunday he feels terrible. You would think men would want to maintain that virility and never let it slip away. For me that would be the greatest loss in my life, to lose my vibrancy.

SS: And also to maintain good brain function. Many middle age women and older are having trouble remembering. When I was low in estrogen I couldn't remember anything. That was awful. The right amount of estrogen solved that problem for me. My brain is sharper than ever now.

HL: I have some powerful businessmen as patients, and I try to motivate them, but sometimes men need something scary to happen to them to motivate them to change. David Deida, who writes on gender-based emotional and sexual differences, says, "A man is like a locomotive going down the railroad; he's going straight ahead and he's not going to change course, he's not going to stop, he's just heading down the track." Then he says, "A woman is like a sailboat on the ocean; it goes this way and that way; the waves go up and the waves go down and the sailboat maneuvers wherever it wants to go." I think that imagery shows that women are flexible and fluid and willing to change and try new things, and men are just going down the track. You almost have to knock them off the track with something big to make them change.

SS: How unfortunate. So they wait for cancer or a heart attack, and either it gets them to change and embrace new medicine or become totally dependent on traditional medicine and pharmaceuticals. How often are you, as a Western-trained doctor, prescribing pharmaceuticals for your patients?

HL: Actually, I would say the ratio of nutraceuticals to pharmaceuticals is probably in the range of 1,000 to 1 or maybe greater.

SS: Wow, wow.

HL: It's rare.

SS: You should be so proud of this.

HL: It's rare that I pull out the prescription pad, except to order hormones.

SS: Well, I know for myself that I haven't had a pharmaceutical in about five or six years.

HL: I don't even take Tylenol. When people are at my house and have a headache all I can offer is an ice pack for their head.

People are taking too many over-the-counter drugs. They don't realize they are decreasing what little stomach acid they have left, which just makes all their digestive problems worse.

The body is incredibly resilient, but we end up poisoning ourselves with these toxic over-the-counter drugs.

SS: What do you suggest for low stomach acid?

HL: I give betaine HCl (hydrochloric acid). Then I suggest stomach enzymes—which are different from probiotics (also important), which are designed to recolonize the gut with healthy bacteria. We need to replace these things because so many people have bacterial imbalances from taking antibiotics or just from eating poorly. Overgrowth of bacteria is called "opportunistic bacteria" and causes bloating, gas, and indigestion. Recolonizing the gut makes the digestive tract healthy, and a healthy gut is tantamount to ideal health.

SS: Is there a test for people to evaluate the GI tract?

HL: Yes, there are two tests. One is a comprehensive evaluation of the GI tract; it's a GI stool test and it goes to a lab called MetaMetrix Clinical Laboratories in Norcross, Georgia. They analyze the digestive tract in a very comprehensive way, looking at digestive enzymes, the pH of the GI tract, bacterial counts as to whether they are opportunistic or pathological, and we look for protozoa, parasites, and worms. We also look at the IGA (an antibody secreted by the cells that line the GI tract) to see if the immune function in the GI tract is adequate. Then we look at food intolerances to see if people are intolerant of wheat, dairy, soy, and eggs.

The other great test is the twenty-four-hour urine test to see how you are metabolizing all the hormones, including cortisol and adrenal metabolites, and based on the patterns, we make adjustments not only in hormones but in lifestyle as well. This test allows me to see how the woman is absorbing her hormones. I had one woman patient who was using huge amounts of estrogen and she needed to put four to five lines (milligrams) on every four to five hours, but then we would do a blood test and her estrogen levels weren't very high. So I switched her to vaginal estrogen, and all of a sudden she had normal estrogen levels and she felt great.

SS: Hmm, bioidentical estrogen vaginally—of course she felt great. I mean, that's a "good time in the old household tonight"!

HL: That's true. How bad is that? We also have a lot of women using testosterone right on the clitoris.

SS: I bet they are happy.

HL: Yes. But mainly it's so that it absorbs correctly, and sometimes it's the only way.

SS: What keeps you going? This is hard work. These are long hours. I know that you and your wife, Dr. Prudence Hall, have worked hard to create such a beautiful experience at your Hall Center.

HL: What keeps me going is that it is so much fun to do this work; being in charge as medical director is the opportunity to constantly be learning new things. Both my wife and I go to conferences or read something that appeals to us as breakthroughs in information, and then we can bring this to the patients the next day without having to go through the bureaucracy of hospitals and having to answer to anyone. I love that I can bring cutting-edge information to my patients, and we are seeing results very, very quickly. Working in the emergency room for so many years is the opposite of what we are doing in our practice today. This is upbeat, enjoyable, satisfying, and I have patients telling me all the time how incredible they feel. In fact, we get letters from patients telling us this is the best medical experience they've ever had in their life.

SS: It must be rewarding.

HL: Very rewarding. I talk with my patients like you and I are speaking right now about health issues. What I teach and what I practice is the way I live my life. It's in my soul. I love to share what I've learned and hopefully inspire them to do the same with their health and lifestyle.

SS: Is there anything in the future you dream about?

HL: I wish growth hormone was less expensive, because there are a lot of people who could benefit from it. I also think stem cell potential is exciting. It gets into a realm that I'm not able to touch, because it's about people who have extensive end organ damage. Once these organs are damaged beyond repair they just need a new organ. Stem cells are able to do that, and it will open up a new realm of possibility for healing people—and the fact that it is no longer necessary to retrieve stem cells from fetuses makes it ethical. Instead, the stem cells are from you. It's your own blood type going back into your body. I think the future is here.

I'm a boomer, and our whole generation has always been a very radical group, and as we age we're going to be demonstrating the benefits *or not* of what we are doing. It's fascinating to be alive in this generation, to be tackling our health this way. It's going to be breaking news for the next generation and generations behind us because it's revolutionary. This type of medicine is not *mainstream,* and it's going against the current, but it is going to open up all new possibilities for people in the future.

SS: And there you will be right in the front of the pack. Thank you so much.

DR. HOWARD LIEBOWITZ'S BREAKTHROUGH BREAKOUTS

- Food should be chewed properly, twenty or thirty times, so that the GI tract isn't barraged with large pieces of food, which causes inflammation over time.

- The digestive tract makes up 75 percent of our immune system; it includes a number of immune-functioning organs, such as lymph nodes, the spleen, and the liver.

- The sugar in regular sodas and the caffeine in both diet and regular sodas is toxic and stresses the adrenal system.

- Growth hormone can be beneficial in increasing muscle tone and in seeing the results of exercise, but it should be added only when all the other hormone systems are in balance.

- Fish oil, which is a very highly concentrated omega-3 oil, treats cholesterol problems, and krill oil in particular is free of toxic mercury.

Dear Suzanne,

I love, love, love your book. It changed my life as I am sure thousands of women have told you because you had the guts to tell your story. I really care about my body, my health, and frame of mind. After reading your book I immediately made an appointment with a very respectable naturopathic M.D. doctor and he took tests that no other doctor ever did and all of my hormones were terribly off including my thyroid, DHEA, D, zinc, and calcium. Wow! I couldn't believe that my family practice doctor told me that at forty-nine I was too young to start menopause and there was nothing she could do but give me testosterone gel, which gave me the worst side effects.

Anyway, to date, I feel great again and am very blessed to have read your story. You have a big fan in me for everything you do for women.

Sandra B.

DR. PRUDENCE HALL

People ask me what I'd appreciate for my 87th birthday.
I tell them a paternity suit.

—George Burns, comedian (1896–1996)

DR. PRUDENCE HALL is my gynecologist and my friend. She and her husband, Dr. Howard Liebowitz, founded the Hall Center in Santa Monica, California. She is a graduate of the famed USC Medical School, but since that time she has moved way beyond the scope and breadth of what one can be taught. She is the rare doctor who goes out of her way to continually educate herself in the next and greatest advancements in medicine, using intellect and the fine "art of medicine" to treat patients with respect and compassion. Dr. Hall is unique in a world when most office visits have been reduced to eight minutes per patient. She has made bioidentical hormone replacement her specialty in order to promote optimal quality of life and health. She is compassionate, enthusiastic, knowledgeable, and best of all (for us women) she is in menopause herself, so she really gets it!

SS: Thank you for your time, Prudence. As a gynecologist, you are unique because you yourself are in menopause and you are a believer in and user of bioidentical hormones. As your patient, I find it is comforting knowing you relate to the passage we are both experiencing. It puts the patients on a level playing field with you because we know you are going to do the best for yourself and then you will pass this on to your patients.

PH: Yes. All day long, it's hormones, hormones, hormones. I see patients from their early teens with hormone problems, often due to birth control pills and sometimes due to conditions such as insulin resistance, all the way to women in their nineties. In fact, my oldest patient is ninety-three.

SS: So you treat the full spectrum of female imbalances, and it can happen at any age.

PH: Most menopausal women are aware that they are close to menopause because they might be having symptoms such as hot flashes, mood swings, irritability, sleeplessness, and weight gain. Those are pretty understood symptoms. But young women come in depressed and don't know what is going on with them. Frequently there's a thyroid problem, or sometimes they have very low estrogen. Thankfully there's more awareness as to what's happening, but some of them have not connected those dots.

SS: Why would young girls have low estrogen?

PH: Well, young girls are in a very highly stressed state these days. They aren't getting enough sleep, they are consuming high amounts of sugar, and a lot of them are taking the birth control pill. Low estrogen can be caused by all those symptoms.

SS: So again, it's diet and of course chemicals, right?

PH: Absolutely it's diet. But it's very easy to be exposed to chemicals at every level. We drink water in plastic bottles; we have pesticides and preservatives in food, especially fast food. Without knowing it we consume rancid oils—we do a lot of deep-frying with rancid oils. The exposure to pesticides and chemicals is just very, very high in today's diet, and children are the most sensitive.

SS: What does it do to children?

PH: Chemicals interrupt the natural functioning of the thyroid gland, ovaries, and adrenals. This can cause inflammation in the body. Toxins like mercury in fish and toxins in the air are actual frank carcinogens, and chemicals affect our ability to detoxify.

SS: Explain what it is you do at the Hall Center.

PH: Our goal is to create health and vitality at every age. Many people fear that getting older means losing what we are and getting sick. It doesn't have to be that way. It can be about being more connected with our wisdom and having a powerful stream of energy. We bring together Western science and new forms of healing. At the Hall Center we have brought together various specialists and created a center where we have different tools to help people be healthy. By doing this we can prevent chronic illness and compress illness actually into the last few moments of a person's life; so what we do is prevention and helping people to feel vital and great at any age.

SS: And hormone replacement is part of aging well.

PH: Right.

SS: There are two distinct approaches to medicine that are happening right now. There's standard of care, and then there is what I call break-through medicine.

PH: Yes, a great deal of energy in traditional medicine is spent trying to make the correct diagnosis. At our center, we care more about the processes that got the person sick in the first place, like hormonal imbalance, neuronal imbalance, toxicity, inflammation, cellular health. For instance, inflammation in the body is responsible for 90 percent of cancer. It's responsible for heart disease, it's responsible for dementia, among other things. It almost doesn't matter what diagnosis you are preventing; by addressing the inflammation and other reasons for why things occur you are preventing all the diseases it would create.

SS: So if a person comes in, has chronic indigestion, can't sleep, has no libido, rash all over her body, itching, plus she can't control her moods and has been on a lot of prescription drugs and is sixty-one years old (by the way, I know this person)—what would you do for her?

PH: When you are mentioning all these symptoms I'm thinking about what processes these symptoms might be related to—what imbalance. First thing that comes to mind with a sixty-one-year-old woman is hormones. I would get good blood levels or a twenty-four-hour urine test and establish that. Most likely we'll see very low estrogen, low testosterone, low adrenals, low progesterone, and, very possibly, low thyroid. But at the same time I'm thinking digestion—what is going on with her digestion? Does she have yeast, or parasites, or food allergies? So I would go over her diet and suggest a change and a shake that would start to heal the gut. Because this woman has so many problems I would want to put her into our detox program for two weeks. It decreases toxins, identifies food allergies, and does a very good job resolving GI problems.

SS: Are these problems just a natural part of aging?

PH: There's a wonderful study coming out of Sweden that looked at 23,000 women for causes of death. They identified twelve major categories. Women on bioidentical natural hormones had a decrease in every single category of death compared to women not using bioidentical hormones. For example, main causes of death were stroke, heart attack, breast cancer, colon cancer. It was incredible: In all the different categories there was a 12 percent to 86 percent decrease in terms of death.

So is it important to balance your female hormones? Absolutely it is. There are a lot of good studies showing there's no increased risk of breast cancer with bioidentical hormones. The Mission study came out last July, looking at 6,700 women in the U.S., and their conclusion was no increased risk of breast cancer in giving transdermal bioidentical hormones.

SS: Why isn't this in the news? All you ever hear are the negative reports on synthetic hormones, and women, not knowing the difference, get frightened, choose not to replace hormones, and then live with the uncomfortable and often fatal consequences.

PH: I don't know why, because it is big news. There was also a study in France in 2003. Frenchwomen have been using bioidentical hormones for a long time; they looked at bioidenticals after ten years of use and connected great benefit to the heart, decreased osteoporosis, and no increase risk of breast cancer. Their conclusion was that there was no reason for women to stop their hormones given these positive results.

SS: I guess the European pharmaceutical companies do not have the hold on their government regulatory agencies like ours do here. In our country, pharmaceutical companies know that bioidentical hormone replacement has such positive and profound effects on women's health, but these studies get buried. If we don't see them we can still be frightened into taking synthetic hormones, which have been proven harmful and fatal. I will never understand how this happened. There is nothing positive about synthetic hormones, and yet they are the only menopause hormones that are approved by the FDA.

PH: Well, the European studies are very exciting and validating. We see the profound effects on our patients who take them, and when these studies come out it gives us peace of mind. Synthetic hormones, such as Premarin and Provera, have been shown to cause three times the amount of breast cancer. It's critical to balance hormones naturally to prevent death and morbidity.

SS: How do you give bioidenticals, and how do you decide who gets what version? There's static dose, there's cycling, and there's rhythmic.

PH: The first rule is you only replace the hormones that are missing. I check estrogen, progesterone, and testosterone. And then I check for adrenal hormones, thyroid (T3 and T4). Of course, we cycle the patient—there is no reason, in my opinion, not to cycle in natural progesterone two weeks of every month. If you give continuous combined (natural estrogen and natural progesterone), you are more likely to cause insulin resistance, which brings on weight gain. Women are hungrier when they are on progesterone combined with estrogen. I try to mimic the natural menstrual cycle as much as possible.

SS: But what if a woman comes to you and says, "I don't want a period under any circumstances. I'm not going to do it." Would you then give her continuous combined?

PH: Well, what I do at that point is respect the needs of the patient. I will have a conversation as to why she feels so strongly about it. Sometimes she has had terrible PMS in her youth and she is fearful that it will come back, or sometimes her cycles were ten days of bleeding each month and she doesn't want to relive that. I try to successfully explain that I am not going to bring back the negatives of cycling. Most likely the reason the periods were excessive or painful was due to hormonal imbalance, and my goal in replacement is to bring back balance. I explain the benefits of cycling that include a good night's sleep, decreased insulin resistance, weight loss, good mood, etc., and cancer prevention; at that point most women are willing to give it a try.

SS: Women are starving for relief from their menopausal symptoms, and I truly believe they are getting the message that synthetic hormones are dangerous and don't do the job. Yet replacing hormones with real ones is an "art," and it takes a little time to get the "cocktail" just right. In my experience a lot of women get frustrated, lose patience, and give up. We have been trained for quick relief with pharmaceutical drugs.

PH: That's the challenge, to reverse the thinking. Replacing lost hormones with real bioidenticals will bring a woman back to her old self, but it does take a little time. Sometimes we get it right away; sometimes it's a little more complicated. We take care of such a wide range of women, and some of them are quite ill by the time they come to our office. The majority of patients, 80 percent, are not difficult to adjust. A couple of visits and they are fine, they feel like their lives have been saved; but the other 20 percent have a lot of complications going on with their hormone imbalances. These women usually have to address and then treat their obesity, usually of 50 to 150 pounds; we have to correct their GI tract; and they usually have adrenal fatigue and deficiencies. I always tell the patients that this may take a few visits, and with the really ill patients it may take up to a year to begin getting good results.

For instance, I have a patient from Texas whom I spoke with today, and she needed to lose eighty pounds and it was going very slowly. I was encouraging her along the way, telling her, "It's happening, but you just don't see it yet!" We had already changed her diet, and now she was sleeping nine hours a night, which is such a huge change for many women; however still she was frustrated. But on the phone today she announced that she had lost forty pounds! You see, once it starts to happen, it happens very quickly. These are the turnarounds that bring such joy to this kind of work. I was so happy for her I could have cried myself.

SS: What an uplifting story. And from my own experience I know what it means to get your life back once you have been to the depths of hormonal despair.

Let's talk about the adrenals. Burned-out adrenals make you feel crazy inside; like you are falling off a cliff. You are exhausted but you can't sleep; you may not have any serious problems in your life but you are depressed, you have no energy.

PH: The adrenals are one of the critical hormones. If you have a severe deficiency it can result in death. Adrenal deficiency is due to stress and we live in a highly stressed civilization. Typically an adrenally stressed person will be exhausted, with hair falling out, weight gain, irritability, and frequently skin rashes and acne.

SS: What causes the skin rashes?

PH: Adrenals help support the immune system, and it's all intertwined in terms of adrenals supporting the different cellular types. Rashes are a very common condition when the cellular matrix starts to break down. We become allergic when we have adrenal deficiencies; for example, adrenal people have asthma or food allergies like intolerances to eggs, or wheat, or milk, or citrus. It also makes the person nauseated and/or bloated.

SS: Are food allergies just part of aging—we just can't tolerate certain foods anymore?

PH: If you have a healthy digestive tract and you're not eating food repetitively, there's no need to develop food allergies. But as soon as we start breaking down the integrity of our GI tract and developing something like leaky gut syndrome, then you can develop a food allergy very easily.

SS: Yes, your husband, Dr. Howard Liebowitz, talked extensively about leaky gut in his interview for this book. What about migraine headaches? I think migraines should be called "menopausal headache syndrome," because women can't seem to connect the dots between falling estrogen levels and migraine headaches.

PH: You are right. Migraines are a classic response to low estrogen or fluctuating estrogen levels. It probably has to do with the inflammation that menopausal women experience, but estrogens can directly affect and decrease inflammation. Estrogen usually blocks a molecule called NFkB (nuclear factor kappa beta), but when you are low or deficient in estrogen there is nothing to block this molecule; that is one source of where your migraine headaches come from. This is a molecule of inflammation, and migraine headaches are due to this inflammation.

There are other causes also. Migraine headaches can be due to GI problems. A typically ill menopausal woman will have bloating and gas and stomach pain. When a woman has normal hormones she usually does not experience problems with digestion. However, hormone imbalances create not only digestion problems, but also cause migraine headaches.

SS: What about perimenopausal women? Do they go through all this hell?

PH: *Perimenopausal women also get migraine headaches due to estrogen levels that fall toward the end of the cycle. When I hear this complaint I prescribe a little bit of bioidentical estrogen right around the time of her period and that usually stops the headaches. I have them put it right on their temples. It's efficient, effective, and it takes the pain away without a drug painkiller.*

SS: Isn't that great? We're so used to the pharmaceutical solution. It's difficult to intellectualize the side effects of taking over-the-counter chemicals, or pharmaceuticals like Motrin or Vicodin, when you are in pain. So I am always thrilled when a natural approach can be used—especially when it is something that really works.

PH: I use over-the-counter painkillers only as an interim solution while getting to the root cause of the pain. That headache, or whatever the pain, is actually your friend. It's telling you that something is wrong, and if something is wrong we want to correct it so it doesn't progress into some terrible condition or disease. We know that hormone imbalances are one of the pathways to cancer; migraine headaches are just one of the results of hormone imbalances.

SS: I see the connections, I absolutely do. When I think about my breast cancer, the hormone imbalances are now apparent to me, but I didn't recognize them at the time: the painful swollen breasts every month in my late thirties and early forties, mood swings, lack of libido, weight gain, sleep problems, twenty-two years of birth control pills (thinking they were safe), short periods of about a day or a day and a half. (I now know that a healthy, hormonally balanced woman needs to have a four- or five-day bleed to ovulate fully.) So the signs were there. I was just blind.

PH: None of us knew back then, but the symptoms *are* signs; they are the body talking to us, telling us that we need to pay attention. Memory loss and lost thoughts are also indicators of hormonal imbalances.

Estrogen decreases beta-amyloid plaquing and also helps prevent Alzheimer's disease; plus, estrogen helps the neurons connect to each other in the brain. So I would say if anyone was concerned about dementia, the best prevention would be natural bioidentical estrogens. It's a first-line therapy for a healthy brain.

SS: What's with all the autoimmune diseases? I mean, five years ago I had never heard of lupus or fibromyalgia, and now I know dozens of women with these diseases. Why the epidemic?

PH: Menopause causes extreme fatigue states and also pain, which gets confusing because these symptoms are also the hallmarks of fibromyalgia in its inception. In order for me to differentiate I must rule out these symptoms as menopausal. I look at adrenal exhaustion and the thyroid. If that checks out okay, then I check for hidden viruses causing a hypercoaguable state. That's when the viruses are hidden in the body.

SS: Are you talking about thick blood?

PH: Yes. A hypercoaguable state is superclotted, thick, sticky blood. Thirty percent of the population was given the genes to have blood that was too thick. It worked great for our ancestors to protect them from bleeding to death on the battlefield. Today, with all the viruses around—Epstein-Barr, microplasm virus, HHV6 (Humanherpesvirus 6), and many more, including cancer—this thick blood works against us.

SS: You mean because the viruses can hide in the thick blood?

PH: Yes. They hide in the blood, which acts kind of like a wall, sort of like the king being protected in his castle. The immune system, which is usually protective, can't get rid of these viruses because they are buried in this thick blood, so they continue to cause problems in the patient. The good news is now we can diagnose this condition (hypercoaguable state) and treat it with something called "transfer factors" that are created specifically for each virus.

SS: How do you treat the viruses with transfer factors? Are they a supplement?

PH: Yes. You see, thick blood (which is dark blood) is starting to be implicated in all the diseases of chronic aging. There is now a lot of research on this and it holds great promise and hope for people who might have the potential to develop chronic diseases long before they even thought of it happening. So this is a long explanation of the seeming epidemic of autoimmune diseases like lupus or fibromyalgia. Check your blood. Make sure it's not thick. Check for viruses. There are blood tests that now tell you if you have viruses, the best one being the Hemex Laboratories test.

SS: And the remedy is to keep your hormone levels at optimum, catching them before they fall or as early as possible to prevent these conditions from happening?

PH: Yes. That's exactly one of the tenets of this new style of medicine: to prevent rather than treat. You see, traditional medicine won't make a diagnosis until the patient is quite ill. For example, with a blood sugar, they will wait until a blood sugar level is all the way up to 120 before they warn the patient that they might have a serious problem. The way we treat is different: Once a blood sugar is above an ideal of 75 we want to intervene and help that patient get back to normal. We look for the ideal state, and not what is sick.

SS: You know, I perform onstage and I have become very aware of throat clearing. It's as though every one has phlegm, and the men make very loud noises. I'm sure they are so used to it they don't hear it, but the women are making constant noises also.

PH: It can be from a couple of different causes. They could be having reflux, which is a result of poor digestion where the food is not digesting completely and backs up a little bit into the lower part of the throat. They could also be suffering from inflammation. Dental health and dental hygiene could cause throat clearing. You don't want to have any root canals or implants in your jaw, and you definitely don't want to have metal amalgams, because it sets up an inflammation in the sinuses and in the head. It causes a postnasal drip. Then a lot of older people are taking Fosamax for their bones and osteoporosis—I've had numerous patients develop a slight cough due to Fosamax. A much better way to deal with your bones and preventing osteoporosis is to replace your estrogens.

SS: Well, I am not a fan of Fosamax at all. It doesn't fix the lost bone situation, it just prevents you from losing any more bone. But hormones (estrogen and progesterone) actually *rebuild* bone and they are not drugs. How does it all get so off base? Why would we take a drug when there is a natural alternative that actually works better?

PH: I, too, am a big believer in going natural as the first line. You see, I believe in vitality at any age. By correcting imbalances in your body before they become a real problem, you could prevent illness until the last few minutes of your life. That would be the ideal; you work until you are a hundred and then you die. But as it stands now, people spend a third of their lives quite ill. They have heart disease, cancers, and this really does not have to be the way we age.

SS: I couldn't agree more, now that we have the knowledge there is a real opportunity to live a long life and die healthy.

PH: Yes. For instance, breast cancer: There are so many ways to prevent breast cancer. Exercise is a huge component, and balanced female hormones. There are new studies showing that women are 28 percent less likely to die of breast cancer when they have balanced hormones. Women can't sleep and that is a contributor to breast cancer. Without sleep, cortisol levels (cortisol is one of your major hormones) won't go down, and also without sleep a woman or man won't produce melatonin. Melatonin is an aromatase inhibitor, crucial in creating hormone balance. I put my patients on curcumin, iodine, and green tea. I put them on melatonin and encourage them not to drink too much wine or alcohol. I help them to prevent obesity. I balance their hormones and treat them with real, natural bioidentical hormones. All of these things add up to feeling good and real, true cancer *prevention*.

SS: It's almost like a recipe, huh?

PH: Yes. It can be something as easy as correcting thyroid levels; if you pick up that the T3 is low, that gives an increased risk for breast cancer. How can I impress upon everyone that you need to be sure that *all* your hormones are balanced to prevent breast cancer and cancer in general?

SS: So it's not just putting back estrogen and progesterone, it's a whole "song."

PH: Yes. You want to be sure that each hormone that is missing is replaced. I find at our center that most patients are low in thyroid, and once that is replaced a whole myriad of symptoms decrease or go away. Hair that's thinning, memory that's off, constipation, depression; this is all low thyroid. Then I correct the GI tract, encourage the patient to sleep eight and nine hours a night, and get them to do smart exercise, where the exercise is not overly exhausting to the patient.

SS: Can people exercise too much?

PH: Absolutely. Too much exercise actually causes damage; heavy exercise causes oxidative stress and creates free radicals. That wears the body down. Smart exercise incorporates doing something called "intervals," where you'll exercise for thirty seconds and then rest for a minute or two, then hit it again. Weights are good, yoga is good, Pilates—these are all good exercises.

SS: There's a lot of buzz about free radicals. Essentially we take in antioxidants to eat up the free radicals, right?

PH: That's exactly right. We make free radicals mainly in the liver, but also in every cell in the body. If a toxin is brought into the liver (as in diet sodas and chemicals), there are two phases of liver detoxification: In phase I, oxygen attaches to the toxin (that is actually what a free radical is—toxin and oxygen); then in phase II molecules like glutathione and sulfur are attached to it to make it *nontoxic*. This is how it is all supposed to work. This is our body doing its magnificent protective healing. But— and here's the big but—if phase II of the liver isn't working quickly enough (because you are consuming chemical-laden food, diet sodas, overexercising), you start developing a lot of free radicals, and free radicals are where we get disease—cancer, etc. If you take in a lot of toxins, the second phase of the liver just can't handle it. This is why I stress my patients take *antioxidants*, plus I stress good diet, good diet, good diet. Then take your anti-inflammatories, curcumin and resveratrol (the kind found in supplements or red wine).

SS: Curcumin is the spice turmeric, and I cook with it a lot.

PH: Yes. Cook with it, cook with all the spices. It's so much better to get your foods naturally if you can. It's difficult these days to get food naturally, but try your best and juice your vegetables. If we did this religiously I'm not even sure we would need supplements.

SS: How do you reach your patients relative to diet? We all hear, "Eat right," but do we really listen?

PH: There is an epiphany in everyone's health where they really look at themselves and their family history and realize that they want to direct their love and care toward themselves. It's an aha! moment. I see this a lot in my menopausal women who are at that stage of life: They've raised their children, lavished love upon their communities and their families, and now they are ready for themselves. When they are at that moment of being "in action," then diet and eating well make perfect sense. When they're not at that place, it's very difficult to try to convince a person, but I consider myself an ally with my patients. They want to be well and get well, and often it's just a matter of convincing them to know how important it is to change their lifestyle and diet in order to avoid disease and poor health. On the other hand, sometimes it's a matter of having to experience suffering and disease before they actually have that epiphany with their own health.

SS: So you become a mentor or a coach of sorts?

PH: Yes, that's a good description; it's being empathetic and really wanting to be of service.

SS: If a woman doesn't choose to change her life, or balance her hormones, or change her diet, or her thoughts, or her bad lifestyle habits, what can she expect?

PH: Having talked with so many women for so many years, and hearing of the abuse, neglect, and betrayals . . . all the things women experience, I realize that I am here not only to redirect their health as their doctor, but also to help them understand they can become loving toward themselves and connected to all love. One of the areas of medicine that is starting to attract attention is energetic healing, how to get to the root core causes of unhappiness and problems. When you address the core issues that stop us in life, we are much more able to move forward to give self-care and self-love.

SS: You are an aberration. Most of us go to the doctor and we get eight minutes and a prescription for an antidepressant. I remember one time I was sitting in a doctor's office and I mentioned that when I ate a lot of vegetables my skin got better. He looked at me and said, "Vegetables are bullshit," and promptly wrote me a prescription for an antibiotic to clear up my acne breakout. So you are a breath of fresh air, and we women want someone like you in our lives. There has to be somewhere we can go to get the answers. As the matriarch of my own family and the mother of a son, I spend most of my time nurturing others. To have a doctor who will go the extra distance is thrilling.

PH: Hormone loss is no joke. Hormones push all the buttons; when they are balanced they make you feel alive and vibrant, and when they are not balanced they make you feel detached, depressed, and unhappy. As the doctor, I have to be understanding of the moodiness and the depression and the overwhelming frustration of weight gain. I can do this because I know if they stay with it they will feel good again. That's why I love this work. It requires patience on the part of the patient and the doctor, but it's constant progress. We are always celebrating at the center because the patient has moved forward.

SS: Energy seems to be the missing component as we age. We just run out of gas. Is this the way it has to be?

PH: This is one of the most common complaints we hear. It happens because we overwork ourselves, our hormones become imbalanced, we are not eating foods that have good value for us, this all adds up to energy deficiency. Some of the medicines we take deplete us of our energy. Statins actually kill the mitochondria that make our energy.

SS: Mitochondria are the power center of our cells, right?

PH: Yes, so if we become energy depleted, that's a fairly big emergency in our life. The only reason we are alive is that our mitochondria create our energy. Imagine if you put a plant into a dark room and you cut off its energy source? It would die.

SS: That's a huge statement, because so many people are on statins.

PH: There are many alternative ways of dealing with high cholesterol without using statins. In fact, I am very, very concerned about the widespread use of statins in our society. This is really the work of my husband, Dr. Howard Liebowitz, but I believe that statins are going to prove that they have not been a good thing in the long run.

SS: Why? What do you see down the road?

PH: When they do muscle biopsies, they are finding that the muscles are dying. The way the muscle gets energy is by these little cells called the mitrochondria, the energy center of each cell. Without mitochondria, that whole cell will die. So statins kill off the mitrochondria, and we are seeing people who are extremely fatigued because they can't create the energy they need.

SS: It's crazy. Let me see if I follow: Statins such as Lipitor inhibit the body from making any more cholesterol, yet the brain and the gut both need cholesterol to reproduce new neuronal cells (brain cells and neurons in the gut). So Lipitor (or any statin) is inhibiting brain cellular reproduction and messing with the GI tract (which is the second brain), preventing it from making neurons in the gut; statins kill the mitochondria, which are our energy source from our cells; and the lack of mitochondria is killing the muscles and draining our energy. What a deal. And Lipitor and all the statins are expensive!

Let's talk about sleeping . . . no woman sleeps. They are up all night reading romance novels.

PH: When women have low estrogen they end up with high cortisol and, of course, cortisol is a stress hormone. Low estrogen causes stress in the female body, and when you correct the female hormones by giving them bioidentical estrogen and cycling with progesterone, plus melatonin at night, sleep returns. Melatonin is actually considered to be neuron protective, and there are wonderful studies showing how it can help prevent Alzheimer's disease. There are also precursors for serotonin such as 5-HTP, which also induces sleep, but again you have to get to the root problem. If the patient is highly stressed, then stress management is extremely important, and usually if the woman is menopausal, her stress is exacerbated because her hormones aren't balanced.

SS: So it's very clear: The backbone of the entire second half of life is replacing hormones with real bioidentical ones.

PH: Yes. Simple as that.

SS: Depression seems to be part of aging—why is that?

PH: There are two large reasons for depression. One of them is hormonal. If you have low thyroid it can definitely cause depression. Low estrogen and progesterone can cause depression, as can low cortisol and low

DHEA. The second reason is the spiritual and consciousness issues that come up with people as they age. We are so busy in the first half of our lives, but in the second half we are given this opportunity to allow for personal transformation and to experience a much richer and stronger life—being filled with gratitude, truly understanding who you are and what has made you who you are, thinking about what you want in life and how to achieve those things, and undergoing transformative processes to obtain happiness. Sometimes this process starts with therapy, and then it can go deeper into stronger kinds of energies, such as connecting with the divine in your life. It's ongoing. As women enter the passage of menopause they ask the same questions: Who do they want to be in life, and what makes them happy? They're done caring for their families, or certainly it's becoming less of a concern, so they are able to look more deeply at their lives. I'm not talking about religion; I'm talking about the mystic, divine connection that makes people extremely happy.

SS: So, this is the whole mind, body, spirit connection?

PH: Yes. You can't leave out the spirit, and if we do the glass is half full. Our consciousness plays a big part in being alive and joyful. As I sit with my patients, I am cognizant of what they're feeling and what I'm feeling, because we're cut from the same fabric.

SS: When I send patients to you they always come back marveling at your compassion; that you listen to them and they feel that you care. I say, "It's for real, she really does care, she really is involved with everyone who comes to her." You are doing the work you were supposed to do, Prudence.

PH: It's a passion. I am so lucky to be alive and to have work that I love to do. We're all given gifts, and to use our gifts to a higher purpose is the best joy in life.

SS: So, red wine . . . what's the deal? Is it good for us?

PH: A glass of red wine from time to time is probably a good thing. It has resveratrol, and there are studies from France—and one in particular, the Lyon Diet Heart Study—showing that resveratrol prevents disease.

SS: But not many women drink red wine; they love white wine, primarily because it doesn't make your teeth red. But there's no resveratrol in white wine, right?

PH: No, just the red. So red wine is actually beneficial to your health in small quantities, or you can take a resveratrol pill.

SS: But not as much fun.

PH: True. I don't tell my patients that they have to give up alcohol. My brother James is the vintner of Patz and Hall, so I appreciate a nice glass of wine. Some doctors are very strict and say alcohol of any type is unhealthy, but there is good data showing that small amounts of red wine are actually beneficial.

SS: Are you excited about the possibilities of stem cells?

PH: Oh yes. Certainly stem-cell research is where great longevity and hope will come for us in the future in terms of chronic illness; in fact, our son's friend's father survived because he received stem cells. Now people can bank their own stem cells when they are young and healthy and freeze them, so if down the road you develop leukemia or lymphomas or a wide variety of diseases, or you need a new organ or you need to grow a new lung or a new heart or a new pancreas you could. Wouldn't that be wonderful? We are now a stem cell collection site at our center and we are very excited about it. The possibilities are tremendous. You could treat menopause by creating a new ovary. So, yes, stem cell treatment excites me. There are other centers that are collecting stem cells from the individual to store for the future right now, and the best part is that you can do this knowing you can help regrow parts of yourself that are sick.

SS: Yes, it's incredible. And you wouldn't have to worry about rejection.

PH: Right, you can't reject yourself. When you start thinking about it, two hundred years is probably a reasonable amount of time that people could live in the next thirty or forty years. There is a lot of research going on as to the extent of our longevity; right now it's clocked at 120 years. But the goal is to live well and feel well, not just live a long time; so it's a matter of correcting all the imbalances to live a long, healthy life with energy and vitality without chronic disease—waking up and feeling vital. The goal is quality life, health, and energy.

SS: And you believe that's possible?

PH: It's possible right now. It's not a fantasy; it's what I teach my patients to do every day.

SS: But I am watching so many people who are becoming "pharmaceutical products." I want to shout *stop!* I feel helpless because I am watching them run out of gas. They have no energy; theirs is just a general run-down, fatigued existence. This accumulation of pharmaceutical drugs is not making them "well"; in fact, it's just a slow, numb death. It's very sad.

PH: It's the mind-set, Suzanne. People everywhere in this country are spending the last years of their lives taking every drug imaginable and therefore have a decreased quality of life. Not enough attention is being put into prevention. We don't have to die sick. We can live until we are old and be in excellent health with vibrant energy. It can happen if you look at the root imbalances that cause the symptoms that eventually cause the disease. If you stay on top of it you never have to develop the diagnosis. You don't have to develop the illness. That's prevention, and prevention is correcting imbalances early on. That's the exciting new medicine and we are practicing it right now.

SS: When you leave your office each day, how do you feel about yourself and the work you are doing?

PH: [laughs] I feel gratitude to my patients who have honored me by sharing their lives, and I am incredibly thankful to be able to live the life that I have: to be connected with life, with love and joy. I can't think of anything I'd rather be doing.

SS: You leave me speechless because I know you and I know you mean it. Thank you, Prudence.

DR. PRUDENCE HALL'S
BREAKTHROUGH BREAKOUTS

- Migraines during menopause are a classic response to low estrogen or fluctuating estrogen levels, in part because estrogen usually blocks NFkB, a molecule of inflammation that among other things causes migraine headaches. Estrogen replacement can relieve the headaches.

- Statins (like Lipitor) inhibit the creation of cholesterol but harm the cells' mitochondria, causing problems both with neural cell development and with energy.

- Autoimmune diseases like lupus or fibromyalgia can be caused by a hypercoaguable state in blood, which can harbor viruses. Have a Hemex blood test to check for viruses and thick blood.

- Heavy and exhausting exercise causes oxidative stress and creates free radicals. Smart exercise incorporates intervals, where you'll exercise for thirty seconds and then rest for a minute or two, then hit it again. Weight training, yoga, and Pilates are all good exercises.

- To reduce free radicals, take antioxidants, eat a good diet, and take anti-inflammatories like curcumin (found in the spice turmeric) and resveratrol (found in supplements or red wine).

- In addition to their physical health, women need to address their mental and spiritual health as they go through menopause, in order to avoid depression. Take time to ask who do you want to be in life and what makes you happy.

20

STEP 5: AVOID PHARMACEUTICALS UNLESS ABSOLUTELY NECESSARY

Sixty-six percent of all department chairs at universities in America have financial contracts with pharmacy device companies, so it makes sense that the pharmaceutical industry in this country is about developing artificial remedies that you can patent. That's why you won't find research on nonpatentable natural cures and healing.

—Dr. Khalid Mahmud

HOW DID IT GET THIS WAY? How is it that every condition or ailment has a magic pill to take the problem away? Why have we so blindly accepted this easy fix? Why have we tried to outthink nature? Why is our present approach to medicine so misguided? We go to the doctor, she has eight minutes to spend with us, we tell her our complaints, and she gives us a prescription for a drug to "handle" the ailment. (Notice I didn't say "heal.")

We spend a lifetime on antibiotics, painkillers, sleeping pills, tranquilizers, synthetic hormones, blood pressure medications, cholesterol-lowering statins, and antidepressants, trying desperately to maintain our health or take care of a problem once we get sick. No one gets *well* on pharmaceuticals. We might get *better,* but drugs don't heal. In fact, the side effects of most pharmaceuticals usually create a need for another pharmaceutical and so on and so on. It's a vicious, unending cycle to nowhere. Pharmaceuticals can build up in our system, leading to a breakdown of our bodies and a toxic environment that is a breeding ground for diseases. The end result? The nursing home.

Breakthrough medicine is not about disease care but about building up our bodies to the point that we never suffer from illness in the first place. Standard medical care involves reaching for a pill to make us better, instead of taking care of our bodies so we don't need pharmaceuticals. The doctors in this book believe in medicine that uses pharmaceuticals as a last resort—sometimes we do need drugs. But our prescribe-a-pill culture is masking our real need to take care of our bodies to avoid illness in the first place, and sometimes makes us more sick in the process. Step 5 to Wellness is about avoiding pharmaceuticals unless absolutely necessary.

Why are we turning so much to pharmaceuticals? You may not realize that drug corporations control health care, including influencing the medical education of most of our doctors. Again, when you have exhausted all natural approaches, particularly in association with pain, infection, or mental illness, then pharmaceuticals are a godsend. But when you can heal a disease or condition, or if your body needs hormone replacement, why would you choose a drug if there is a natural way to approach the problem?

The largest political lobbying force in Washington is the drug companies. These drug lobbyists are able to manipulate legislation that highly favors their abilities to sell their expensive brands. It is in the best interest of drug companies to create an environment where we have no choice but to take their drugs. Their bottom line is business, and they work closely with the FDA to regulate their pharmaceutical drugs and to rule out natural nonpatentable medicines. Their reasoning is that nonpatentable medicines have not gone through rigorous double-blind studies (which is not true; there are many studies done on bioidentical hormones).

One example of this happened in early 2008. The FDA actually started the process whereby women would not have access to natural bioidentical estriol, the component of estrogen, which protects women from breast cancer. It is difficult to understand until you realize that Premarin and Prempro, the FDA-approved menopause drugs, do not contain estriol. Wyeth Pharmaceuticals filed this complaint with the FDA, and the FDA sent out warnings to five major compounding pharmacies in America warning them to stop selling estriol. Taking out the breast-protective component in the bioidentical estrogen compromises its effectiveness and takes away our protection. Doctors tell women that bioidenticals and synthetics are the same thing, which is untrue, but this makes natural hormones unappealing to women, so they would be more likely to resort to Premarin and Prempro.

Let's talk about Premarin and Prempro. If I convince you of one thing in this book, it is to run, don't walk, from these two drugs. As I discussed in my chapters on bioidentical hormone replacement, these hormones are unnatural drugs, shown to increase cancer and vascular risks. They are made from pregnant mare's urine. A horse has thirty-four different estrogens not including estriol, and none of these are compatible with a human woman, yet these two drugs are approved by the FDA, even though the Women's Health Initiative in 2002 declared that "it would be better for women to take nothing at all than to take these dangerous, harmful, and even fatal drugs." So why is Wyeth Pharmaceuticals selling over two billion dollars' worth of these dangerous drugs yearly to unsuspecting women? This is a serious question, particularly in light of some recent court cases regarding Wyeth.

If you Google "Wyeth and hormone drugs" you will see many articles such as "Wyeth Hit with $134.5 Million Hormone-Replacement Verdict." The jury ruled that "Premarin and Prempro were defective products and Wyeth concealed a material fact about the safety of the product." The jury also answered yes to the question "Did you find by clear and convincing evidence that Wyeth acted with malice and fraud?" Wyeth is fighting some 5,300 similar lawsuits in state and federal courts across the country. There has never been a lawsuit regarding bioidentical natural hormones. Why would a woman take fake synthetic drug hormones when real, natural bioidentical hormones are available?

Drugs do not have to be the answer for most conditions. There are numerous natural alternatives and supplements that are effective and provide healing to do the job in lieu of many of the most common drugs that people begin to take from the time they reach middle age.

For instance:

- Instead of Ambien for sleep problems, why not take melatonin? Melatonin is a natural over-the-counter hormone intended for sleep and is also an effective antioxidant made in our own bodies until we reach middle age.
- Instead of diuretics, why not take natural progesterone, which is nature's natural diuretic?
- Instead of statins, why not take over-the-counter niacin and or nattokinase, a natural blood thinner?
- Instead of antidepressants, why not go on a bioidentical hormone regimen that regulates your mood and replaces your declining endocrine system daily?

The list goes on—the doctors in this book talk about so many natural, breakthrough alternatives to drugs. Whenever we can heal ourselves without taking drugs, allowing nature to take its course, we are better off. We know this intuitively, but a simple pill seems so easy . . . and fast!

Take, for example, inflammation. At its most basic level, inflammation is a defensive reaction to a specific infectious agent, toxin, or injury. Inflammation is the heat of a fever, inflammation is what turns the tissue around a splinter red or causes swelling in an injured toe. Inflammation is the body's natural healing mechanism. It activates a defensive attack the instant a deadly microbe slips into the body. Once this process subsides, healing begins. But the moment we experience recognizable inflammation we run to the doctor and demand to be given something to stop it, whether it is the swelling of a sprained ankle, a toothache, a sore throat, or a sunburn. Inflammation is an indication of proinflammatory cytokines at work, helping our bodies—in other words, this kind of inflammation is our friend in disguise. But in today's allopathic medical protocol, a natural response to any condition in most cases is not allowed to exist, yet inflammation importantly disables pathogens and repairs damaged tissue.

After a serious injury or surgery, high levels of inflammatory chemicals in your blood are elevated. Once the healing process is under way the inflammation subsides and the levels of inflammatory chemicals in the blood return to normal.

Nature has it figured out. Nature has the inflammatory process hardwired into our systems and brains, yet we prefer to take painkillers and other drugs to do the job. The sad part is that everyone from middle age on (commensurate with declining hormones) experiences bodily decline. This creates a variety of symptoms, from sleeplessness, weight gain, anxiety, depression, high cholesterol, autoimmune diseases, high blood pressure, cancer, heart disease, and dementia.

For every one of these conditions there is a drug waiting to be sold. Soon the patient has a virtual tackle box of pharmaceuticals, and the interaction of prescription drugs often creates an inability to think, and in many cases a brain fog, which makes taking care of oneself impossible.

Think about the alternatives to every bodily response before you jump onto the pharmaceutical bandwagon. When we stop the inflammation process with a drug, we leave our bodies confused. By trying a natural approach to pain, by using natural methods of replacement and regeneration, you will be better off, you will be healthier, you will live longer, you will not have devastating side effects, and you will retain your life as you know it. Right now is your chance and your hope. . . . You can turn the tide of your health and educate yourself about other methods of natural medication. Pharmaceutical drugs do not have to be abandoned, just minimized and used only when absolutely necessary. This is an essential element in the 8 Steps to Wellness.

The next few chapters talk about three big issues—high cholesterol, cancer, and hysterectomy. In all three chapters you will see that the standard-of-care approach to illness—such as taking statins, undergoing chemotherapy, or undergoing hysterectomy for bleeding—is often ineffective at best or even harmful. It is important to go through all options with a knowledgeable doctor, so you are not taking a pill or having surgery unless it is absolutely necessary. Remember, there are alternatives!

21

STATINS

If Nietzsche were alive today, he could be pitching antidepressants for Pfizer.

—Jan Morris, *Guardian*, March 27, 2004

ARE YOU ON LIPITOR, or any of the many statin drugs? How has it happened that virtually everyone at age fifty-plus suddenly needs a statin drug? By following the path of this phenomenon, it clearly began when traditional medicine concentrated on cholesterol as the supposed culprit in arteriosclerosis (hardening of the arteries) and atherosclerosis (plaque in the arteries). This was a big bonanza for the pharmaceutical companies, and they were ready; they decided that the simplest way to lower cholesterol was to "cut it off at the pass."

Sounded logical, so everyone bought into it—the patients (my husband included), even the doctors themselves. Everyone was thrilled when their blood tests came back and their cholesterol levels had lowered. Whew! Now we didn't have to worry about heart attacks. Statins were declared a "miracle," and everyone from middle age on was urged to start taking them. They were expensive but "worth it." After all, if you have to spend a little money not to have a heart attack, why not?

Now that half of all adults in America are on this type of drug, we are learning (and as most of the doctors interviewed in this book have stated) that cholesterol manipulation may be irrelevant to removing plaque in the arteries, and irrelevant to stopping heart disease. As I'll explain, cholesterol is not really a bad thing, and statins not only do not necessarily stop heart disease, but they can also lead to a host of problems that are truly frightening—from nerve dysfunction to muscle-wasting disease to dementia and memory loss to lack of sex drive.

THE SCIENCE:
HOW STATINS INHIBIT CHOLESTEROL

Cholesterol is produced in the human body when *glucose* (the fuel of our bodies) is converted into a two-carbon molecule, "the building blocks of life," which are known as *acetyl-CoA*. These two fragments combine to start the cholesterol pathway.

Next, three molecules of acetyl-CoA combine to form the six-carbon *hydroxymethyl glutaric acid*, which is part of the intermediate complex known as *HMG-CoA*. When two molecules of HMG-CoA combine to form *mevalonic acid*, the resulting cholesterol enzyme is inhibited.

Researchers jumped for joy when they discovered this information, realizing that the "weak point" was finding the inhibition of the important enzyme. They never stopped to think that inhibiting cholesterol would affect the rest of the body's systems.

They forged ahead and suddenly the multibillion-dollar statin industry was born. They had it . . . the development of HMG-CoA-reductase *inhibitors*, which stopped the cholesterol enzyme and became known as all the various statin drugs, including Lipitor, Mevacor, Zocor, Pravachol, Crestor, and Baycol. They all use this same mechanism and are merely variations of the same theme.

HEART DISEASE AND NERVE DAMAGE

First let me explain why statins don't stop heart disease. It's a series of events. Aging people overexpress a molecule called nuclear factor kappa beta (NFkB), which then ignites a lethal cascade throughout the body. NFkB acts like a switch to turn "on" inflammation if you live an unhealthy lifestyle with a poor diet, but it turns "off" the inflammation switch if you are in good health.

NFkB in the body acts like a smoke sensor. It detects dangerous threats such as free radicals and infectious agents. So to recap: NFkB works *for* us if we practice a healthy lifestyle and eat a good diet, but in the presence of poor health, bad diet, and unhealthy lifestyle, NFkB works *against* us, turning the inflammation switch to on. Inflammation, not cholesterol, is the primary culprit in heart disease.

Now, here is where it gets complicated. Statins *do* inhibit NFkB, which is why the drug apparently works, but by inhibiting NFkB, it also inhibits the effectiveness of our immune system, which matters because the immune system is our defense system. Because of this, inflammation can run out of control, causing among other things . . . heart disease.

It gets worse. Statins inhibit our vital $Co-Q_{10}$ (coenzyme Q_{10}), which is our most important essential nutrient. $Co-Q_{10}$ is responsible for the body's production of energy and is present in its highest concentrations in the heart and liver. Supplementing with $Co-Q_{10}$ capsules is one of the primary ways to keep our heart healthy. Inhibiting $Co-Q_{10}$ can lead to heart attack for many statin users.

Dr. Peter Langsjoen, a well-known cardiologist, has published several articles reporting that reducing or removing statin drugs from heart patients' protocol *improves* their chances of surviving.

$Co-Q_{10}$ is found in all cell membranes. It has many vital functions, including keeping the lining of each cell membrane elastic. Statins are responsible for the breakdown of cell walls, and, because of that, are suspected to be the potential cause of neuropathy, a condition in a nerve or a group of nerves that causes pain and dysfunction, and myopathy, a muscle-wasting disease that is now rampant in middle-age adults.

Polyneuropathy (pain in more than one nerve area) is reported among long-term statin users and should be of special concern to diabetics, many of whom have been prescribed statins because of their high-risk status.

Doctors know that a very common outcome of longstanding diabetes is peripheral neuropathy, a loss of nerve function, causing tingling, numbness, and pain. To prescribe statins to these patients because of their predisposition to heart attack and stroke is a serious decision. It requires a delicate balance of judgment that should be undertaken only after painful soul-searching on the part of the doctor.

There's more (a lot more). Statins are also associated with an inflammation of the muscles called myositis and rhabdomyolysis, a condition where the breakdown of the muscle fibers results in the release of muscle fiber contents into the bloodstream, causing blockage of the kidneys.

A popular statin has already been removed from the market primarily because of muscle cell breakdown. Unfortunately, many people died before the pharmaceutical company took action. The breakdown of muscle fibers, which can lead to death, still occurs because all the currently "approved" statin drugs share the Co-Q_{10}-depleting side effects, but to a slightly lesser degree. It seems FDA-approved ain't what it's cracked up to be.

Read Dr. Jonathan Wright's interview (see chapter 2) regarding one of the statin manufacturers that had actually obtained a patent for combining a statin with Co-Q_{10} but withheld the drug from the marketplace because it would be forced to make the shocking admission that the statin drug was doing serious damage that needed offsetting with Co-Q_{10}.

Curtailing Co-Q_{10} production with statins leads to other problems besides breakdown in the muscle fibers. Co-Q_{10} feeds the mitochondria, the energy centers of the cell—adequate stores of Co-Q_{10} act like a powerful antioxidant with a free-radical-quenching ability fifty times greater than that of vitamin E. Without adequate stores of Co-Q_{10}, our cells lack the necessary repair mechanisms. Just remember, antioxidants eat up free radicals. Free radicals are the little "home wreckers" in our bodies responsible for disease, including cancer and heart problems. Statins inhibit Co-Q_{10}, which is our body's most powerful free-radical-quenching mechanism.

THE CASE AGAINST STATINS

Statins can:
- alter the immune system
- inhibit Co-Q_{10} production (our most important nutrient), which leads to loss of nerve function, muscle disease, and pain in more than one nerve (neuropathy, myopathy, and polyneuropathy)
- cause inflammation of the muscles (myositis and deadly rhabdomyolysis)
- lead to breakdowns in muscle fiber and the release of myoglobin, which blocks the kidneys
- cause brain damage, dementia, and "memory lapses"

MEMORY LOSS

The brain is composed of neurons and neurotransmitters. Each neuron in the brain requires cholesterol to replicate. If we are taking a statin drug that inhibits our body's ability to manufacture any more cholesterol, then our brain is left without the necessary tools to continue replicating new healthy brain cells.

It starts with "senior moments": forgetting who you are going to call when you reach the phone, losing a thought midsentence, or forgetting what you did yesterday. These things are most often laughed off as part of the onset of aging, and usually they have much to do with declining hormones, which is easily rectified with hormone replacement. Most everyone becomes aware at some point in his or her life of the vagaries of memory; it is frustrating, but a long life is filled with lots of memories and experiences and it is natural that some would have faded away.

But in memory loss with statins we are talking about complete failure of the imprinting mechanism: an inability to formulate new memory, having no recall because there has been no memory processing. Like a newborn, each experience is brand-new except there is no *accumulation* of new memories . . . just one new memory after another, with nothing being saved—essentially being "brain dead."

It takes time, years sometimes.

I know of two friends whose mother has been on a combination of statins, diet soda, chemotherapy, and radiation. She is a beautiful, vibrant woman who now can't remember a moment ago, who gets lost routinely, who leaves the oven blazing away, who asks the same question over and over. The stress on the grown children and their families is overwhelming. She appears "fine" to the outside world, maybe a little repetitive but functioning, but the brain loss is accelerating, and it is clear she will follow in the template of today—overdrugged and finally confined to a nursing home. There is no going back, just a long, lonesome, frightening road to the end.

We have come to expect statin side effects such as liver damage, muscle pain, nerve damage, and heart failure, but the increasing cognitive side effects from statin drugs are completely unexpected by both patient and physician.

Sometimes symptoms begin within weeks of starting medication; in other cases several years might pass before the onset of symptoms. The symptoms are a full array of cognitive side effects, ranging from amnesia to severe memory loss, confusion, and disorientation.

To *tamper* with one's memory is unconscionable. When medications that are prescribed for a patient go way beyond their intended purpose, when memory is destroyed or distorted, the medical community needs to investigate what went wrong and then correct it. But this medication is a ten-billion-dollar-a-year business. I am not hopeful that the pharmaceutical companies will examine what has gone wrong with statins and put their profits at risk. The situation is ripe for someone else to come in and expose the pharmaceutical companies, like *The Insider* (starring Russell Crowe) did with the story of how tobacco companies were complicit in withholding information from the public concerning the deadly consequences of smoking.

STATINS AND SEX DRIVE

There are a variety of reasons why the libido diminishes as we age; most often it is due to hormonal decline, which again is easily rectified by a qualified doctor who specializes in bioidentical hormone replacement. Emotional problems also contribute to sexual dysfunction and usually that is hormonal in origin unless you are clinically depressed, yet even clinical depression is often hormonal in origin.

Women who have had a hysterectomy, especially those who have had their ovaries, uterus, and cervix removed, will not be able to ever "feel" sex again (women are rarely told this before the procedure) unless they restore their bodies to full hormone replacement, which means estrogen and progesterone taken in a "cycle" to mimic nature. Rarely do women get an informed doctor who understands this necessity, so most women are put on synthetic estrogen, with no progesterone, and told to have a nice life (and a sexless one, I might add).

Men with prostate removal can no longer enjoy sex.

People who have been overmedicated, those who have endured chemotherapy as well as various other medications that impair function, and those suffering from extreme stress can have lower sex drives, too.

What about statins? Cholesterol, which we have been taught to fear, is our sole source for our sex hormones: testosterone, estrogen, and progesterone. Cholesterol is the parent from which these hormones are derived. Statins inhibit cholesterol production, and we now know that statins deplete testosterone. Testosterone is essential for a sex drive (for men *and* women), as well as for building bone and muscle.

According to Dr. Duane Graveline (spacedoc.net), who is a huge opponent of the use of statin drugs, "Testosterone levels are depleted by statins. Drug company researchers are well aware that testosterone blood levels correlate poorly with sex drive. Every student of this area knows that a high serum testosterone may be associated with a complete lack of sexual interest, and a low level for this testosterone is not at all unusual in sexual 'athletes.' There is an extremely wide range of 'normal' with respect to testosterone levels. The key, according to drug company researchers and primary care MDs counseling on ED and low-libido patients, is 'how your current blood levels for testosterone compares with what it used to be twenty years ago,' and, of course, most people do not have this on record."

Bottom line, according to Dr. Graveline (please notice his cynicism), "There is a consistent tendency for decreased testosterone biosyntheses once statins have been started but the thinking of the pharmaceutical companies is that testosterone correlates poorly with sexuality therefore you can feel comfortable about using it." . . . Researchers have done their duty; the data is presented "honestly," meaning pharmaceutical tracks have been artfully covered, and as the patient takes his first statin pill his thought is "it can never happen to me."

So now ask yourself the question . . . why would we take a statin drug that doesn't protect us from heart disease and deprives our bodies of their ability to manufacture the hormones that give us our sexual pleasure, as well as helping us in other ways? Why, when a person is put on a statin, are they not told that in time their sexual feelings and drive will simply go away?

Sex is what keeps us vibrant and alive, it gives us our edge, our glow, it brings us happiness, it is calming and thrilling. Little by little the information is coming out—sexual dysfunction, including erectile dysfunction (I bet you've noticed they have a drug for that), can be brought on by statin use. Then you have the dilemma—you can't "get it up," but you don't want to have a heart attack—that is, if you have the belief that statins are the only thing that will prevent you from having a heart attack. But cholesterol is not as relevant to heart disease as finding the source of inflammation. Your loss of libido brought on by statin use is a waste of your beautiful human experience. Men without a sex drive lose something vital. Pheromones attract; you can feel it when you are around a sexual person.

It absolutely boggles the mind why adults everywhere are gobbling these pills daily (ten billion dollars' worth a year) when they are causing so much havoc in the body. The medical establishment has made us all crazy about cholesterol, and we are in a panic about reducing it. If you feel the need to lower your cholesterol, there are more natural ways to try to control it than by taking pharmaceutical statins. Nature has already provided us with a simple yeast from the Orient that is a completely natural HMG-CoA-reductase inhibitor called red yeast rice, and it can be purchased at most health food stores. It is a natural control for cholesterol if accompanied by a healthy diet that includes omega-3 oils and fish oil supplements, but Merck got there first. They were able to obtain the first-ever filed patent on a naturally occurring substance. Mother Nature's cholestin (red yeast rice) would never be able to compete with Merck's identical product, lovastatin, which has the trademark of Mevacor. Merck rushed to patent this because researchers identified the HMG-CoA-reductase step as a natural control point for cholesterol synthesis.

It is important to note that red yeast rice, although natural, is also indeed a statin. It contains numerous active constituents, including monacolin K, dihydromonacolin, and monacolin I to VI, all of which have the same HMG-CoA-reductase-inhibitor effects as our modern statins. When you take red yeast rice, there are purportedly the same side effects as pharmaceutical statins, including the same muscle disease and even the dreaded rhabdomyolysis, but the difference is that it is not a drug and the molecular structure has not been altered.

It is crucial that your doctor understands the importance of getting the right dosage for *you* personally and how red yeast rice intermingles with other drugs. The difference between pharmaceutical statins and red yeast rice is the latter comes from nature and has not been tampered with to get a patent. It is the better choice.

Cholesterol is controllable by good nutrition and bioidentical hormone replacement (BHRT). If we are lax in our dietary approach we can make the necessary adjustments in our diets, cut back on saturated fats, trans fats, and omega-6 fats, cut out chemicals, and take red yeast rice supplementation under a qualified doctor's supervision in appropriate doses until our cholesterol is under control. I am able to control my cholesterol with my healthy Somersize diet. I love the way I eat: I eat fresh delicious food until I am full, and I am never hungry. I use good fats liberally in my diet and eliminate sugars and chemicals as best I can. It's going well . . . I do not take one pharmaceutical drug, my weight is perfect, and you would have to pry my mouth open and hold me down to make me ever, ever, take a statin drug.

We have to stop looking at cholesterol as the sole culprit in heart disease. Inflammation is more directly linked to heart problems. We can't live without cholesterol and we need an abundant supply in our bodies for proper functioning. Cholesterol is the precursor for a whole class of hormones, known as steroid hormones, that is critical to life. These hormones determine our sexuality, control our reproductive process, and regulate blood sugar levels and mineral metabolism. Cholesterol is required to replicate every cell in the body.

Statins may lower cholesterol, but we have to ask, at what cost are we trying to lower that which is so vital for our body to function well? With all the negative side effects associated with statins, the entire strategy for dosing of statins needs to be rethought.

Once again, we are looking for a "cure" instead of focusing on prevention. Let's find better ways to prevent heart disease. Let's throw in the towel and all agree that statins were a bad idea. Ironically, even when presented with this negative information, many people refuse to believe that this is not the miracle drug originally touted. I've thought about this and I believe it's because it would mean admitting that putting trust and faith in our longtime doctors' ability to take care of us was not a wise decision. We tend to be very loyal to our doctors even if we are led down an irreparable path. Sad.

Dear Suzanne,

I am sixty-three years old and have been on Premarin and Provera for eleven years. I read your book Ageless, *and then I went and bought* The Sexy Years *and now I am feeling so worked over because I trusted that the FDA and my doctor were keeping me safe.*

I have been bleeding excessively for quite some time and I have been petrified that I have cancer. Now that I realize I have been taking horse estrogen all these years, and that progestins in Provera are dangerous, I knew I had to make some big changes in my life. I have chronic breast tenderness, and bloating . . . I feel stuffed all the time. My sex drive doesn't exist (when you are bleeding constantly who feels like sex) and I feel badly for my husband who loves me but is having a difficult time understanding my mood swings. I just don't feel like myself.

I went to Dr. Hall in your book and for the first time I feel that there is a doctor who knows what she is doing and she also has great compassion. She told me (like you said in your book) to stop the synthetic hormones and make the switch to bioidenticals. She also told me the bleeding is from too much estrogen and not enough progesterone. So we tried a new combination with bioidenticals and now after only a few weeks the bleeding has gone back to normal and the bloating is going away, and best of all I am feeling happy again. I feel like my old self.

It's important that you write these books, Suzanne. We women don't know where to go or who to believe. There is something about the way you speak to us in your books that feels reassuring.

Thank you. I'm going to be okay. I am very grateful.

Joyce A.

22

DR. KHALID MAHMUD

There is no scientific evidence that food or other nutritional essentials are of any specific value in the control of cancer.

–American Medical Association, 1949

AS WITH MANY OF THE DOCTORS in this book, Dr. Mahmud had an awakening. Born and raised in Pakistan, he came to America as a young man and was able to have a tremendously successful career as a practicing oncologist. Twenty-five years into his practice, he felt uneasy. He wasn't happy with the Western model for disease care. He had to accept the fact that people were not getting better, that the traditional standard of care wasn't geared toward prevention but rather focused on finding a cure. He decided that he needed to leave his traditional practice and devote his life to the prevention of cancer.

His book *Keeping aBreast: Ways to Stop Breast Cancer* is a must-read for all women. Dr. Mahmud's thoughtfulness and compassion will give hope to all those who fear the dreaded diagnosis of breast cancer. Dr. Mahmud truly believes cancer is preventable, and this interview will tell you why. I enjoyed speaking with him and consider his work to be truly groundbreaking.

SS: Good evening, Dr. Mahmud. Thank you for your time. It's unusual for an oncologist to make a switch to antiaging medicine. Why did you do that?

KM: I realize it's an unusual switch, and the irony of all of this is that practicing oncologists have zero interest in looking into antiaging as a means of prevention of cancer. But let me digress: I began my training in the specialty of hematology–oncology about forty years ago. I came to America from Pakistan and settled in New York at first, and then moved to Minnesota. From the very beginning I was distressed with the emphasis in this country on things that were artificial: margarine instead of butter, baby formula instead of mother's breast milk, chemicals instead of real food. America is a wonderful country full of opportunity, but this was discouraging. I finally became the medical director of oncology at my medical center, and many patients with all types of cancer came to me. Some died right away, others were cured, yet others went into remission for variable lengths of time. As I followed those in remission, it became more and more difficult to maintain a strict doctor-patient relationship. I found myself attached to them. When and if they died, a little part of me died with them. "Duration of complete remission," "prolongation of survival"—the usual oncology jargon—meant less and less with time.

SS: Was your practice successful?

KM: Yes, very. I was financially secure, but deep inside I was restless. I started a van service to treat the sicker cancer patients in their homes, and a "cancer link program" in rural areas to give chemo to patients in their own hometowns so they wouldn't have to travel to the big city and be sick on their way back home—and at the same time it would create good business for my hospital.

But I remained troubled: troubled with losing my friend-patients and troubled with the fact that overall cancer statistics had not changed appreciably over the years in spite of all of our new therapies. I was burdened with the suspicion that we could not adequately assess the real value of time that we added to our patients' lives. And I was bothered by the wastefulness of American medicine, which was number one in the world on spending but twentieth on life expectancy, while providing no coverage for one-sixth of its citizens. I mean, it's crazy; America spends 25 percent of its health care dollars during the last six months of life; more than $300 billion a year to finance every conceivable treatment for every possible condition—without adding an iota to quality of life! I realized that America was doing nothing to correct problems early because we were not spending anything on *prevention*.

SS: Is that the problem, that we have put very little effort into understanding prevention of disease? Does prevention not fit into the profitability of business?

KM: We are a capitalistic society and everything is run by and for profit. Industry is based on profit, so they have developed technology and drugs that can be used to provide temporary relief and, unfortunately,

everyone wants the quick fix. You have to understand that these technologies are expensive. Profits pay for them, and also (this is the amazing
part) 66 percent of all department chairs at universities in America have
financial contracts with pharmaceutical device companies, so it makes
sense that the pharmaceutical industry in this country is about developing artificial remedies that you can patent. That's why you won't find research on nonpatentable natural cures and healing.

SS: Well, there's the dilemma with bioidentical hormones. This
means that our medical schools are compromised. They *can't* teach about
natural remedies or natural hormones because they will lose their financial grants. This is shocking; this means pharmaceutical companies are in
control of our universities, our government officials, our airwaves, TV and
print media. No wonder we are all on so many drugs. Frankly, it's a brilliant business model, but it is the demise of *us* in the process.

KM: Absolutely. When I start patients on bioidentical hormones they
then go to their regular doctors, who tell them not to take them because
there are no studies. I think to myself, well, whose fault is this? Bioidenticals have been available for fifty, sixty years, so why don't they fund studies? Europeans are more open to natural hormones and have done many
positive studies.

SS: We know the answer: Bioidentical hormones are not patentable
and businesses are not interested in promoting a drug, no matter how
beneficial, if they can't own the patent.

KM: You are correct. And they ignore the European studies like the
Fournier study and others because they don't want us to have that information. But it's also another problem, and it's a sociological problem. In
Pakistan, when you grow older you become the responsibility of your
children. You move in with your children and they take care of you. You
are not lonely, you are not depressed, and you are part of a family system.

But in America the children are scattered all over the place because
their lives are so busy. Then something happens to one of the parents
(and they are already feeling so guilty that they haven't been there to see
them often enough), so they say to the doctor, "I want everything possible under the sun done for my mom."

SS: Sad but true.

KM: Right there you have the reason why we spend so much money
during the last six months of life. As a cancer specialist I saw that over
and over. In crisis the family gets together; half the people come from
New York, the other half are from California. While the mother is lying
in the hospital I always have a conference with the family and tell them

the truth, as in, "She does not have a very good type of cancer. We treated her with chemo and she's only got a twenty percent chance that she's going to respond." Inevitably the family will agree that "we've got to try everything possible."

SS: But what do we do? Do we go home and let our parents die? What is more humane: letting the disease win by doing nothing, or trying any of the many poisons that are available to allow us to slowly and tragically die? When the results are the same, what *is* more humane?

KM: That is not for me to answer for any family member. I know what I would do for myself, but I cannot make up anyone else's mind. You see, Suzanne, everything in this country is focused on the CURE. There's Susan G. Komen, which is spending millions and millions of dollars and funding treatment options and new protocols to treat breast cancer, but there is no emphasis *at all* on preventing it.

SS: In your book *Keeping aBreast*, you write about 101 ways to prevent cancer.

KM: Yes, and it's all based on scientific evidence. It's not something I concocted. Everything in that book is supported by some reference in scientific publications. But nobody talks about these ways of prevention. We have a race for the cure, but no one knows enough to promote my book or any book like it, which is how to *prevent* cancer.

SS: We are hooked on drugs as the cure for everything in this country. I am often criticized for not marching for breast cancer, but I do not believe the answer lies in drugs. I, too, believe in *prevention* of cancer, and I am trying my best to live that way through diet, bioidenticals, sleep, and good thoughts. Let me ask you—how do we get cancer?

KM: First of all, you have to understand that breast cancer develops in the cells that line the milk ducts or in the cells that form the glands that drain into the milk ducts. An essential event that has to occur is some sort of an assault on the DNA located in the nucleus of the cell.

SS: That "assault" you speak of could be chemicals in our diets or in our homes, right?

KM: Yes, you are correct. You see, DNA is the biological version of a computer code contained in a hundred thousand genes and is the master controller of all cellular functions. It is rare that a cell gone bad survives to become a full-fledged cancer because our defense system has amazing capacity, but in the breast there is an unappreciated mechanism for the formation of free radicals.

SS: What would that be?

KM: The formation of free radicals can happen in the fluid that accumulates and gets pent up in the milk glands and ducts. Studies have shown that this fluid eventually breaks down and forms free radicals. Right next to this fluid are the cells lining the ducts and glands, which bear the brunt of these free radicals. These are the cells that commonly become malignant in the breast.

SS: So you're talking about ductal cancer.

KM: Yes, and it is the most common type of breast cancer.

SS: So how do we avoid or get rid of free radicals in our breasts?

KM: Chemicals constantly enter our bodies, and most of these common toxins are organic compounds, meaning that they are soluble in fats rather than water and tend to accumulate in body fat such as the breast. When the body tries to get rid of them they can become activated and cause damage. Also, estrogen that is made in the breast stimulates a cancer cell that is already there. It doesn't make new cancer cells, but it stimulates the existing cancer cells.

SS: Wait a minute. Are you saying that estrogen made in the breast is a dangerous estrogen, but when you apply external bioidentical estrogen it doesn't do the same thing?

KM: Right. It doesn't cause problems, but I need to get a little technical to explain this: Because the estrogen is made in the menopausal breast, its level in the breast is many times that in the blood. So increasing the blood level of estrogen by giving a bioidentical hormone does not increase the breast estrogen level that is already there.

SS: How does the body deal with chemicals?

KM: Phase I enzymes change these chemicals into intermediate metabolites. These intermediate metabolites are extremely reactive, like free radicals; they cause DNA damage and damage other molecules. These reactive molecules have to be removed immediately before they can cause harm. That's the job of phase II enzymes. These phase II enzymes quickly convert the intermediate metabolites into harmless entities that can be easily excreted from the body via the intestinal or urinary tracts. But these detoxifying enzymes can be impaired with age, poor health, alcohol, and certain pharmaceuticals, including Premarin, which has been used by millions of American women.

SS: Once again, it's about diet and chemicals. Tell me for the sake of my readers, tell me for the sake of young women who have never had cancer, how they should live their lives so they would not get cancer.

KM: For a young woman, the most important thing she can do toward prevention of breast cancer is breast-feed. I came from a poor country and I was breast-fed for two years and so were all the other kids in the neighborhood. You never heard of anyone getting breast cancer. Breast-feeding is nature's way to prevent getting cancer, and besides, breast-fed kids are healthier in every respect and also their children are healthier. Studies from thirty different countries have proven that the breast cancer rate is lower in women who breast-feed their babies.

SS: What about birth control pills—especially these new ones that give a woman four periods a year?

KM: This is an artificial approach. Going against nature is something we should all avoid. Human knowledge is incomplete and it's always going to be incomplete. Only Mother Nature knows everything, and we need to try to learn from it and try to replicate nature. Taking hormones so you can get your period only four times a year will cause a menopause-like state that will confuse a woman's hormones. Surely, down the road these women are going to have problems.

SS: What else?

KM: Change the American diet.

SS: Amen! Dr. Hertoghe told me that when he arrives at the airport in America he is astonished at what he calls the deformed bodies of the American people.

KM: It's a tragedy. Americans are the heaviest people on the planet. Sixty percent are overweight and thirty percent can be categorized as obese. This is a problem because obesity can lead to breast cancer.

SS: How can that happen?

KM: Fat cells contain the enzyme aromatase, which converts testosterone into estrogens; overweight and obese women have more estrogen, and the more estrogen produced in the breast, the more chance of stimulating the growth of breast cancer cells. In my book I show how there are eight different ways body fat causes breast cancer and many other problems like diabetes, heart disease, arthritis, and joint problems. In fact, when you take a look at degenerative disk diseases and back problems for which people have surgeries and fusions, no one realizes how much a good diet and exercise could prevent these conditions. If people truly understood nutrition, everyone would be so much healthier and would not experience these problems.

SS: Everybody says change your diet. We laypeople hear it over and over, but it doesn't seem to sink in. We like our chemicals and diet sodas.

KM: I used to tell my kids, try to make your life simple, "Eat God-made foods, not man-made foods," but it's difficult to make an impact that these artificial things that we eat are making us sick and killing us. Refined foods and the confusion from the medical establishment didn't help when they posted the food pyramid and scared us against fats, while increasing carbohydrates. We know there are good fats and bad fats, but the body needs monounsaturated fats as in olive oil, and the other omega-3 fats like egg yolks (if they say omega-3 on the package) and salmon are probably the best source. Wild game is good, wild turkey, wild deer, animals that are free and wild have omega-3s naturally. But you can also supplement with omega-3 fish oil capsules. It's just so important that my patients know that good health cannot exist without a good nutritious diet, and the healthiest diet comes from food that is organic and comes in an unaltered form. Artificial food is not going to promote good health, and poor health leads to disease, and cancer is a part of that.

SS: There is a lot of controversy about mammograms and self-exams. What are your thoughts on mammograms and the exposure every year to radiation? Some of the doctors I have interviewed said that if you start out with no cancer and you have mammograms every year for ten years, by the end of ten years you'll have developed cancer as a result of the radiation. What do you think?

KM: The rads you get with mammograms are minimal, between 2 and 5 rads over ten years. Compare that with radiation in the atmosphere all around us, and personally I don't think the small amount of rads in mammograms will make much of a difference. So my feeling is they do more good than harm.

SS: With all due respect, I tend to think every little bit hurts, but I'm not a doctor or a scientist. One other theory out there is that flattening the breast has the potential to crack a tumor in the breast. Is that theory for real?

KM: There's never been a study that shows that trauma to the breast can crack tumors. So I don't think that can happen.

If people would have their breasts stimulated or massaged regularly, especially when they are young, there is actually scientific evidence that it increases the secretion of oxytocin, which not only helps remove pent-up secretions from the breast ducts but also fights breast cancer in several ways, and besides, it reduces stress.

Of course, such practice should be nontraumatic. This is not an opportunity for a woman to be taken advantage of. . . .

SS: Well, I have to tell you, in my household you are a big hero. I told my husband he has to do this to keep me healthy, and he is more than happy to oblige. He always says, "Dr. Mahmud told me to do this." [Laughter] He said he'll do it for ten hours—anything to keep me healthy.

KM: Well, it's one of the things that help, but I don't want it to be misconstrued.

SS: No, but as you were telling me this I said to myself, "Here goes nature again." Nature has created breasts that are pleasurable to men and women, and stimulation is a part of it. Nursing is also a part of it.

KM: It's a fine line—I believe it is an important function, but I don't want it to come across as my main message. It's part of the course of prevention that I feel is important. Stagnant fluid in the breasts contributes to breast cancer. Nipple stimulation gets things moving. Oncologists don't know any of this. This is from my own investigation: the fluid in the breast duct becomes stagnant; the contents break down and release free radicals. Breast ductal fluid has a lot of free radicals and the job of these radicals is to cause DNA damage to the cells, and then DNA damage occurs because the cell becomes abnormal.

SS: Thus the reason we all should eat a healthy diet and take antioxidant supplements, which kill free radicals.

KM: You are quite right. Now, the body's immune system will try to remove cells like that, but every once in a while it fails and a cell like that, which has abnormal DNA, could possibly be the beginning of a cancer. So that is why I stress breast massage and nipple stimulation to keep the fluid moving. Then the second part is all of the chemicals we are exposed to from pharmaceuticals, from the environment, and from the food industry. In fact, industry as a whole brings us harmful materials, like organic chlorines, dioxins, etc. I list them all in my book and explain that the chemicals that are all around us act as free radicals and cause damage.

SS: So let me get this straight. You feel that the causes of cancer are, (a) clogged-up breast fluid, which creates free radicals, and (b) the chemicals in the environment. And *prevention* is breast massage, nipple stimulation, and avoiding chemicals by switching to a healthy chemical-free diet full of antioxidants (which kill free radicals)—and then we could expect to avoid cancer.

KM: That is what I think. And, of course, breast-feed. There are other factors, as in genes. We have genes that protect us and genes that have gone haywire, and with those we tend to see more cancer. Some of those genes are BRCA1 and BRCA2, which are hereditary mutations pertinent to breast cancer. When working normally these genes are "cancer suppressor genes," meaning they prevent normal cells from becoming cancerous. Women who inherit either of these abnormal genes have a 70 percent chance of developing breast cancer by age seventy. Those with BRCA1 mutations have an additional 40 percent chance of cancer of the ovary by the same age. But overall these gene abnormalities are responsible for only 5 to 10 percent of all breast cancers in women.

SS: Yes. My husband's ancestors were Ashkenazi Jews and they carry the BRCA1 and BRCA2 genes. There is a blood test you can take to see if you carry the gene, and it's called the BRCA1 and BRCA2 blood test.

KM: The other risk factors are women whose mothers or maternal grandmothers had breast cancer; they have an increased risk for developing cancer.

SS: I know of a woman whose family was burdened by breast cancer. It seemed to hit every generation, and they thought it was genetic. But when they did testing for the gene, it wasn't there. Then, in putting two and two together, they realized that all these women had grown up near a chemical plant in Pennsylvania and that that was probably the reason and not a genetic predisposition. Chemicals again, nasty stuff.

KM: Normal genes protect us, but if they are mutated then you get more cancer. Now with genomics they are discovering more genes, tiny ones that contribute to this, so there are many factors. It's not as simple as I put in the two steps, but those two steps can have a profound effect on cancer prevention.

SS: What are other ways to get free radicals?

KM: Eat fried foods and you will get free radicals; with infections or inflammatory disease you will have more free radicals; overeating creates free radicals. Smoking is the worst; you get a lot of free radicals with smoking. Our lifestyle habits and nutritional habits are way off in this country. Refined foods have created havoc.

SS: As in white flour, white rice, breads, pastries, cakes . . .

KM: Yes, yes, and yes.

SS: Let's talk about bioidentical hormones. Do you think they are the backbone of antiaging medicine?

KM: Yes, very important. But I am talking about all the hormones in the body, not just the sex hormones estrogen and progesterone and testosterone; I'm talking also about thyroid, DHEA and adrenals, cortisol and insulin. There are three organs in the body for which sex hormones are essential; the first is the heart, and estrogen is extremely important for the heart.

Estrogen dilates our coronary arteries and increases our good cholesterol. I mean, think about this: You rarely see a forty-year-old woman drop dead of a heart attack, but you do see men dying of the same thing at that age. Women have a lot of estrogen still at forty, and that estrogen is protecting them.

It's when women lose their estrogen that they start to get heart attacks. The issue with men is that they start losing their good cholesterol early on. Good cholesterol is like a garbage truck that goes through your arteries and cleans out all the debris. A typical woman in her forties has twice the amount of good cholesterol than a man the same age, and men tend to inherit more cholesterol abnormalities from their parents for some reason.

SS: But men make testosterone, which builds bone and muscle. The heart is the largest muscle in the body, and there are more testosterone receptor sites on the heart than any other muscle. Doesn't testosterone protect men from heart attacks?

KM: Yes, that's true. Testosterone is an important hormone for the heart, which is why it is important to keep testosterone levels at optimum with bioidentical testosterone replacement. So, managing a man's cholesterol through good nutrition and replacing his missing or low testosterone are both protective, preventative measures.

SS: What about progesterone?

KM: Progesterone augments the good effect of estrogen on the heart and blood vessels. Men don't have as much progesterone as women, but both are essential for the heart. The other organ that is protected by hormones is the brain. Estrogen is very important for your memory and for multitasking. Estrogen acts in the part of the brain where it makes connections in the hypothalamus and the memory sensors, it repairs the damage to nerve cells, *and* it fights the beta peptide that causes Alzheimer's disease. On the other hand, if you don't have enough progesterone you tend to be more irritable, so progesterone calms the brain.

SS: Progesterone calms the brain, and testosterone has an important effect on the brain. Is this in both males and females?

KM: Yes. Testosterone gives a sense of security, it creates competitiveness, and it gives you hand-eye coordination so you can play golf better. I have a lot of women patients who come back and say, "I'm hitting the ball better than my husband now." So it's not just for their sex drive (which it helps), but it is for overall improvement of muscle tone when they work out. You can work out with a trainer all day, but if you don't have testosterone you can't get anywhere. Testosterone makes muscles tighter, and you can gain muscle with testosterone. But you have to be careful not to go overboard.

SS: Yes, I understand. Too much is too much. Too little is too little. I have said this in all of my books. We strive for our perfect individualized needs and not more.

KM: You see, conventional medicine never monitored blood levels of these hormones. You can go overboard with DHEA and testosterone and then these wonderful hormones become bad for us. I constantly stress that you create a balance with a patient and then check these hormones on a regular basis.

Hormones are important for the brain and the heart. Suzanne, we have our nursing homes full of women, 40 percent of whom are there because they broke a bone, and the other 60 percent are there because either they can no longer be trusted to take care of themselves (their brains stop working correctly) or they've got heart problems. If only these women could have received bioidentical hormones, they would have reduced their risks for heart disease, dementia, and osteoporosis. It breaks my heart that whoever was taking care of them didn't have the new information.

SS: Well, all I know is we women (and men) seem to do fine until we start hormonal decline.

KM: Yes, science has proven that before menopause women are producing estrogen in their ovaries, but after menopause they produce estrogen in the body fat mostly. That body fat becomes your endocrine gland and it produces estrogen. So if you were to measure estrogen in the breast duct fluid, it will be anywhere from ten to fifteen times higher than what's in the woman's blood. Everybody is focused on the blood (blood tests for estrogen levels), but no one is paying attention to the breast itself that is making all the estrogen. A blood test might say the estrogen level in the blood is 20, but in the breast it might be 100 or 200. So if you give bioidentical estrogen to most menopausal women with fatty breasts, it is not going to increase estrogen in the breast and, therefore, would not increase the risk. On the other hand, when women who come to me with shriveled-up breasts with little fat, who are in menopause, are given estrogen, it may enter the breasts and their breasts could enlarge again. So you have be careful and work on a case-by-case basis.

I tend to give menopausal women iodine supplementation, because the iodine creates estriols, and menopausal women don't have too much estriol. So, with iodine supplementation the estriol increases, which will block estrogen receptors on the breast and protect them from breast cancer.

SS: Do you think bioidentical hormones prevent breast cancer and breast cancer recurrence?

KM: In my most recent presentation, I talked about this. I spoke of three published studies of women who had had previous breast cancers who went on bioidentical estrogen hormones afterward and had no increase in breast cancer. As a matter of fact, breast cancer seemed to be decreasing in women on the hormone. Recently I came upon a study of baboons (who are very similar to humans) where they removed their ovaries. When you remove ovaries, the breast starts to produce more estrogen, because as I said there is an enzyme, an aromatase enzyme, that turns on very high and overproduces estrogen in the breast. They measured the aromatase enzyme in a baboon without ovaries and the aromatase was very, very high. Then they gave the animal estrogen. The effect was amazing: It turned off the aromatase overproduction in the breast of this baboon. In other words, it's like another endocrine system: When we provide something from the outside, the endocrine organs stop making what was missing. This is called a negative feedback loop. So you give these baboons estrogen and it acts like an aromatase inhibitor. Giving bioidentical estrogen to females who are no longer making estrogen because they are in menopause reduces the production of estrogen in the breast. And that's my point: You've got to pay attention to what is happening to the breast. In my book, I also talk about a large study of 23,000 Swiss women who took mostly natural estrogens. The breast cancer risk was reduced by 25 percent.

SS: Let me try to understand this for me and my readers: When a woman is not making any more estrogen from her glands and ovaries, she starts overproducing estrogen in the fat, and the breasts are prime fat for estrogen; but when you give the woman bioidentical estrogen from the outside (transdermally), she stops overproducing estrogen in the breast and the body is protected from breast cancer.

KLM: Correct. Bioidentical estrogen replacement is essential. In addition you must replace progesterone. Progesterone is anti–breast cancer. And you also must replace testosterone in moderate doses, because testosterone has been shown to have its own receptors from breast cancer cells that inhibit breast cancer.

SS: This is wonderful news. Bioidentical hormones replaced correctly can be anticancer! That's profound. I realize you are not saying that it cures breast cancer, but when used correctly, *can* prevent cancer or a recurrence.

I always feel relieved when I hear this because, as you know, this is the choice I made for myself at a time when no one was doing this. My doctors were horrified. But I knew from writing my books and from gathering a lot of information and doing research on my own, plus my inner logic, that it made sense to put back what was missing that had given me the cancer in the first place. But you know and I know that when a woman is diagnosed with breast cancer, the first thing she's told is to stop all hormones.

KM: Hopefully, studies will be done to prove what we in the antiaging business are seeing daily. It's a long shot, because American academia and department heads have never and are not planning on ever doing any studies on bioidentical hormones.

SS: I have to say that this makes my blood boil. We are being forced to live in a pharmaceutical world because our professors and universities take money and grants from pharmaceutical companies, and in order to keep this money they cannot teach or study any natural measures. I guess it's up to you and me and the thousands of other doctors who meet regularly to discuss the predicament of modern medicine. I admire all of you who have stepped out of the box to treat patients in a way that doesn't involve unnecessary drugs. One day your voices will be heard. Is there anything else we can do for ourselves that is preventative?

KM: I go into great depth about this in my book. Yes, there are natural anticancer measures you can take: Green tea extract kills breast cancer cells in ten different ways. Vitamin D is anti–breast cancer, especially vitamin D$_3$; you should take a minimum of 1,000 units daily. Lycopene, at 15 milligrams a day, enhances the effects of many of the good genes that are antibreast cancer. Folic acid should be taken at 600 micrograms a day, especially for women who drink alcohol.

SS: I saw in your book that if a woman does drink, red wine is the best choice.

KM: Yes. Red wine has benefits from resveratrol and is much healthier than white wine or hard alcohol, and it has antioxidants. Red wine also tends to be an aromatase inhibitor rather than a stimulator. It's important that if you drink any alcohol that you should take folic acid. A large glass of alcohol will increase your risk of breast cancer by 7 percent; however, if you take enough folic acid you can reduce that. Selenium is necessary as a supplement. Indol-3 carbinol supplementation is equivalent to a pound of broccoli a day, and we all know the benefits of broccoli; Indol-3 carbinol kills breast cancer cells. And vitamin E gamma-tocopherol is vital for its anticancer and anti–heart disease activity. Melatonin is important especially for women from age fifty on. Sleep is vital to hormonal balance and disease prevention. Melatonin is not only necessary but will also help you sleep, so you take it at night before you go to bed.

SS: Yes, but so many women can't sleep. Just can't sleep.

KM: Then they should be on bioidentical hormones. You slept when you were young, right? You were making all your hormones then. Now that their hormones aren't balanced, women can't sleep. It's a simple equation: Put back the hormones and your body begins to function properly again. Sleep is proper body functioning.

SS: Yes, but women go to their doctors and tell them they can't sleep and are depressed, and as a result the doctor gives them Prozac or Ambien.

KM: Because most doctors (and they are a million strong) have been trained like that. It's a very difficult situation we are in, and the patients are the losers. It's like a big ship is going in one direction and a small tugboat wants to change its direction, but it's very, very hard.

SS: I take my hat off to you for doing your part.

KM: And I take my hat off to you. Your voice is very important. I'm doing this because I feel it's my duty. It's not a field where I make a whole lot of money, but if I leave this planet and feel I had contributed a little bit and people got on the right track so that there are a few less cases of cancer and Alzheimer's, a few less broken bones, then I feel I would have done my job.

I know for myself, embracing this new medicine, antiaging medicine, that I'm vigorous; at sixty-five I passed the American Board of Anti-Aging Medicine, when all my partners have retired. I'm working in this incredibly exciting field. I'm discovering new things regularly, I feel more fulfilled, and I don't have the fatigue that I used to have. I'm hitting the golf ball longer and harder than I ever did at fifty-four when I started, and I'm sixty-nine now . . . and also, I have passion.

SS: How great. What is your hope for the future?

KM: My hope for the future is that these new ideas about prevention will take hold and the younger docs will adopt this information and gradually medicine will change over. I love antiaging medicine. It's like going into a diamond mine. You're not going to see the walls covered with diamonds. There will be a lot of rock and dust and things. It's your job to find the diamonds in the rough, because the diamonds are certainly there. Each patient can have their antiaging medicine customized to their particular needs; they just have to know going in that the diamonds will be there and that by working with their doctor the patient will indeed find their diamonds.

DR. KHALID MAHMUD'S
BREAKTHROUGH BREAKOUTS

- Women in their twenties and thirties should breast-feed as long as possible. It is protective against breast cancer for her, and her baby will be healthier and have a higher IQ.
- Women should avoid birth control pills.
- If young women have infertility problems, they need to have their progesterone levels checked. If progesterone is consistently low, you are at great risk for breast cancer. It should be watched and controlled by someone who truly understands bioidentical hormones. Progesterone should never be replaced by progestins, or progestagen, the artificial, synthetic, and harmful hormones.
- Women with risk factors for breast cancer should consider estrogen replacement delivered transdermally.
- Cancer prevention is achievable through exercise; sleep; good nutrition and eating real food; supplementation with multivitamin and mineral supplements, including vitamin E, folic acid (600 micrograms daily), vitamin D, and green tea extracts; as well as breast massage and nipple stimulation.

23

CANCER IS PREVENTABLE

It is now evident that plant chemicals, vitamins and minerals can attack cancer cells at all levels, but at the same time have no harmful effect on normal cells while powerfully protecting normal cells from becoming cancer cells.

—Dr. Russell Blaylock, *Natural Strategies for Cancer Patients*

CANCER, CANCER, CANCER. It's everywhere. I remember as a child not knowing a single person who had cancer. Now we all know someone with cancer or, worse, have or had the dreaded disease ourselves. It's one of the things we fear most in life. What's feared even more than cancer is its *treatment*. In fact, it seems that more people die from the treatment of cancer than of the cancer itself. Chemotherapy in many cases kills cancer. We know that, but chemotherapy also destroys the immune system, and unfortunately cancer can grow back faster than the immune system can repair itself. That is why so many who go "standard of care" with radiation and chemotherapy have a recurrence. The immune system just wasn't there to help out.

And what of the consequences and devastating side effects of poisoning one's body with chemicals? Most people never really think about the word "chemotherapy" for what it is—chemical poisoning. Poisoning ourselves with chemicals in any form, whether with traditional medicine like chemotherapy drugs, or with chemical-laden foods, or with household cleaning products and pest killers, or with diet sodas, can have deadly consequences. Personally, I believe that in the future we will look back at chemotherapy treatment and wonder, What were we thinking?

Those who believe in antiaging breakthrough medicine are asking these questions now. How can we build *up* our bodies as we need to do to be strong and healthy if we treat illness by breaking down our bodies with chemicals that in most instances do more harm than good? As I discussed in the last chapter, we have to look outside standard medical treatment to find the most effective ways to fight disease, and that can include cancer.

When I was diagnosed with breast cancer in April 2000, I refused chemotherapy, based on information I had garnered from writing my books on health and hormones, and the understanding that a hormonally balanced body rarely gets cancer. Young people do not get cancer unless there is some genetic aberration, or an environmental cause, as in ingesting chemicals through poor-quality food or being exposed to household chemicals or pollution. One of the greatest decisions I made for myself was to refuse chemotherapy. I felt that if I could replace my missing hormones with nondrug bioidentical hormones to optimal levels, and take nutrition seriously, I could effectively keep the cancer at bay.

The brain recognizes a reproductive body as a healthy body. We are here (biologically speaking) to reproduce—"perpetuation of the species." A person with perfectly balanced hormones is a reproductive person. With bioidentical hormone replacement you can actually trick your brain into believing you are still a reproductive person. Reproductive people rarely get cancer, because they make a full and balanced complement of hormones. Bioidentical hormone replacement was my first line of defense. I put back the hormones I had lost in the aging process to exactly replicate my youthful hormonal output. Just doing that so improved my outlook and disposition that I became emotionally intact again and able to make better choices for myself. Plus, I started sleeping again, a good eight or nine hours a night, and that was healing. The hot flashes stopped, the itching subsided, and my libido returned. Being in the mood for love while battling cancer helps the healing process. I was doing well. I was happy. I felt I would win this war.

There was only one bump in my recovery. In 2000, I was still educating myself. I had enough information to know I wanted to refuse chemo, but I got frightened into taking radiation. Today I don't believe in either of those treatments (this is just my opinion, of course, but many of the doctors in this book concur), but at that time I was too frightened to refuse radiation.

I'm sorry that I did that. My health these days is perfect except for the consequences of this radiation. It burned and scarred the insides of the top of my digestive tract, which has given me serious acid reflux, and it compromised my lymphatic system. Because of that I need to work regularly with a lymphatic specialist to unclog my lymph system or face serious problems down the road. This is the weakness in Western medicine.

The treatment for cancer causes other serious complications in the body. It's like trading a headache for an earache, but of course the consequences can be much more deadly than that when we talk about cancer. We have more lymph fluid in our bodies than blood. If that fluid is compromised and congested we have a dangerous scenario. No one told me about the complications, no one told me that nausea would have me in a fetal position all day long for six straight weeks. No one told me the skin on my chest would turn black and burn like it had been charred, and no one ever mentioned that radiation was going to create scar tissue in my lower esophagus and congest my lymph fluid. Lymph fluid is what transports hormones throughout the body, and it also exports the "garbage" and toxins out of our systems. Pretty important stuff.

A cancer diagnosis is the scariest information anyone can share with you about yourself. Being diagnosed is so frightening, so horrifying, so out of control that it is easy to do exactly what your doctor tells you. And if you have the misfortune of having a doctor who has not kept up with the latest information, it is easy to fall into the standard of care trap and go with radiation and/or chemo. We're now learning how futile and downright dangerous these options can be. If you choose standard of care medicine, at least be informed of every option, whether it be pharmaceutical or alternative, then you will have the peace of mind that you did your homework.

Two to 5 percent of the 350,000 people a year who undergo in-hospital chemotherapy treatments die as a direct result of the toxicity of the treatment itself. Think that doesn't sound like many? That's between 7,000 and 17,500 people who die from this treatment every year. What if one of those was you or a loved one? Another study found that it was higher, that 21 percent of patients receiving high-dose chemo die as a complication of the treatment.

Here's worse news. The two most popular chemotherapy drugs used to treat women with breast cancer have now been proven ineffective. The names of these drugs are Avastin and paclitaxel, a generic drug. According to the FDA, the Genentech drug Avastin (also called bevacizumab) "did not help women with breast cancer live meaningfully longer, and it caused significant side effects." My oncologist sent this report to me and said, "I die inside thinking of all the women I have poisoned for no reason." He also said, "If you had agreed to chemotherapy, Suzanne, this is what we would have given to you." That was pretty sobering. All these women suffered needlessly. The drugs did *nothing* but bring pain, suffering, and false hopes.

As we've seen, chemo and radiation, despite being the standard of care options when confronting cancer, are dangerous and not always effective, as they destroy and poison so much of the body that often cancer has a chance to come back. But what if I were to tell you there is an alternative way to fight cancer, "a third way"?

Here it is—the third way is simple and doesn't involve drugs or poison or radiation. The third way is . . . nutrition! The doctors and oncologists I have interviewed believe the answer to fighting cancer and cancer *prevention* lies in nutrition.

Yes, nutrition. Numerous epidemiological studies have shown that people who eat a lot of fruits and vegetables have much lower cancer rates than those who eat few or none. Scientists have learned that various components of plants, including vitamins and minerals, can affect cancer cells in such a way as to cause them to stop growing or even die. Other studies have shown that certain plant chemicals called flavonoids (see page 199), especially when combined with vitamins and minerals, can attack cancer cells at all levels but at the same time have no harmful effect on normal cells. In fact, they powerfully protect normal cells from becoming cancer cells. This is not only important in preventing cancer from forming in the first place but especially important in preventing secondary cancers that can be created in the wake of chemotherapy and radiation treatments.

Cancer is a formidable opponent, and fighting it is like war. Fighting cancer requires rolling up your sleeves and a shift in your thinking. It requires a belief that by eating real food, good food, and by learning what bioidentical hormones, supplements, vitamins, minerals, herbs, and spices enhance your health, you will be taking advantage of the most forceful and beneficial way to fight cancer before it has a chance to develop or recur.

It is a fact that overall cancer rates were reduced 50 percent (!) in a recent study for people who ate the most fruits and vegetables, with the greatest reduction being in cancers of the esophagus, oral cavity, larynx, pancreas, stomach, colon, rectum, bladder, cervix, ovary, endometrium, and breast. To better understand and appreciate the power of phytochemicals, a study done in Japan found that people eating the most yellow-green vegetables had a 65 percent lower stomach cancer incidence than those eating significantly fewer of these vegetables. Another study found that people who ate citrus fruits only twice a month or less had a sixteen times *higher* incidence of developing stomach cancer than those who ate citrus at least once a week or more.

Risk of pancreatic cancer (which has a mortality rate of more than 90 percent) can be reduced by eating vegetables and fruits high in beta-carotene and especially lycopene, the red pigment in tomatoes, pink grapefruit, and watermelon. This same red pigment plays a leading role in preventing prostate cancer, with the risk being lowered 35 percent to 45 percent in those eating a lot of such fruits and vegetables. Vitamin E, especially when combined with selenium, also dramatically reduces the risk of this cancer.

> Eat God-made foods, not man-made foods.
>
> –Dr. Khalid Mahmud

It's diet, diet, diet. No fooling around. We are what we eat. And the only loser in this is us if we don't take our diet seriously.

Dr. Russell Blaylock says, "I always try to tell my patients that if they try to depend on supplements alone and not change their diet, they will ultimately fail. It is estimated that as many as 70 percent of all cancers are related to diet." Imagine! Foods contain extremely powerful cancer-causing and cancer-promoting substances. According to Dr. Blaylock, "The typical Western diet, high in red meats, bad fats, food additives and carbohydrates, is a perfect cancer brew. This brew not only causes cancer, but can promote the growth of existing cancers as well."

In terms of health benefits (mainly considering antioxidants) eating fewer than five servings of fruits and vegetables a day does very little good. The health benefits of eating these valuable foods begin at five servings (a serving is a half a cup) a day, and for people below age fifty reach a maximum at ten servings a day. That makes you stop and think.

Several studies have shown that eating large amounts of fruits and vegetables, especially vegetables, not only retards the growth of cancers but can also convert very aggressive cancers into much more benign tumors. This is remarkable information and needs to be taken seriously. Newer studies are showing that some cancer cells can be changed into normal cells using specific nutrients. So instead of scientists figuring out how to kill cancer cells without harming normal cells, they now know that changing cancer cells back to normal cells is possible . . . by consuming a true healthy diet.

Nature has provided us with all that we need. We spend so much time and money trying to find the cure for cancer when the answer appears to be right in front of us. Every year, tens of billions of dollars are spent on the war on cancer, and still we have not found a cure for the disease. Perhaps we are looking in the wrong place. In A.A. they say, "Keep it simple, stupid." Perhaps that wisdom should apply to cancer, too. If we stop using chemicals in our everyday lives, if we stop eating junk and chemically laden foods and start consuming the foods nature has provided, we would all be much healthier. Maybe the cancer epidemic would quietly fade away. We have to stop trying to outthink nature.

> It is estimated that as many as 70 percent of all cancers are related to diet.
>
> –Dr. Russell Blaylock

Fruits and vegetables are rich sources of antioxidants that quench free radicals. They contain hundreds of bioflavonoids (plant chemicals) that have anticancer properties, including the fact that they turn on phase II enzymes that rid our bodies of cancer-causing toxins. They also provide fiber that binds the toxins excreted into the intestine, so that these toxins are not absorbed back into the system. It is an overall consensus, worldwide, that fruits and vegetables not only reduce the rate of cancer but also prevent atherosclerosis and heart disease. Fruits and vegetables are lifesaving foods.

Changing your diet is a difficult thing to do. Most people are so used to grabbing bags of Doritos (40 percent chemicals), ranch-flavored chips (contain high levels of MSG), crackers, cakes, muffins, donuts, biscuits, rolls, peanut butter crackers, potato chips, taco chips. All of these so-called foods contain procarcinogenic oils and high amounts of sugar, methionine, and food additives. These snacks are also high on the glycemic index release and promote cancer growth. Most chips are cooked in omega-6 oils (read Dr. Russell Blaylock's interview for more on these dangers) so you get a concentration of cancer-stimulating additives and ingredients. And we wonder why cancer is an epidemic.

Increased body fat can manufacture estrogens. Obesity is one of the factors known to increase the levels of 16-alpha-hydroxyestrone, the metabolic product of estrogen breakdown that has been shown to powerfully stimulate the growth and spread of breast cancers.

The more you understand the mechanisms of phytochemicals and nutrition, the more you will appreciate why even minor variations in your diet can have significant effects on cancer. In time, your taste buds will readjust to good nutritious food and then chemically laden, poor-quality food will actually taste bad to you. No one knows for sure if cancers are ever really eradicated in your body. If they are not, then sticking to a nutritious diet becomes even more important, since the dormant cancer can be *reactivated* by a bad diet. Think about that when you reach for that next diet soda.

> If people don't supplement, consume a nutritious diet, apply homeopathic therapies, and pay attention to their bodies, they are going to continue to get sick.
>
> –Dr. Steve Nelson

24

DR. MICHAEL GALITZER

Once a physician starts doing energy therapies, that's the point of no return. When you see how dramatically patients respond, you can never practice medicine the same way again.

–Dr. Milton Hammerly

DR. MICHAEL GALITZER AND I go back a long time. He has graciously written the forewords for many of my books. I practice energy medicine with him, and here he will explain the healing aspects of his work. I send many friends and patients to him, and each and every one of them can't say enough good things about his approach. He makes people well. He is able to pinpoint what other doctors can't, and as a result chronic conditions and diseases other doctors have given up on are healed or brought under control. Whether it is bioidentical hormones, thyroid problems, adrenal problems, a lack of energy, autoimmune disease, or cancer, his approach to all conditions is the same: Gently, naturally, people get well.

I always look forward to what he has to say, and his medicine keeps progressing, keeping up with the damaged world in which we live. Dr. Galitzer understands the toxic assault on all of us and what we need to do to stay healthy in spite of it. From his years in the ER to his antiaging energy medicine practice in Santa Monica, California, he is a doctor who is truly cutting-edge.

SS: Thank you again, Dr. Galitzer. How would you describe your specialty?

MG: I work in energy medicine, electrical medicine.

SS: Okay, this needs explanation. It sounds like you work on cars.

MG: Well, traditional medicine basically looks at the body from a physical point of view; X-rays, CT scans, biopsies, MRIs, mammograms—those are all physical ways of looking at the body. Medicine also looks at the body from a chemical point of view; blood tests are a great example of chemical analysis of the body fluids. But there is very little electrical medicine being practiced, except for the EKG of the heart, the EEG of the brain, and the nerve or muscle EMG. So I would say that our kind of medicine looks at the body from an energetic or electrical point of view. I am concerned about the energy level of the liver, pancreas, kidneys, and adrenals.

SS: But I have to say if I weren't practicing this kind of medicine with you and feeling the amazing results, this would sound like gobbledygook.

MG: Okay. For instance, anger is an emotion that affects the liver, but if you did a liver scan you wouldn't see it physically; if you did liver blood tests you wouldn't see that chemically. But the anger would manifest in some symptoms, such as migraines or insomnia. These are electrical or energetic changes.

SS: Is it German in origin?

MG: Yes, it came out of the fifties and the sixties with Dr. Reinhard Voll, who had an extensive background in acupuncture. In acupuncture there are meridians that traverse the body, and there are twelve major meridians. He was able to measure skin resistance along these different meridians, which allowed him to correlate these meridian channels to different organ systems. So, for instance, the large intestine meridian would start on the index finger and end up at the nose. The different points along this large intestine meridian would correlate to different areas of the large intestine. He could demonstrate that when a point had a change in skin resistance, there existed a weakness in the large intestine that was associated with symptoms that the patient was experiencing. His great discovery was that he was able to show that when he added a natural substance to return the skin resistance to normal, that substance helped the patient feel better.

SS: This is not easy for us laypeople to grasp, but I think I get what you are saying.

MG: The real value of this type of medicine is to discern what substances work for people, and at the same time do no harm. For instance, a great example of something that is effective but not tolerated is cancer chemotherapy. It kills cancer but also harms the body. My kind of medicine makes sure I give the patient everything from an antibiotic to an herb, a vitamin, or a mineral, and to be sure it is effective and tolerated. I think this is one of the great advances in this kind of medicine. I actually feel if you're not testing at this level you're not as complete as you could be as a physician.

SS: When people come to you, are they well or are they sick?

MG: Most people aren't well and the major complaint is that they feel fatigued. After analyzing their blood tests, which are frequently normal, I utilize electrical tests such as bioimpedance analysis, heart rate variability, applied kinesiology, and electrodermal screening to determine where the energy weakness is located.

SS: Why is everybody so tired?

MG: I think it's a combination of lifestyle, unhealthy nutrition, toxicity in the environment, and a lack of understanding of how to get rid of these toxins. The liver, kidney, and lymph systems are the organs of elimination. These organs get rid of the toxins. When they are overwhelmed they put in a call to the hormonal systems: adrenals, thyroid, etc. Hormones aid the liver, kidney, and lymph systems, but eventually the glands that secrete these hormones get tired, and at that point you've got a toxic person with tired hormonal glands, which are the setup for being fatigued and not feeling well. People are on the go all the time. Right now the goal appears to be to work as hard as you can and be as successful as you can. This allows for huge amounts of stress, ultimately resulting in poor sleep and, most likely, eating fast foods. Travel takes its toll: airplanes with recirculated air and ionizing radiation, too much coffee and alcohol, too many soft drinks, too much sugar, and not enough water. Add to this mix that people are not taking enough vitamins and supplements, and when you put it all together this person doesn't feel "well."

SS: So, they're not exactly sick, as in they can't get out of bed, but they aren't exactly well. Why are men so reluctant to see what's available with this new medicine that you and others are practicing?

MG: Men don't really want to show their vulnerability, and frankly most men would rather take Viagra and Cialis before they would take testosterone. You see, men don't want to appear weak. Even when you look at the whole issue of obesity in men, they are never described as obese, they are "big." Big is viewed as strong, skinny is viewed as weak.

SS: But women are "fat."

MG: Right. But there are more overweight men than women. However, men seem to overeat with happy emotions, and women crave with negative emotions. Appearance is important to women, but confidence is important to men. For a man even to want to lose weight it's got to be viewed as a problem. He's got to see that it's linked to diabetes or heart disease. So knowing this, you see that men are resistant to this whole element of testosterone for the same reason.

SS: Is it any different if the man is younger? Is a young man easier to convince?

MG: It's no different, but I do personally believe that the key to testosterone is to start it as early as possible.

SS: Which would be when?

MG: Early fifties. An article recently came out saying that low testosterone levels were linked to earlier death, meaning that people with the lowest testosterone levels had a 33 percent greater increase of dying from any cause for the eighteen years of the study. It's obvious that testosterone is a key. It's a heart protector, it stimulates the bones, it's a brain stimulant, and most important, it helps generate excitement and passion.

SS: What can a man who has a poor diet, doesn't exercise, is a type A executive, is stressed, drinks, smokes, and doesn't sleep expect by following traditional medicine?

MG: Definitely a lower quality of life and greater incidence of premature death. A man who is living this lifestyle doesn't feel good at all, and he will definitely be susceptible to chronic cardiovascular disease and sudden death.

SS: Have you had male patients come to your office who you were able to completely turn around?

MG: Numerous, numerous men. I've had the fortune to attract a lot of men who are interested in this kind of work and are ready to follow a program. I put them on a detoxification program, including liver, kidney, lymph drainage, searching for heavy metals. I have often sent them to the dentist to take care of the mercury fillings, and to look at infected root canals and cavitations in their mouth. I give them the right supplements, nutrients, and lots of vitamin C. I test their hormone levels, including testosterone, and the result is that these guys are feeling great. They are very grateful and thankful.

SS: Do these men come in already sold, or do you convince them?

MG: Most are not sold, but thanks to your books, their wives are dragging them in. But they've seen the change in their wives and they've become extremely curious about how much better their wives look and feel and want the same for themselves.

SS: Well, I know my life and health have turned around by embracing your kind of medicine. You've got me feeling great and my energy is fantastic. I leap out of bed each day. Let's talk about your intravenous treatments. I remember the first time I looked into your IV room and it was like some kind of science fiction movie. Of course, now I am one of those people in the IV room. Why are these IV treatments so important?

MG: When I was an ER doc, we all knew in the emergency room the effects of intravenous fluids and intravenous medications, because they work fast to save lives. Intravenous nutrients are very powerful, because they facilitate the excretion of toxins and can rejuvenate organs, such as the liver and the brain. Intravenous vitamin C detoxifies chemicals, cleanses the liver, and strengthens the adrenals. The same goes for intravenous phosphatidylcholine for its liver and brain effects. I give chelation when appropriate to get lead, mercury, and cadmium out of the body.

SS: I was surprised you found high levels of cadmium in my system. How does cadmium get into our systems?

MG: We've all been exposed to lead in the gasoline that used to be in the pump, and then paint in our homes and old lead pipes, and cadmium is also a by-product of cigarette smoke and automobile exhaust; secondhand smoke is probably where you, as a nonsmoker, got exposed. All those years when you were a nightclub performer you were breathing in everyone's cigarettes.

SS: Yes, but that was so many years ago—maybe twenty years.

MG: Right.

SS: Well, I do remember at that time they were starting to make showrooms in Vegas smoke-free, but I never pressed it, being the pleaser that I am. I do remember coughing up black stuff every morning when I was working nightclubs full time and thinking it was ironic that I didn't smoke and that I was taking in so much each night. But I never thought it would stay in my tissues for this long.

MG: They've done studies that show our bones have a thousand times more lead than a hundred years ago. Mercury is a by-product of coal, and it's been proven that in our country we get more mercury from the Chinese, who burn their coal and then the trade winds bring it over, than from the coal that's being burned in the United States. It is impossible to avoid the amount of pollution with which we are assaulted, so it is up to each of us to stimulate our own elimination systems so we can better deal with the massive insults of chemicals that are in the environment.

SS: Talk about a bad neighbor. My God, it shows you the dire consequences if anyone were ever to detonate a nuclear bomb anywhere in the world. We are truly global.

MG: Right, depending on how the wind is blowing.

SS: Okay, but why do we care if we have mercury in our systems?

MG: The EPA ranks mercury either number one or two, depending on who you are talking to, with arsenic being the other one, as one of the two most toxic substances in the environment. Mercury has been linked to illnesses involving the kidney and the prostate. Mercury blocks enzymes, and there is a lot of information that it plays a big role in autism. There is the mercury that was in the preservatives in vaccinations. I really don't understand why anyone would want to vaccinate a kid for hepatitis on the first day they enter the world. There has been major mercury contamination in our environment.

SS: When I was a kid we used to have those thermometers that we would break on purpose to play with the mercury. The other great fun was to look through your feet in those X-ray (radiation) machines in the shoe store.

MG: Some people can be exposed to mercury and can excrete it, but most people are nonexcreters; they just can't get rid of it, and it can stay in their bodies for thirty years.

SS: It is a silent killer?

MG: I'd say it's a silent weakener of the body. Absolutely.

SS: So it's systemic: the blood, bones, organs?

MG: Everywhere, and it is dangerous for the central nervous system and the brain.

SS: How does it rear its ugly head?

MG: For me, it's usually when people complain of fatigue, then right away mercury is suspect. I also see it in the thyroid, especially in regard to teeth, because mercury leaks out of old fillings and the thyroid isn't very far from the lower jaw. Often we come across something called Hashimoto's thyroiditis, which is an autoimmune disease where the body attacks the thyroid gland with antibodies. I frequently neutralize the mercury with selenium, and then at some point down the road, when they're less toxic and feeling stronger, I have them take their mercury fillings out. Thyroid issues are huge with mercury, as are blood pressure and mercury, high cholesterol and mercury, heart disease and mercury, kidney disease and mercury, and prostate disease and mercury.

SS: Should everyone be taking selenium?

MG: Yes. Selenium is an antioxidant, and selenium neutralizes mercury and also has anticancer effects; 200 micrograms a day in tablet form is what I usually recommend.

SS: Let's talk about the other heavy metals. I think my readers will be very interested in this. What about aluminum, and how does it get into our systems? What damage does it create? For years my deodorant had aluminum in it and they bragged about it.

MG: We've all stored our food in aluminum foil; we've been drinking soda in aluminum cans. Aluminum is all over the place. They found aluminum in the neurofibrillary tangles in the brains of Alzheimer's disease patients. Tangles are nerve cells that have become bunched together and knotted. Many of these heavy metals affect the neurological system. So whether it's Parkinson's or dementia or slow thinking or forgetfulness, I look for heavy metals first. Working in ER medicine taught me to look for "horses not zebras."

SS: What does that mean?

MG: In our kind of medicine, heavy metals are the horse that's most likely associated with neurological deterioration, so I look for aluminum, cadmium, lead, and mercury and then I start the detoxification of those substances from that person. Horses are the most likely diagnosis, whereas zebras are the ones you hardly ever see.

SS: What about acetylcholine levels? Would they be any indicator of neurological problems?

MG: Acetylcholine is a neurotransmitter, and low levels have been linked with Alzheimer's. But levels could be low due to the presence of heavy metals, so you would first want to eliminate the heavy metal before you attempted to increase levels of acetylcholine.

SS: New medicine—or, as I call it, breakthrough medicine—is more complex than ever, yet it all seems to be about restoring the deterioration. The world we live in today is stressful, polluted, and chemicalized, plus our enormous stress pushes hormonal imbalances earlier, so no one is feeling quite right. Am I imagining this, or were we always this sick and out of whack?

MG: Two things: We're living longer, and we're exposed to many more chemicals and toxins than ever before. And then there are the electromagnetic frequencies that we are exposed to. A person with mercury fillings in their teeth generates electrical currents in the mouth due to the presence of saliva. Electrical currents can also be generated by the presence of two different metals as fillings, such as mercury and gold. Those electrical currents can override the currents in the brain and therefore lead to symptoms such as insomnia, headaches, and irritability. Now, if this person has a BlackBerry attached to his body twelve to eighteen hours per day, those electrical currents will be amplified. And if he now sits in front of his computer, there is even greater generation of electrical currents. It's almost like sticking your head in the microwave oven in terms of the potential damage. I mean, I'm not going to tell people they can't use their cell phones, but our parents were not subjected to this amount of electromagnetic radiation, and these are some of the big issues that are undermining people's health.

SS: Plus, our parents weren't eating fake food.

MG: Right. And adding to this whole problem is that the soil doesn't have the proper minerals. The selenium is depleted, the water isn't as healthy, and we're drinking less water as well, and we're eating food that isn't as nutrient dense as it once was, plus we're exposed to toxins and electromagnetic radiation as never before.

SS: Do you ever feel overwhelmed that people are coming to see you in such deteriorated states, or do you feel with your type of medicine that you can restore anyone?

MG: I really feel I can bring anyone back if they are willing to work with me and believe in it. I have an underlying faith that people are more resilient than we are led to believe, and with proper guidance, education, and tools, we've got everything we need to help these people. The key is getting these people to come in and get going.

I've worked in this arena of medicine for twenty years and I know there are statistics that say one woman in eight will get breast cancer. But in my practice it's more like one in a thousand. So the question is why? Is it because of what I know? Is it because my practice attracts a health-conscious patient? Is it because of the synergy between myself and my patients? These people really want to get better, and consequently the levels of diseases in my practice and those of my fellow practitioners are much lower than in the general population.

SS: That's true. I enjoy that I go to you when I am well, and frankly, when I think about it, I am almost always well. Yet we have found things deep within me that I never would have known were there until they had reached a disease state. Your medicine is proactive, which I like. For instance, we found tiny amounts of plaque in my small arteries, which was profound. I had been feeling cocky because my tests showed zero plaque in my heart and large arteries, yet you had me take a new blood test and we found small amounts of plaque in my small arteries. This was significant for me because I come from an Irish family—we have high homocysteine levels, and my family dies of heart disease and stroke. I remember the day we received the test results, and you said this was huge relative to preventing a stroke. I can't think of anything worse than a stroke, as I have watched it so often debilitate my loved ones.

MG: The best example is coronary artery disease. There are the large coronary arteries—the left anterior descending, the left circumflex, and the right coronary artery. Over time these arteries slowly get occluded or obstructed as the process of atherosclerosis continues. The patient will complain of chest pain and then they'll get an angiogram, and usually by-pass surgery is recommended or stents. But frequently in medicine it is a small artery within the heart that gets inflamed, cholesterol and platelets rush to the site of inflammation, and suddenly you can go from a 10 per-cent to a 90 percent occlusion. We call this "vulnerable plaque." You can't see it on a CT scan—you can see it on a CT angiogram, but that's a test that costs several thousand dollars. The test I gave you, the CV Profilor, for the early detection of vascular disease, basically measures the elastic-ity of the arteries; it's an office test, it takes ten minutes, costs $150, and is actually reimbursed by insurance companies—it's FDA approved. And it was with that test that we were able to pick up what we call small ar-tery disease or vulnerable plaque. Under the right set of circumstances, this vulnerable plaque could lead to a heart attack or stroke.

SS: And that is why I love this kind of medicine.

MG: But these tests are an indicator. The first thing that comes to mind are heavy metals or viruses. As I recall, we actually found the heavy metals and treated them with chelation, but it didn't change the artery test at all. It was only when we went to this other test, through a lab called Hemex, which looked at abnormalities in blood coagulation, that we found that you had some blood coagulation problems, most likely due to viruses. When we started treating the viruses, that's when your artery test improved. Very few cardiologists use this test, and it's a great screen-ing tool.

SS: Why is everyone on some form of statin?

MG: Well, for some people they make a lot of sense, but for the ma-jority of people there are probably better ways to take care of that issue.

SS: Is niacin the alternative?

MG: I think niacin is great. I usually combine it with garlic and red yeast rice, baby aspirin, and fish oils. Fish oils lower your triglycerides; they have anti-inflammatory effects. They help improve blood flow, be-cause they keep blood thin, and in medicine we prefer that the blood be like red wine as opposed to ketchup.

SS: So thick, sticky blood is not a good thing?

MG: No, it's not. Thick, sticky blood is caused by inflammation. Lots of saturated fats in the diet cause it, chronically high levels of microbes in your body such as viruses and yeast cause it. The major cause of thick blood is chronic viral infections and a poor diet. Too much sugar results in inflammation and then thick blood.

SS: How do we get these viruses, and how do we know we have them?

MG: Think about all the people you meet and shake hands with. People are carriers. Other reasons may be the people who are not vigilant about washing their hands. You have to live a healthy lifestyle and pay attention to hygiene. Viruses are everywhere, and they stay hidden in your blood, making it thick and sticky, until your body is weakened by poor diet or stress or just being run-down—then one or more of these viruses can be activated. Fish oil helps tremendously. The pharmaceutical companies have realized this and have created capsules with high, high levels of fish oil. It costs about $150 a month, which is very pricey, but most people don't care because their insurance will pay for it. You can see how the rising cost of health insurance happens. But you can get great fish oil for about $30 either from your physician or from a high-quality health food store. It's the one thing we doctors who embrace natural strategies for health have in agreement with mainstream cardiologists. We all recognize the importance of fish oil and that it should be a part of every man's and woman's diet.

SS: What about Co-Q_{10}?

MG: Co-Q_{10} is another great supplement that helps with energy production within the body. The five nutrients that improve energy production in the heart are Co-Q_{10}, fish oils, magnesium, carnitine, and a sugar called D-ribose. Regarding the heart, it doesn't matter what heart disease you have—valvular, cardiomyopathy, or hardening of the arteries—what's happening is that the heart isn't making enough energy.

SS: Explain.

MG: The heart is a muscle and the muscle has mitochondria or "energy factories." Each cell has mitochondria, but the heart muscle has a hundred times as many mitochondria as some of the other cells in the body. But if your mitochondria are impaired with one of the heart diseases, your heart is not making enough energy. Co-Q_{10}, magnesium, carnitine, fish oils, and D-ribose increase energy production, which will help all people with heart disease.

SS: And they haven't taken a drug. Ah, I just put it together—this is ENERGY MEDICINE! This explains what you do. So, you do this not just for the heart but for the whole body.

MG: Yes.

SS: But instead everyone is on a statin, which inhibits the body's ability to produce any more cholesterol and depletes the patient of their energy. But our bodies need cholesterol for our brain and our gut. I know we have neurons in the brain and in the gut, and these neurons are made in part by cholesterol, so for those taking statins it seems to me that down the road we're going to start seeing severe dementia and GI problems.

MG: Right. Statins reduce levels of cholesterol. Cholesterol has many valuable uses in the body. We don't want our bodies to be without it. Cholesterol is the building block for all the steroid hormones. Steroids are any hormone made by the adrenals, ovaries, and testes. Cortisol is a steroid hormone, DHEA is a steroid hormone; estrogen, progesterone, and testosterone are steroid hormones. So, if you are a guy and trying to reduce your elevated cholesterol with a statin, you definitely should be taking testosterone and DHEA, and women, estrogen, progesterone, testosterone, and DHEA.

SS: But men have a huge fear that testosterone is going to give them cancer.

MG: A man deficient in testosterone isn't going to have a healthy prostate, but that doesn't mean he is going to get cancer. An unhealthy prostate makes men have to urinate a little more and they might develop conditions like BPH (enlarged prostate), so the first thing to do is get the prostate healthier, which is very easy to do. When you get the prostate healthier, then testosterone can be optimized. Red meat, excessive coffee, and excessive alcohol irritate the prostate; whole grains, vegetables, and fruits like pomegranate help the prostate. Removing mercury fillings is important because mercury has an affinity for the kidneys and the prostate. The two front teeth, above and below, are energetically connected to the prostate, and sometimes there is a root canal in those teeth. When I have their root canal cleaned out, or if a lower tooth has to be pulled if it is extensively infected, the prostate gets healthier. The prostate can be strengthened by taking saw palmetto, giant redwood, vitamin E, selenium, fish oils, vitamin D, zinc, and other minerals.

Lymphatic drainage in the abdomen, pelvis, and groin has been shown to help the prostate get healthier. Sex helps to keep the prostate healthier, and very important are Kegel exercises—the same ones women do for pregnancy. So, instead of like when having a bowel movement, you push out, you push in with your internal rectal muscles, and in doing so you are using your internal sphincter to massage the prostate. You can do ten of these sitting in your chair, or in your car, two or three times a day.

SS: Well, I hate to be commercially crass, but there is no better way to do Kegel exercises than with a ThighMaster. Let me just throw that out there.

MG: All right, well, there you go. You're probably right.

SS: I just happen to know where you can get one!

MG: I try to encourage men. I tell them, I can get you ultimately healthy and we can make testosterone work as well as possible by getting your prostate healthy.

Now there's one other issue: The prostate represents the ability to give of yourself to your sexual partner; it's the same issue with women and their uterus. The emotional aspect needs to be addressed and very early on in our work together. It's the whole deal—mind, body, spirit—and there are sometimes deeper issues, rather than toxicity and hormones, that are causing the prostate to act up. When you look at the prostate from these different perspectives, you can address the issues and get the prostate healthier. Then when you put the man on testosterone you can explain to him why he is not going to get cancer.

SS: In your opinion, is testosterone an antidote to prostate cancer? Would you give a man with prostate cancer testosterone as the remedy? You know this therapy is being done in Europe.

MG: I would stay away from testosterone and prostate cancer. There are too many issues with men at that point, and cancer is the result of a toxic accumulation within the body. Cancer represents a state where the hormonal systems are at a very low level.

SS: Well, with all due respect, wouldn't it make sense that you optimize the hormonal levels and return the body to its optimal hormonal prime, including testosterone?

MG: We just don't know that yet. I do find in *all* cancer patients that their pituitary gland is not making enough growth hormone. Now, this is anecdotal, but I've looked at hundreds of people with cancer and you can generalize that in cancer there exists an extremely high level of toxicity, and that the key hormonal systems, such as adrenals and thyroid—all the hormones including testosterone—are very *low*.

SS: Well . . .

MG: When I am looking at cancer I *first* want to see how we can reduce the toxicity in the body. How can we strengthen the adrenals? How can we strengthen the thyroid? How can we optimize nutrition? What intravenous therapies, such as vitamin C, could help detoxify the patient? I personally believe that toxic people in weakened states are not going to be turned around with testosterone. There may be a point, or a place, for testosterone, but I'm not convinced it's anywhere in the beginning of the treatment. I'd be very hesitant to replace testosterone in proven prostate cancer patients.

SS: Well, I'm not a doctor, but if I were a man with prostate cancer, I would do all of the above, all the detoxification, all the IV treatments, I would strengthen the adrenals and thyroid and the other hormones. I would do everything you mentioned, but in connecting my own dots I would also roll the dice and replace the testosterone. My thinking would be that when I was young and making a full complement of hormones, including testosterone, I didn't get cancer. But I'm a risk taker, and I'M NOT A DOCTOR.

MG: You are just one of those patients that think for themselves and you have done very well for yourself. There are theories that the primary cause of cancer is a lack of oxygen use by the cells of the body, that they instead turn to fermentation of sugar in order to create energy. This is called "anaerobic metabolism." The normal body cells meet their energy needs by using oxygen (aerobic metabolism), whereas cancer cells meet their energy needs by fermenting sugar.

SS: Ah, now we're getting back to your kind of medicine, energy medicine.

MG: Yes, this may be one of the key issues in medicine. I would first ask how we get cells to start utilizing oxygen and not fermenting sugar to produce your energy before I went toward hormones. Energy may be the biggest issue we have to pay attention to and, also, how do we change people's beliefs about cancer?

SS: What do you mean?

MG: How do we get rid of the fear? How can you live with cancer for thirty or forty years without dying a slow, painful, torturous death? I think that may be one of the huge issues facing medicine in the future. How do we change the mind-set and reduce the fear? Frequently, people are told that they have cancer, and they have six months to live, and to get their affairs in order. Very often those people end up dying at that six-month time frame just due to the fear. Just getting the diagnosis of cancer greatly depresses the immune system. As doctors we have got to be very tender with people when we tell them they have cancer.

But I feel the big issue—and it is where medicine has to make a big jump so people will get to live to be a hundred—is to get our patients to get over the fear that they don't have to die from cancer and that they can live a fairly normal life with the disease. This is where the global belief system kicks in that we can live normal, happy, healthy lives even with cancer. It's going to require a multipronged treatment protocol on many different lines, which might include pharmaceutical medication, like RNA interference technology where you can silence certain genes in cancer.

SS: Okay, what's RNA?

MG: It's called RNAI and it stands for RNA interference; you basically create chemical products that can actually stop certain genes from expressing themselves.

SS: I get nervous whenever I hear the word "chemical." Isn't it our chemicalization that has gotten all of us in such trouble?

MG: I'm saying that we use all the tools. We have pharmaceuticals, intravenous nutrients, homeopathics, enzymes, nutraceuticals. We know how to eat healthfully if we would just do it, and I think the time has come for us to put it all together, for East to meet West in medicine and try to figure out how we can use all treatments together.

One of the problems with alternative medicine is that there are many practitioners who tell their patients, "Don't do that drug, we can do it better our way." Maybe they can, maybe they can't. It's certainly difficult in the area of hypertension not to use pharmaceuticals and just use alternative medicine. Not to take advantage of drugs when they might be the answer does a great disservice. It alienates traditional medicine and I don't think you have to do that. There is so much in alternative medicine that works. I'm saying that when called for, traditional medicine has its place, especially as we go into the future.

SS: Well, I do find all the new areas—stem cell possibilities, nanotechnology, biotechnology, neurotechnology, mapping DNA profiles and linking that knowledge to prevent illness—are all new ways to radically change medicine by making it predictive and progressive. These truly are exciting new measures on the horizon, and I know I will be taking advantage as they become available and feel safe. I already take advantage of nanotechnology and I have banked my stem cells.

What I like right now is that there is a groundswell, a movement or "a knowing," that present traditional medicine is not adequate or relevant to today's world. Those of you who are thinking outside the box, call it alternative or whatever, know that traditional medicine is not making the cut. We see it every day and that has contributed to this groundswell. That is why I am so involved. I did not like the treatment offered me when I was diagnosed with breast cancer. I realized that *I* had to think outside of the box until I could find a doctor or doctors with whom I could work creatively.

What you are describing is the "art of medicine"—the highest form of medicine, where thinking is required. This has to happen. Right now, testing has replaced thinking. You and I were talking the other day about how, because of technology, we are able to see a teeny little spot and immediately everyone jumps on it as cancer. Right away, surgery and violent "after treatments" of poison trying to kill a "spot" that actually could have been there for twenty years not bothering the person. I had a friend like that; even when they went inside his stomach and could no longer find that little spot, they gave him chemotherapy and radiation "just in case." That body is put in a violent state and maybe that spot could have sat there not bothering him for his entire life. Now he is sick as a person and will never be the same. This is the kind of medicine that bothers me.

MG: Some of these cancers take twenty years to grow, but right now we use our technology and pick up that cancer and decide we have to start treating that cancer next week, and that probably isn't correct. I believe that instead we take that same patient and build up that body, strengthen that body, and then decide how to treat the cancer, but now we do it with a strong body. Treating a cancer patient with a weak body is not a recipe for success. It is to the benefit of the patient that we first utilize alternative treatments. "When is the ideal time to treat any illness?" is referred to as chronobiology; trying to respect the natural circadian rhythms within the body. There is an ideal time to treat any person with any disease, and we doctors have to decide if it is prudent to treat it at the time of diagnosis or better to treat it six weeks later after putting the patient through a program that increases overall health and reduces the toxicity.

SS: What are the five or ten things we each should do to live a healthy life?

MG: I'd start by impressing upon you that it's not your fault that you're exposed to high levels of toxicity. I liken this toxicity to a toilet bowl that doesn't flush well, so there's always junk left in there.

SS: Eew!

MG: But you get the picture of toxicity. I tell my patients that you've got to wake up your liver. Most people don't even know where their liver is located. Remember this, the first four letters of liver are LIVE, and the liver sits under the right breast, right behind the lower ribs on the right side. You've got to increase drainage within the liver, lymph, and kidney system. You've got to take a lemon every morning and drink the juice, with six ounces of water, first thing on an empty stomach. Lemon is very alkaline and neutralizes acidity. Lemon also helps to cleanse the liver.

You've got to consume certain liver foods in your diet. You can juice them, cook them, eat them raw—carrots, beets, zucchini, squash, watercress, and artichokes are all liver foods. Drink as many vegetable juices as you can. One day a week try to fast from dinner one night to dinner the next and drink raw vegetable juices.

To strengthen the kidney system, you've got to be drinking healthy water. It can't be distilled. Distilled water is dead water, because it has no minerals. Volvic water is great because it is slightly alkaline, has lots of electrons, and has the right amount of minerals. It's active, vibrant water. You've got to take care of your lymph system through exercise, and decrease dairy intake.

This is about getting toxins out, and recall drainage. You want to unclog the drain to make the liver, lymph, and kidney systems more efficient and more miraculous in eliminating the junk that we are all exposed to. This is where I'd start.

Then, you must understand the importance of nutrition. You've got to eat healthy foods; you've got to eat live foods and exercise. You've got to look at your body as a high-efficiency Ferrari that needs high-octane fuel, so you must put good fuel into your car to get optimal performance. The body is no different. Everyone needs to be on healthy supplements.

Next, I'd look at the stress in your life. Look at what's really important to you. Your internal emotional health is a major part of your wellness. Are you happy in your relationship? Are you happy in your work? What excites you? What are you grateful for and what is the purpose for your life? Why do you think you are here? I try to get people to align themselves with their own purpose as opposed to just going to work every day. For instance, most people say to me, "I'm doing this job because it makes sense and I've got to make money so we can support our family." People who have that outlook on life are not the healthy people. Healthy people are the ones who know where they are going and have a purpose in their lives. Whatever that purpose, it doesn't have to be to save mankind, it can just be to feel happy, to get to know yourself a little better. Whatever that purpose, allow it to guide you. You will do better if you live a purposeful life with excitement, passion, and gratitude. These are the building blocks of life.

People need to have more fun in their lives. People who are not having fun in their lives get sick. These people don't know why they are here, they're not excited about anything, and they are not very grateful for their lives. Of course, when you are feeling lousy, it's hard to be grateful, but when the attitude changes, the excitement of life comes back and so does health.

SS: And where are hormones in this?

MG: Yes, hormones, thank you for reminding me. The hormonal system modulates our detoxification and metabolism by interpreting our internal and external environment through the release of messenger hormones from the hypothalamus and pituitary glands in the brain. I obtain information about my patients from blood, urine, and saliva tests, where we look at the adrenal and thyroid hormones, then the sex hormones: estrogen, progesterone, and testosterone. These are all key, but the granddaddy is growth hormone (GH). Growth hormone is like turbocharging your car. You've got to have four wheels before you can even think about turbocharging it. The four wheels are insulin, sex hormones, thyroid, and adrenal. Once those wheels are on the car and once your body is less toxic, that's the place to turbocharge. You wouldn't want to turbocharge it in the beginning, it would be too much, and you've got to do all these other things first.

To determine growth hormone deficiencies we check the IGF-1 level (insulinlike growth factor). Unfortunately, growth hormone has been misrepresented because of its name. It's not really just about growth; it does cause kids to grow, but it's really a metabolic hormone. It stimulates protein synthesis, burns fats, and conserves carbs. If you are taking growth hormone you are obligated to exercise. Plus you must eat protein at each meal. You can't just inject something and not do the other necessary things in your lifestyle that will support it. Growth hormone should not be given until the body is less toxic; then with exercise and with protein at each meal, you will get the maximum benefits from growth hormone. When you add growth hormone at the right phase of restoration, when everything else is in balance, when you are less toxic, you will get great benefits.

SS: Absolutely. And it's so satisfying to see muscle definition come back and amazing to see your body respond to exercise so beautifully. To me growth hormone is just another missing piece of the hormonal "song." It's like making a cake; you don't put the frosting on top until the cake is finished and cooled off.

MG: I never give growth hormone to my patients until their livers are cleaned up.

SS: I'm glad you said that. People look to GH as a magic bullet. You've got to get the rest of the "song" in tune before you add the GH; then when you do it, it makes you feel healthy—very healthy. You have to exercise, and you will enjoy working out because the body responds like it did when you were young. But I think what is giving GH a bad name is that so many people are buying inferior brands online, and also athletes are overusing it. In some cases, athletes are injecting a hundred times more than the body ever required, plus they add to their cocktail synthetic anabolic steroids, which are very dangerous.

MG: It's all about timing, doing the right things at the right time. With growth hormone we know it is something you do at the end. Timing is key.

SS: In the field of antiaging, in terms of the future, what excites you?

MG: There are two areas. Antiaging will be useless in the future if we don't get our children on track. Soda machines in school, junk food, sugar, Gatorade, which has yellow dye #5 in it—these are just some of the factors that are creating a generation of children in poor health. We've got to stop the autism epidemic, we have an overload of children with ADD, we have adults with ADD, we've got to get a handle on vaccinations and educate our children so they truly understand the value of nutrition. Adults need to be role models for them not only in life lessons but as it pertains to health.

SS: I so agree. We cannot continue to let children eat their usual diet of nonfood and expect them to grow up healthy.

MG: And the second area is getting a better handle on cancer. We've got tremendous technology, and if we can combine this with antiaging medicine we can change people's beliefs about cancer. In the not-so-distant future a person will be able to place a hand on a machine and it will tell you how much energy your cells are making.

SS: And then as a doctor you would know how to build up that energy?

MG: We'll be able to measure energy fields. We all have energy fields; patients have energy fields and so do doctors. I know it sounds a little "Star Trekkie," but say, for instance, in choosing a doctor you will be able to put your energy field in the machine along with the energy field of the doctor to find if there is a compatibility.

SS: But why would we want this, why would we care?

MG: Matching people's energy fields with energy fields of healers, practitioners, and physicians will improve treatment. You will be with the right person for the right circumstance.

I also believe there will be a lot greater use of homeopathy in the future. Homeopathy represents information, and the key to healing is to combine information with energy. Kids have tons of energy and respond dramatically to homeopathy because you are combining information with their inherently high levels of energy. The real problem with sick people is they don't have enough energy, and that's why I use intravenous nutrients. That's also why we use hormones. Intravenous treatments and hormones raise energy. The reason homeopathy doesn't work well in older people is because the information is great, but there's no energy to kind of suck it in. In the future homeopathy will be used with more success because more and more people with serious illnesses will find their way to doctors who practice this kind of energy medicine and will be able to increase their energy. Once you increase their energy you'll get them back to health.

SS: You know, homeopathy is not understood by many of us. Could you in a sentence describe homeopathy?

MG: Well, you know about herbs. Herbs are plants. Homeopathics are dilutions of herbs, and also dilutions of substances from the mineral and animal kingdoms. Homeopathics can help balance the emotional and mental energy of a person.

SS: And what would you say to men who are reluctant to cross over to this new form of medicine that integrates hormones, detoxifying and increasing energy?

MG: *If men want to work hard, play hard, stay hard, and stay healthy, if men want to keep their hair, then this is the kind of medicine they would want to practice. The boomers get the concept of exercising. I even think the bulk of boomers know how to eat correctly. If they add to that this new approach to medicine, of increasing energy, building up with intravenous nutrients, replacing lost hormones and growth hormone, then men and women can expect to live a long, healthy, quality life.*

SS: Sounds good to me. Thanks.

DR. MICHAEL GALITZER'S
BREAKTHROUGH BREAKOUTS

- Mercury has been linked to illnesses involving the kidney, thyroid, and the prostate, it blocks enzymes, and it may play a role in autism. It can be neutralized with selenium, 200 micrograms a day in tablet form.

- Niacin lowers cholesterol, and when taken with garlic, red yeast rice, baby aspirin, and fish oils can lower your triglycerides and have anti-inflammatory effects, contributing to improved heart health.

- Five nutrients that improve energy production in the heart are Co-Q_{10}, fish oils, magnesium, carnitine, and D-ribose.

- Once insulin, sex hormones, thyroid, and adrenals are in balance, your doctor might add growth hormone to your regimen to turbocharge your health.

- Intravenous treatments such as chelation, glutathione, and vitamin C can detoxify the body and improve energy and vitality.

Dear Suzanne Somers,

Bet you've never heard this one before . . .

I'm forty-eight, my husband of twenty-three years has flown the coop and has started his new family, my kids won't talk to me; they come home at the end of the day and run upstairs and lock their bedroom doors to keep me out. I don't know how they survive, since they don't eat with me anymore.

Me on the other hand loves to eat and I do it really well. At school, I was captain of the cheerleading team, blond, trim, tight and frisky. Now I am a size 18, I don't know what color my hair is, and frisky left the building years ago. I really feel like a great big mushy bag of s—t!

Then I saw you on TV and what you said made so much sense to me and you looked great. I called and ordered all your books not knowing the title of the one you spoke about and about seventeen books arrived.

How did you find the time to write all those books and still look great? Is it really all about real hormones?

You are a wonderful inspiration and I expect to look like you someday. When it happens, I will send you a picture of me in my old cheerleading outfit.

Until then,
Doris B.
Ms. Bag of S—t!

25

DR. STEVEN HOTZE

America spends 25 percent of its health care dollars during the last six months of life, more than $300 billion a year to finance every conceivable treatment for every possible condition—without adding an iota to quality of life!

   −Dr. Khalid Mahmud

THIS TEXAN DOCTOR is going to steal your heart. He has so much energy he can't wait to get to his office each day. He has built up a practice that is the envy of doctors everywhere. The reason it works is that he gets people well and rarely, if ever, resorts to pharmaceutical drugs.

Dr. Hotze is an honorable guy and a renegade. He learned as he went and saw that bioidentical hormones made men and women alike feel good again. You are going to love him. He is a pioneer and he is fearless. He is the founder of the Hotze Health and Wellness Center in Houston, where he works finding the underlying causes for the conditions that plague people from middle age on. He can be heard regularly on his radio show "Health and Wellness Solutions," on Houston's KSEV 700, and has been on the air for six and a half years. I loved talking to this guy.

SS: Good morning, Dr. Hotze. How did you get involved in today's new cutting-edge natural approach to medicine?

SH: My patients weren't getting well. They were chronically sick all the time, and then one day one of my patients said to me, "You know, ever since I quit taking all the medications you were giving me, I feel like a million dollars." I knew she was right. I knew she was smarter than me and all the other doctors, because as my daddy had been telling me for years, "Some of these doctors will kill you with all these drugs. Don't do that to your patients. Those drugs kill people." And he was right.

Then my dad had a severe heart problem, and two weeks after surgery he handed me a letter by Dr. Julian Whitaker. It said, "Here's the deal on heart disease: If you have not had heart surgery, the mortality rate is 5 percent; if you have had angioplasty, you have a 15 percent chance in 100; if you don't do anything but take vitamins, exercise, and lose weight, you only have a 1 percent mortality rate." So I realized right then that my daddy was right: Don't let the doctors get a hold of you, it increases the chances of them killing you. I didn't want to be one of those doctors.

That's when I decided I was going to make a change and literally asked God to give me direction in my life. I had eight kids at the time. I said, I want to be able to help people get well, and I want to be able to make a living to feed my family.

In 1992, one of my colleagues said to me, "You've got to take care of your women with thyroid problems. In the coming years you are going to see a ton of women with thyroid disorders, but if you don't look for it, you won't find it." I started looking and found about a third of the women, and about 20 percent of the males, had antibodies to their thyroid gland that adversely affected their bodies' ability to utilize thyroid, which governs the body's metabolism.

I started using Armour thyroid and people started getting well. There was still a group of people who didn't get well, and it was women who were saying, "You know, I had a hysterectomy and that's when I started having health problems." Or they would say, "Since I started birth control pills, I just haven't felt the same." That got me thinking.

Putting that together with what Dr. Julian Whitaker was saying about natural hormone replacement and then reading his newsletter on hormones and thyroid, I knew I was on track. Lack of hormones was making people feel bad. So let's put them back the right way. Simple!

SS: Yes, I know of Dr. Whitaker and am a big admirer. He was one of the first to embrace this type of medicine. And what about Dr. John Lee? Do you know of him?

SH: Oh yes, he is the first doctor who talked about bioidentical progesterone. You know, when the student is ready, the teacher will arrive . . . and it was Dr. Lee. He made sense. That's when I realized that I had to get all these women off of counterfeit hormones, these synthetic hormones, and get them on bioidentical natural hormones. And gosh, the women did awesome. At the time I only had eight people on staff, now we have eighty people on staff. We also have a compounding pharmacy and a vitamin business. That is how I can maintain control and quality. That's how I got into the bioidentical business.

The first woman I prescribed them to was a pastor's wife, and she had always been edgy. But when I gave her bioidenticals she got better: The edge went away, her headaches went away. We found out she was allergic to corn. We got her energy up, but the biggest deal was taking her off of Premarin; that made the biggest difference. She had had a hysterectomy at age thirty-three and had been unhappy, unhealthy, and in a bad mood ever since. A month later the black cloud had lifted. She could not believe the way she felt. She had been a recluse for years, hadn't even been out of her house for ten years. She then wrote a letter to her son and said, "I'm sorry I've been such a grouchy mother all of these years, but it was the Premarin that made me feel that way, and I apologize." That's pretty dramatic.

SS: Did word get out that something pretty dramatic was happening over at Dr. Hotze's office?

SH: Yes, and we started getting phenomenal results with women who were coming from all over the country. Then I met Dr. William Jeffries and learned about the natural uses of cortisol, and that kind of rounded things out. Today the success we've had is just amazing. Our goal is to help our patients obtain and maintain health and wellness. We get the immune system healthy and we get the energy level up. We treat for airborne allergies, we treat for yeast, we use natural thyroid hormones, we use bioidentical hormones for sex hormone replacement, we treat for adrenal fatigue, we use vitamin and mineral supplementation and a nutritionally balanced eating program. These steps put our patients on a path to good health and wellness.

SS: So you mainly deal with women, or do men come to your clinic?

SH: We're geared toward women, but we also take care of men. We treat men with testosterone, and it's been dramatic. But men also need to take care of the rest of their hormonal system. By the time men and women come to me, they've been to five or ten other doctors. They've been mistreated, misdiagnosed, maltreated, and treated like they are hypochondriacs, neurotics, and hysterics. They come to me as a last resort and they get better.

What we do is give them their lives back. Most women who come here are loaded up on antidepressants, sleep medications, a whole host of drugs that their doctors have poisoned them with over the years. Our goal is to get them off those drugs, especially the antidepressants. Those drugs ought to be banned; they are criminal. There's a cartel that pushes them legally through the system. It's horrible. The effect they have on women and men is just terrible.

SS: Is it difficult to wean women off of antidepressants? I think it would be difficult for them to follow a comprehensive program, knowing what antidepressants do to the mind.

SH: The biggest problem is their other doctors who say things like, "Don't go on those bioidentical hormones." I mean, ever since Adam and Eve we've had bioidentical hormones in our system that have worked. That's why there is a human race. It's like saying, "We don't know if water works, or if food works."

SS: You make me laugh. But it's true, what are they all so afraid of? Do these doctors think the patients' problems are all in their heads?

SH: Usually it's the husbands who are convinced their wives are crazy, and they are sick of them spending money going all over the country trying to get better. So these women don't have support at home, which is unfortunate.

SS: Do you find when women have balanced hormones they have less yeast?

SH: Yes. Yeast is a problem, and you've got to clean it out or you will have problems. But it's from all the antibiotics they didn't need and have been taking all their lives—another crazy overuse of drugs. Antibiotics have been used for so long "just in case," but they kill the healthy bacteria in the vagina and the colon. And too much yeast depresses the immune system. Then you get a cycle of illness, so you've got to clean out the yeast. We put them on a program of nystatin (an antifungal medication) and probiotics for several days, and it will usually clear up. Women on the counterfeit hormones (Premarin and Prempro) or estrogen alone are going to have worse problems. These drugs propagate yeast. And, remember, the counterfeits are not even hormones. Birth control pills are not hormones; they are drugs that mimic hormones. Hormones exist in nature and in our human bodies. Those are the only things that are true hormones. And drugs like BCPs (birth control pills) have hypereffects; they are hard to clear from the system, and they cause a host of side effects.

SS: Do you think birth control pills are one of the causes of breast cancer?

SH: I would say that's a huge contributing factor. We all know the Women's Health Initiative (WHI), 2002, showed that the combination of Premarin and Provera was harmful to women. The WHI said it would be better for women to take nothing at all than to take these dangerous drugs that are made of horse estrogen, which is then made into a chemical, and medroxyprogesterone, which is not real progesterone, and the real tragedy is that most doctors don't know the difference.

SS: That's the part I can't understand. If I was a doctor and I heard all this talk about real bioidenticals, I sure would educate myself just so as not to look stupid.

SH: I agree. I was talking to one doctor who said, "You can't give women progesterone because the WHI said it was dangerous," and I said, "That's medroxyprogesterone, not a real progesterone." I then asked that doctor, "Would you give pregnant women medroxyprogesterone?" "No," he says, "because of the detrimental effects on the baby." Then I asked him, "Would you give natural progesterone to women who are having problems with infertility?" "Yes," he says, "all the time." So let's think about this: Real progesterone exactly replicates what nature made in a woman's body. Medroxyprogesterone cuts off the natural progesterone that puts a woman in a state of estrogen, which is exactly what birth control pills do—and that propagates cancer. Real progesterone protects against breast cancer; that came out in a study by Johns Hopkins in 1981. In this study it proved that real, natural progesterone protects against cancer and that a progesterone deficiency dramatically increases your risk of breast cancer.

SS: And I am one of those estrogen-dominant women who got breast cancer. If I had known, if doctors had known this, as little as a decade ago, I could have protected myself from cancer by increasing my progesterone to the perfect ratio with estrogen. This is why it is important, crucial, for women to educate themselves at this point. Until doctors and med schools catch up, women will get sick and die needlessly because of the pervading attitude about nonpatentable medicines. Unfortunately, at this time, there are not many doctors around such as you who have taken the time to learn about the hormone mystery.

SH: Progesterone is vital to a woman's well-being. Progesterone is crucial for everything from brain function to skeletal function to libido. If a woman has symptoms of low estrogen—vaginal dryness, hot sweats, night sweats, migraines—then we give estrogen to relieve the symptoms.

SS: What about a woman who has had a hysterectomy?

SH: If she's had a total hysterectomy, then she's got to have complete hormone replacement. I don't care if she's thirty-five, forty-five, or whatever—she has been surgically thrown into menopause. The misconception is about total hysterectomy: A total is when the uterus is removed; a partial is when the cervix is removed, leaving the uterus. And if they remove the ovaries you have cut the circulation from the uterus to the ovary, cutting off the blood supply; you will then get significant atrophy of the ovaries and your ability to produce hormones is dramatically reduced.

SS: And then that woman is left without her beautiful hormones to keep her feeling happy and balanced—and she'll have headaches, I might add.

SH: And, by the way, hysterectomy doesn't solve the problem. The problem is hormonal imbalance. The problem is not with the uterus. Usually if a woman has dysfunctional uterine bleeding, you put her on progesterone and the problem clears up. You can save her from a hysterectomy.

SS: Why are so many hysterectomies done each year?

SH: You know why: Ob-gyns are trained as surgeons. Surgeons see all problems as surgical. "You're bleeding too much, honey. We'll take care of it, and we'll cut it out." But it doesn't treat the underlying hormonal problems, which by the way do not affect only the uterus; they affect every cell in her body, including her brain cells. She's no better off; she still has a hormonal problem. So you really haven't solved the problem, she's just not bleeding.

SS: Are hormones the backbone of your program at the Hotze Health and Wellness Center?

SH: Absolutely. The backbone of antiaging, and health in general, is hormonal replenishment. You have to do that to stay in the game. Then you need to exercise; you've got to clean out, as in detoxification, and if you have allergies, we treat for that. These are all the things that plague people in today's world but are usually treated with pharmaceuticals—which as you know won't get them better.

Our regimen basically takes care of 80 to 90 percent of people, but there are some folks who have toxic injuries from chemicals they've been exposed to and they need to be detoxified. For instance, mercury in fillings gives many people adverse effects. Mercury is so toxic that if you throw it into a lake, they condemn the lake for toxic waste, but then they go and stick it in your mouth. Go figure.

Another problem is root canal, which can lead to sublingual abscesses in the jaw and in the teeth. You've got miles and miles of little cavities inside one tooth. Bacteria can get in there, but unfortunately these bacteria don't breathe oxygen, so they can create subclinical abscesses in the jaw. But the dental society doesn't promote getting rid of root canal or mercury fillings, because they hold the patent on root canal.

So you ask, Why doesn't the government get involved? Well, who is the government? Who controls the government? It's the pharmaceutical companies and big insurance, and these companies wine and dine our officials with vacations, limos, and then the payback is approval of some drug that is not going to hold up.

May I say this to you? I want to commend you. I think you've got more courage than anyone I've seen to take this on. I'm proud of you to go up against these idiots, all these powers that be, to go on national TV and be ridiculed by these morons. You have a tough skin, and you've got the message, and the women who hear you know that you ring true. They know you know what you are talking about. This is a huge movement of wellness that you are spearheading and getting people off of drugs.

SS: Thank you, but it's all of us. Once you realize the health that is available, once you realize how off-track our medical approach has been, once you realize the damage that is being done by overuse of pharmaceuticals, it's pretty difficult to sit and be quiet.

SH: Half of the funding for medical schools comes from drug companies, and they fund most of the professors, and these professors get grants from drug companies to speak at their conferences. Do you think they want to encourage natural healing? No way! That's antibusiness as far as they are concerned. You've heard of Dr. Thierry Hertoghe?

SS: Yes, he is a friend of mine, and he was interviewed for this book. He is a giant in the field.

SH: I work closely with him also. He has written several books about hormones, and in the back he has listed thousands of references on every one of the hormones. So it's not that there haven't been studies done, it's that they have never looked for the studies. But even if there weren't any studies, deductive reasoning would tell you. You have to use what your body makes rather than something that never existed before in nature. And we've shown that it works. We've had thousands of patients who are successful in their hormone balance today because of bioidentical hormones. Most of them came to me having been on the counterfeit hormones and feeling like crap. With bioidenticals they get well, they lose weight, they feel good, and they are happy. They tell me, "You gave me my life back." It's simple: They come in sick, they leave well.

SS: I hear it all the time. I am living it. I am a bioidentical-ed woman and I feel great.

SH: *Toxins are the other big problem. How about Splenda? It's sucralose, which is chlorinated hydrocarbon, which is toxic. Any chlorinated hydrocarbon in the world is toxic, carcinogenic. Splenda was originally made as a pesticide— go dump it on your ant beds and come back tomorrow to see all the dead ants. If you have to have sugar, just have a little sugar. It will be a lot better than eating poison. If it's in a bag or a box, it's going to be bad for you. They've all got food additives and chemicals and dyes, and these things cause ADD in kids.*

SS: And we wonder why kids are going on "shoot-'em-ups."

SH: We are learning the hard way.

SS: What's with all the enlarged prostates and prostate cancer in men? What is going on?

SH: Most doctors don't realize that men need to have their *progesterone* levels checked. Men can get estrogen dominant, which needs to be balanced by progesterone. Estrogen dominance in men can lead to prostate cancer. Dr. Lee has also written about the fact that men make as much progesterone as women do, interestingly not in their testes but in their adrenal glands. Progesterone balances estrogen; as males get older they convert testosterone to estradiol, and that can affect the prostate gland and cause it to swell. Prostate cancer is not caused by testosterone. If that were true, every young buck in town would have prostate cancer. People get prostate cancer when they have little or no testosterone. Again, simple: Let's keep the testosterone levels at optimum so this doesn't happen.

SS: Don't you feel that prostate cancer is way overtreated and excessive?

SH: Every man who dies over age eighty dies with prostate cancer—not of it, but *with* it. In other words, it's been there for years. My feeling is, leave it alone. You know, if you go in and kick the ants, the ants will spread all over the place. Same with prostate cancer. When doctors get aggressive with men and their prostate cancer, they ruin their lives. I don't even check my prostate anymore. It may get checked on a test, but I don't even care about it.

SS: Checking for prostate cancer in men seems knee-jerk to me. As soon as the PSA is up, they want to take it out or give them the nasty drug Lupron, which makes them a woman. My male friends on Lupron are in menopause: hot flashes, can't sleep, their breasts grow, their stomachs enlarge, and they generally feel miserable all the time.

SH: Yes. A doctor friend of mine came to me and said, "I had prostate cancer; they took out my prostate, and in doing so they took out my soul. A man's soul is his prostate; my life is ruined." So that's why I say, leave it alone. In Sweden, if men are diagnosed with low-grade prostate cancer, they don't do anything. The studies show that they live longer than the men with prostatectomies.

SS: So what's the rush in this country?

SH: Fear—it's the fear gig. You've got cancer, we've got to do something with it. It's the surgeons: "Let's cut it out." That's the way they make their money. There's no money in making a living helping people be well. If people were well we wouldn't need near as many drugs.

SS: So when is it too late?

SH: Well, we can always help people to a degree. The longer you've had problems, the older you are, the less chance there is that you are going to get the maximum benefits from any regimen of bioidentical hormones. But it is going to help you. You will feel better. In a perfect world it would be great to get on a path to health and wellness as soon as you can. Bring your kids up right. Teach them how to eat. Warn them of the dire consequences of chemicals. Get them on vitamins when they are young, get them off of junk food. We are now obligated to teach our young people the truth.

I'll tell you a story: About five or six years ago a woman comes in who was seventy-eight years old. She had emphysema in her lungs, she had allergies, and her thyroid was way off. She told my girl up front that she was going to die if Dr. Hotze didn't see her. She had cash in hand, she was serious. I worked with her and I know we've given her five years or more of her life when she could hardly take a breath. So it's never too late.

SS: Do you feel hopeful about the future?

SH: Well, we're confident in what we do. We have a fight ahead of us and we've got to fight socialized medicine, we've got to fight the insurance companies. But in my practice I see miracles every day, and usually it's as simple as restoring lost hormones with bioidentical real ones. People feel and look so much better when their hormones are restored; if you do that, you can live a long time. They can come up with these obscure treatments and expensive technologies, but you're not getting to the basics. Coach Vince Lombardi once said, "Guys, we're going to win football games, because we block and tackle better than anybody else." That's how I feel about bioidentical hormones. They block and tackle better than anything else, they correct problems. Hormones, eating right, exercise, mineral supplementation, and you are in good shape.

SS: What does it mean to you that you have created this environment, this practice that has been so well received?

SH: First, I give thanks to God, and credit to my wife for staying with me, and I love my wonderful staff. I love what I am doing. I get up every day and look forward to my work. I love the Stallone movies . . . Rocky. That's an inspiring character. I love his attitude. He never quit. They could knock him down, but they could never knock him out. He always got up. That's what this movement is about. Big business wants to knock it down, knock it out, get rid of it. I refuse. Bioidentical hormones are the right thing to do for my patients. I know they work, I know Americans are on too many pharmaceutical drugs. I'm never going to give up. They'll never knock me down.

SS: Good for you. I'll be rooting for you all the way.

DR. STEVEN HOTZE'S BREAKTHROUGH BREAKOUTS

- A rounded-out program for health and wellness includes treating for airborne allergies and for yeast, using natural thyroid hormones and bioidentical hormones for sex hormone replacement, treating adrenal fatigue, using vitamin and mineral supplementation, and implementing a nutritionally balanced eating program.

- A program of nystatin and probiotics for several days will usually clear up a yeast infection.

- Women on the artificial hormones Premarin and Prempro, or estrogen alone, are more susceptible to yeast infections.

- According to a 1981 Johns Hopkins study, natural progesterone protects against cancer, and a progesterone deficiency dramatically increases the risk of breast cancer. Men with a hormone imbalance can prevent prostate cancer with treatments of progesterone.

- Men who are diagnosed with low-grade prostate cancer might benefit from not doing anything to treat it. Studies from Sweden show that they live longer than men with prostatectomies.

26

HYSTERECTOMY IS PREVENTABLE

THERE ARE SOME CASES where hysterectomy is necessary and these usually involve cancer. However, as I've discovered, many women end up having hysterectomies when they are not necessary. The medical establishment resorts to hysterectomies when there are many other things that can be done to save a woman's uterus. Today in this country, over one million hysterectomies are performed a year. I highly doubt that many women really need to lose an organ or organs.

It is important to know the ramifications of losing your uterus—many doctors don't tell women everything they need to know.

Losing your uterus is not a simple matter. Most women have their uterus removed because of uncontrollable bleeding. That is why my uterus was removed, and also I had what was called severe hyperplasia and atypia, which is a precancerous condition.

Why would cancer be dancing around me again? I asked myself. Well, let's think about this . . . I took birth control pills for twenty-two years. (None of us knew better back then.) It is very possible that because I never fully ovulated (no woman does on birth control pills) all those years, my body thought I wasn't reproductive and did its best to try to get rid of me.

I believe these birth control pills have led to my many little bouts with cancer in my life: two bad Pap smears in the seventies indicating possible cervical cancer, one melanoma on my back, several other skin cancers, severe hyperplasia and atypia in my uterus indicating a precancerous condition, and then the topper . . . full-out breast cancer.

When my uterus started bleeding and acting up I didn't have enough information to go against the grain. Emotionally, I felt awful the day of my surgery. I knew in my heart there had to be another way. Nature would have had a better plan than this.

All those years of hormonal imbalance were the culprit for all these cancers, but I didn't know that then. We all have cancer in us, but when hormones are in full balance the brain perceives us as reproductive and the cancer stays at bay. It is only when the hormones get imbalanced that women begin getting their cancers. That is why young women who make a full complement of hormones rarely get cancer unless it is genetic, environmental, a result of poor nutrition, or a stress-induced hormonal imbalance.

The worst news about birth control pills is the new pill that gives women only four periods a year. Can you think of anything crazier than going against nature in such a violent way? I fear this group will have cancer in unprecedented numbers.

Since my surgery I learned about rhythmic cycling, which is taking your hormones in a rhythm. This means the dosages change by looking at a calendar and your doctor works out a program for you to provide rhythmic cycling.

I have written about rhythm extensively in *Ageless*. The rhythm allows for the estrogen receptor sites to open, receiving the progesterone so the normal monthly bleed can happen. Some women take their bioidenticals in what is called a "static dose," as I did (the same amount of estrogen every day of the month, the same amount of progesterone two weeks of each month). If these women start to bleed (as I did) it's because they are usually no longer making any estrogen at all in their bodies, so the endometrial lining keeps building up and building up like a motor on rev, but the receptor sites don't open up to receive the progesterone. When this happens the lining gets thick and the woman starts to bleed every day.

I explained this form of hormone replacement in *Ageless*, and many women, my sister being one of them, have written to tell me that switching to rhythmic cycling stopped the bleeding problem and then became normalized.

The women who report bleeding are most often my age or older and have estrogen-dominant bodies. We are the curvy ones, but the reality is that we probably never made enough progesterone, which caused our estrogen dominance in the first place, and it's likely one of the many reasons

for the epidemic cancer rates of our generation. We were hormonally imbalanced. Hormonal imbalance is a breeding ground for cancer. Take it seriously.

Losing your uterus and other female organs is a true loss. What no doctor ever mentions is that once the uterus is gone you will never again be
able to enjoy those delicious, deep uterine orgasms. No uterus, no uterine
muscle, no deep orgasms.

When the cervix and ovaries are also removed, then your sexual feelings
are gone forever. No more feeling . . . at all. Women have total hysterectomies and they are told, "Take them out and then you will never have to
worry about cervical or ovarian cancer again." Nothing is further from the
truth. Without your ovaries, you no longer have your main estrogen-making
gland, and if you are young when you have this procedure, you go into
instant surgical menopause. This is an awful scenario, so in your face;
instant and drastic (much more intense than the suffering caused by normal menopause, which is significant). Hysterectomy causes immediate
night sweats, hot flashes, sleeplessness, and often tremendous weight
gain.

Most women I speak with had no idea they would never feel right
again after their hysterectomies.

Real natural hormone replacement is the answer to most so-called female problems. Usually when there is excessive bleeding it's because the
hormone-making abilities of your body are starting to decline. Or if you
are young it could be due to chemicals in your diet, workplace, or environment; or it can be from stress. Stress blunts hormone-making action in
your body. If you're in your early thirties, stress and overwork are accelerating your aging and speeding up menopause.

By embracing hormone replacement with BHRT, you can protect
yourself from disease, save your female organs, and improve your mood,
your happiness, your weight, and your quality of life.

Dear Suzanne,

I can't tell you how great my life has become. Well, first you must know that I was miserable. Truly miserable. I went from doctor to doctor, telling them about my horrible symptoms; I wasn't sleeping, I gained thirty-five pounds, my stomach was bloated constantly, my sex drive went away, my hair got stringy, my vagina dried up, I was depressed, and I felt ugly. No one knew what to do about it. I was given antidepressants and sleeping pills, but I knew that was not going to save me. I took them for a while and then finally gave them up, which was very hard. They are addictive.

I bought your book Ageless, couldn't believe that someone finally knew what was going on with me, and went to Dr. Paunesky in Atlanta, the kindest, sweetest woman I have ever known, and she got me all straightened out on bioidentical hormones and I have never looked back.

I feel happy all the time. My weight is back to normal and my stomach isn't bloated and I am loving sex with my fantastic husband again.

It saved my life . . . changed my life. I have you and Dr. Paunesky to thank.

So thank you, thank you, thank you.
Bernadette F.

27

STEP 6: SUPPLEMENT YOUR DIET

IN TODAY'S WORLD we are no longer able to obtain the proper nutrients, herbs, vitamins, and minerals we humans require for survival without additional supplementation. Our food supply is largely deficient, contaminated by pesticides, herbicides, cold storage, early picking, "beautifying" at supermarkets, nonorganic soils, contaminated water, acid rain, and much more. After reading the interviews in this book, you now realize the importance of nutrition; each doctor has addressed the problem and stressed that lack of proper nutrients in our diets is having a serious negative effect on our health.

Every cell in the body requires good nutrition to replicate, and without these vital nutrients we cannot operate at maximum. Breakthrough medicine is dedicated to optimal health and lifestyle. Even when consuming organic foods as often as possible it is still necessary to add to the "nutritional pot" through supplementation. Up until now it has been a fiasco. We would go to the health food store and hope the person behind the supplement counter knew what they were talking about (they usually didn't), and together we would try to guess at what might be important for our bodies, but this approach is no longer advisable or acceptable.

Supplementation is now extremely sophisticated. There is no guessing, there is no "one-a-day" vitamin that can do it all. To properly put back the missing nutrients and protective supplements we now need on a daily basis, we have companies that will individualize a supplement regimen just for you through blood work, meaning your blood results can show your exact deficiencies. No more guessing.

This kind of supplementation makes sense; putting back into your body *exactly* what has been lost through toxicity, stress, or normal aging assures that you are getting not only the missing ingredients but also protective modalities such as the magical resveratrol to protect against disease, curcumin to eliminate free radicals, pomegranate extracts to protect against heart disease and prostate cancer, green tea extracts to increase fat burning and improve insulin sensitivity, essential fatty acids such as fish oil for cellular membrane strength, nutrients like mesozeaxanthin and lutein that are designed to protect against macular degeneration, GliSODin for aging arteries, or D-ribose for energy metabolism for people with cardiac and other debilitating health problems.

Supplementation is lifesaving, disease protective, and essential to ward off the toxicity of our present environment.

Life Extension magazine is one of the best suppliers of supplements. Life Extension is a nonprofit organization and uses most of its revenues to research the best possible way to ensure that you are getting the highest-quality vitamins, herbs, and supplements with the greatest abilities to absorb. There are many tests available at low cost through the magazine. In addition to being a member you have access not only to high-quality supplements but will also receive their fantastic magazine each month. I am not involved with this magazine, I am just a huge admirer. And the purpose of my books is always to expose you to the most cutting-edge approach to today's health.

In addition to Life Extension there are two other companies of note. New Chapter sells excellent herbs, vitamins, and supplements made with love and care. The owner and founder, Paul Schulick, whom I interviewed in *Ageless*, has been a dear friend of mine for twenty years and is so very meticulous about his ingredients that he personally oversees his farm in Costa Rica to be sure you are getting the very best and purest ingredients. Once a year he goes on retreat to "pray for the world," so you know that supplements made by a man with this capacity to care are going to be of top quality.

Another company I greatly admire is Designs for Health. The interview that follows is with nutritionist Cristiana Paul, an independent nutritional counselor, who introduced me to the concept of blood and stool testing to determine your exact supplemental needs.

These three companies are dedicated to bringing quality, life-restoring good health to all of us. It is vibrantly clear after interviewing all the doctors for this book that supplementation is definitely a backbone to today's breakthrough life and a necessary step to wellness.

When I stopped taking my supplements for a few weeks a couple of years ago (just to see what would happen), I experienced a severe depletion of my energy, my skin did not glow in the way it usually does, and my system did not work as well. It was an experiment that convinced me that the good food I was eating still was not enough.

You will enjoy hearing from Cristiana Paul about the essentials of supplementation. After reading what she has to say, you will be more convinced than ever that to remain healthy today we need to augment what our bodies require for optimal health.

28

CRISTIANA PAUL, M.S.

RECENTLY, I HAD THE OPPORTUNITY to meet Cristiana Paul, M.S., a nutritionist and an independent consultant who provides education to health care practitioners and their patients. She is also involved in research support for Designs for Health, one of the companies that makes high-quality vitamins and supplements.

In other words, she is the one who teaches the doctors and their clients about nutrition. I sat down with her and asked her how we can optimize our health through supplementation, and how we can know we are getting the right supplementation for ourselves.

I think what she has to say will help you considerably in choosing for yourself the regimen that would best support your health.

SS: Tell me why and when we need nutritional supplements.

CP: Think about your body as if it were a car. We know a car needs good maintenance: checkups, tune-ups, high-quality gasoline, oil, and water in order to function with high performance. The difference between our cars and our bodies is that we can trade in our cars when they get run-down, but not our bodies (not yet anyway). The good news is that your body, unlike your car, tries to renew and repair itself all day and all night long, but you need to give it the right materials in the right amounts and at the right times.

SS: But how do we know what materials (or supplements) we need in terms of nutritional supplementation?

CP: For example, we now have tests that can measure the levels of nutrients in the blood or nutrient metabolites in the urine, which indicate if we have enough of any particular nutrient for our individual metabolism's needs. If a person is really committed to maximizing his or her body's function, health, and longevity, then he or she needs to be very smart about how to get the absolute best combination of nutrients from food or supplements. The only way to know for sure is to take these tests; unfortunately, these are not tests that your regular doctor will order for your physical. Most doctors just aren't aware these great tests exist.

We need to analyze blood, urine, saliva, and stool samples. My Web site is www.CristianaPaul.com, and I can give your readers a list of the practitioners who perform particular nutritional tests.

SS: How long have these tests been available?

CP: Ten years ago, when I received my master's in nutrition, they were not mentioned in my academic training, and very few of them were available. But in recent years more and more of them are being offered, and the technology is getting better.

It's so important to evaluate your nutritional deficiencies; I see nutritional deficiencies even among people who consider themselves healthy eaters and who already take basic multivitamins, minerals, fish oils, and some antioxidants.

These tests can tell me if a person has trans fats in his or her system, and this is important because trans fats can create cardiovascular problems or may get into various tissues—like the brain, for example—and interfere with optimal function.

If I had my way, I would perform these tests on every patient who walked through my door. Nutritional support can create optimal health and healing.

SS: Well, this is exciting. It's great to know that by simple blood, urine, and stool tests you can pinpoint exactly what you need nutritionally. This is a designer regimen of vitamins, customized to the individual. I know, having taken these tests myself, that I feel secure knowing I am supplementing with exactly what I need. There's no guessing.

CP: Tests tell me one thing, and then there is the interaction with the individual. For example, if I have a patient who is depressed, and I look at her diet and see that she is not eating fish but only chicken and turkey, I know that she probably has a major deficiency in fish oils. My recommendation would be to put her on six soft gels of fish oil daily, and I can prove it to her by taking her blood work and showing her the low levels of DHA (the fatty acid in fish that is essential for her brain to work). This way she sees the connection and will willingly take the fish oil supplements. As a result, I know there is a good chance that her depression will be partly alleviated or resolved.

SS: What are the other important supplements that are a must for everyone?

CP: Well, besides omega-3 fish oils, there is the fatty acid GLA (gamma-linolenic acid), which is an essential fat important for reducing inflammation, optimal immune function, and skin health, to name a few.

Essential fatty acids are found in the outer layer of every cell in our bodies, and it's important to understand that they have a very profound effect on how our bodies work. This influences how well cells communicate, how well they respond to hormones, the levels of inflammation, blood clotting, blood thinning, blood vessel dilation/constriction, immune activation against infectious agents, cardiovascular plaque buildup, and the risk of plaque rupture.

Next would be a multivitamin/multimineral, but not a one-a-day.

There is a test called the Comprehensive Metabolic Profile (CMP by DFH & Metametrix), which can uncover a person's needs for B vitamins, Co-Q$_{10}$, lipoic acid, and magnesium. If people knew they could benefit so greatly from burning energy more efficiently and having less energy stored, I believe they would take supplements more often. This test will also show if you have rancid fats in your body from fried or unstable fats and if you have bacterial overgrowth in the intestinal tract (this can give you "brain fog").

SS: Well, yes, if a need can be shown, as in a deficiency, I am sure people would be more than willing to supplement. How do we know which vitamins really work? Which ones are true to their label, which are bioavailable and which are not?

CP: Most over-the-counter vitamins are tablets, because it is an inexpensive way to produce them, and you can press a lot of material into one pill, which makes the formula look good on the label. "One-a-day" is not optimal. It is similar to drinking all your daily requirements for water in one sitting rather than distributing them throughout the day. Same for vitamins: You want to spread them out as evenly as it's practical to do.

What we want is chelated forms of minerals (like glycinates, for example), which have two to three times better absorption than all other available forms and do not interact with other food components in the stomach. Oxides, citrates, carbonates, gluconates, aspartates, hydroxyapatite: These are forms of minerals that are poorly absorbed.

Minerals are not affected when pressed into tablets, but some vitamins are fragile and may be destroyed during this manufacturing process.

SS: But why—if we are eating well, as in good organic food, and really thinking about nutritional support from the food we choose—why do we need to supplement?

CP: There are many reasons:

1. Seemingly nutritious food may be coming from insufficient soils or from long, improper storage or be cooked too long or cooked in temperatures that are too high.
2. If we do not chew our food well, it doesn't digest. Or it could be that we don't have enough stomach acid or digestive enzymes or we do not absorb nutrients well due to an irritated intestinal tract. This could be due to aging, stress, yeast, or parasites present in the colon, or allergies, celiac, or inflammatory conditions of the intestinal tract. This is why a periodic stool test is helpful (Metametrix offers one called GI Effects).
3. We do not eat at regular and even intervals throughout the day. We skip breakfast or lunch and then eat a huge dinner that we cannot possibly digest adequately. And you have to remember that what is left undigested, the bacteria, yeast, and parasites in our colon will use for food to grow and multiply (yummy left-overs for them). So that is how we support their overgrowth, which then irritates the colon, causes gas, and suppresses the local immune system of the gut.
4. As we age, our cells do not operate as efficiently as when we were born. Imagine our cells making Xerox copies of themselves, and then the copies get less and less accurate as we age. These tiny imperfections may be due to mitochondrial deletions, and may require that the energy pathways in our cells increase their need for B vitamins, Co-Q_{10}, lipoic acid, and magnesium. So, as we age, our requirement for these nutrients may increase over that of a younger person.

It is essential to eat as healthy as possible, but as we age, we need to add every trick in the book to compensate for age-related changes in our systems. If we give our bodies the right amount of nutrients, they can help it to function almost as good as new.

SS: So, it's the same as we do with bioidentical hormones: identify the deficiencies, then replace what is missing.

CP: Absolutely. Bioidentical supplements go with bioidentical hormones and, of course, a bioidentical lifestyle and diet. This is how we harvest the maximum potential from our bodies.

SS: Bioidentical supplements?

CP: Yes. I would call bioidentical those supplements that contain substances that have an essential physiological role in the human body's physiology: vitamins, minerals, essential fatty acids, and others such as Co-Q_{10}, R-lipoic acid, fish oils, creatine, carnitine, phospholipids, and GPC (glycero-phospho-choline).

These nutrients should be provided in their naturally occurring form— or at least a form that is easily usable by the body—and in amounts similar to what we get in natural foods or is made inside our bodies. Sometimes we need to use higher therapeutic doses of these nutrients, but only under a health care practitioner's supervision.

Then there are additional substances found in nature from which we can greatly benefit such as fiber, grape seed, resveratrol, curcumin, and green tea.

We should never forget where we came from and what our bodies have adapted to for millions of years: lots of fruits and vegetables, roots, nuts, seeds (raw, not fried, roasted, or salted), and animal fats from animals that are grazing on natural pastures or fish that are eating algae and other fish as opposed to what they feed them in the fish farms.

When animals eat grass, their fat is high in omega-3 oils, and when they eat corn, their fat is high in omega-6 oils. Farm-fed fish are low in EPA/DHA, which is what wild fish have and are preferred.

SS: And it has been said over and over in this book to avoid omega-6 oils like, for instance, corn oil. Besides, corn is fattening. I guess that's why they feed it to the cattle—fatten them up. Do you eat perfectly all the time? I mean, do you ever go crazy with cake or desserts?

CP: I try to eat right most of the time. But I throw in some forbidden desserts once in a while . . . chocolate. The trick is, I know how to compensate with supplements when I eat nonoptimal foods. I would take R-lipoic acid, carnosine, benfotiamine because these help process the sugar in a way that reduces the typical damage that occurs after eating starch and/or sugar. I take fiber before a nonoptimal meal with refined sugar and flour, so that at least I slow down the sugar absorption by mixing it with fiber in my stomach.

SS: Then please tell my readers the core supplement regimen, even before they do any testing. What do they need to get through the day?

CP: I would recommend a multivitamin and multimineral of high quality. Do the best you can for about three months with your diet, then take the nutritional tests to see if you need extra minerals, B vitamins, antioxidants, and whatever is relevant for your goals and health problems.

SS: What about the gut? Everyone is bloating; everyone has food allergies and intolerances. Are there any supplements that can alleviate this discomfort?

CP: Fiber is important in reducing the risk of constipation and helping the body get rid of the toxins that the liver pulls out of the blood. Fiber is also great for reducing appetite because it sends a "full signal" to the brain. When you get enough fiber in your diet, your intestinal muscles actually get a good workout.

Gas may be an unwanted consequence of having too much fiber, so you have to find the right amount for you gradually. But fiber does not make the gas on its own; the excess bacteria and yeast (your personal brewery) in your gastrointestinal tract make the gas when they use fibers as food, especially the soluble fiber. Excess bacteria and yeast are a result of eating too much sugar and carbohydrates. There are herbal compounds (for example, grapefruit seed extract, bearberry, caprylic acid, and black walnut—Designs for Health offers these in the GI-Microb-X formula) that can kill and reduce the numbers of problematic microbes in the colon. Also, a lack of stomach acid and use of antacid medications can create bloating and allow for too many of these gas-producing creatures to take residence in our guts.

SS: I think if my readers walk away with anything from this book, it would be the misconception of antacids. Bloating and discomfort in the gut is almost always a result of not enough hydrochloric acid, yet doctors and people treat this discomfort with exactly what they don't need: They take an antacid to take away acid, when what they need is more acid called HCl.

CP: Yes, and you also need probiotics if there are not enough probiotics in your diet, like yogurt or fermented cabbage.

SS: I would say most of us are probably not pigging out on fermented cabbage.

CP: Probably not. But it's important to understand the importance of probiotics, which are like your personal army of soldiers that defend the intestinal borders. Those are entry points for approved citizens (like food), and are constantly under the attack of terrorists (like unfriendly bacteria, yeast, parasites, and toxins). One problem is that nonorganic animal foods and dairy contain antibiotics. So when you eat these foods, it's like you are taking antibiotics. These antibiotics kill probiotics in your gut, they wipe out your gut defense system, leaving a void where the terrorists (the bad bacteria, yeasts, and parasites) can take over. That's why we constantly need to take in probiotics—unless what you are eating is strictly organic, in which case you need to take them less often.

SS: What other supplements do you recommend?

CP: For aging joints and back pain, you need glucosamine two to three times a day, spread evenly. Joints can wear out due to overuse and/or excessive inflammation, so if you do not take your fish oils and watch your arachidonic acid intake (from corn-fed animals and dairy), your glucosamine supplements cannot repair the damage done by the inflammatory compounds derived from arachidonic acid fast enough.

Until you've accumulated enough fish oils in your cell membranes to keep inflammation under control, you may need a hefty dose of anti-inflammatories like green tea, curcumin, and resveratrol.

SS: Now . . . let's talk about resveratrol. This is the new wonder supplement.

CP: Red wine contains resveratrol; white wine has hardly any. Resveratrol has shown that it may reduce the risk of many diseases and extend the health and survival rate (in animal studies), even when someone is not on the perfect diet and/or is overweight.

SS: That sounds like you can have your cake and eat it, too.

CP: No. You can't go ahead and commit nutritional sins thinking the resveratrol will wipe out all the consequences. Resveratrol may help people who do not have perfect diets, but for people who do have relatively good diets, then the effects are dynamite.

Supplementing with resveratrol essentially fools the body into thinking it needs to do everything available to preserve function, rev up defenses, and keep us in top shape.

SS: There is something powerful in this resveratrol molecule. It turns on a gene called SIR-1 that makes our bodies rev up our defenses to protect us from disease. I see it as ninja warriors sitting at the entrance saying, no way!

CP: Yes. It signals the body to inhibit cancer development and improve sugar metabolism and cardiovascular function; it protects the brain and arteries from plaque by stabilizing it in a way so that it is less likely to rupture, reduces the risk of excessive blood clotting, reduces excessive inflammation and cholesterol, and improves energy production. It also has antiviral and antifungal and antibacterial (*H. pylori*) effects. I never imagined one substance could do all this, yet there are thousands of studies supporting it.

SS: What red wine is the best source of resveratrol?

CP: Pinot Noir and wines that are made with the muscadine grape. Plants (grapevines in this case) make more resveratrol when they experience tough conditions . . . excessive cold or drought or when attacked by mold.

One study this year on Medline (which I check all the time) shows that it may help the body destroy breast cancer cells and reduce their invasiveness. Another study shows that it reduces glucose metabolism in ovarian cancer cells, thus helping the immune system kill them. Keep in mind that sugar fuels cancer cells like gasoline on a fire, but our friend resveratrol helps inhibit that fire.

SS: This is an amazing new discovery. I take resveratrol every morning and evening. I have been doing so for the past year. Many companies are making it. I get mine from Life Extension.

CP: Yes. Resveratrol is available now from many nutritional companies. Designs for Health offers it in a product called Resveratrol Synergy, with 200 milligrams per capsule with Quercetin. Other companies offer it in the powder form, if you want to dose it higher and minimize the number of pills you take.

Resveratrol is a very powerful molecule. It thins the blood in a good way, and it is a powerful anti-inflammatory. If you had cancer, it claims to offer great protection from a recurrence.

SS: Have you felt the benefits since you've been taking resveratrol?

CP: My brain feels more focused and clear; I feel more brain energy.

SS: Me, too. Since I have been taking it, my brain is operating top-notch. What else do you recommend? What about vitamin D?

CP: Vitamin D is very important. We now recommend doses ranging from 1,000 IU to 10,000 IU per day, based on sun exposure and blood levels; readers should not dose themselves without a health care practitioner's supervision, due to the potential toxicity of excess. People are no longer sitting in the sun, and as a result we are deficient in vitamin D. This amazing prohormone reduces osteoporosis, osteoarthritis, cancer risk and progression, inflammation, fibrinogen (which influences blood clotting); it normalizes blood pressure, improves insulin sensitivity, supports the health of the arterial wall, and may reduce cardiovascular mortality. It may also improve mood and help relieve some symptoms of PMS.

Vitamin K is the new superstar on the nutrition horizon. It has shown reversal of calcification in the arterial plaque of rats, and I feel we will be seeing a reduction of calcium deposits in the arteries in humans who have adequate intake of vitamin K. I need to mention here that people taking anticoagulants should not take vitamin K. Vitamin K supports bone building and has amazing potential for reducing the risk of kidney stones, cancer, inflammation, and arthritis; it helps the myelination of nerves and the brain (so it may help with multiple sclerosis), and supports the pancreas in producing adequate levels of insulin. As if all of this was not enough, vitamin K seems to have other roles involving skin, sperm, salivary glands, and sex hormone receptors.

Co-Q$_{10}$ is a well-known energy supporter, antioxidant, and immune booster. I would not go one day without it. It's that important. Co-Q$_{10}$ was shown to improve life span in rats.

Curcumin is anti-inflammatory, anticancer, anti-Alzheimer's, antiallergy, anti–cardiovascular plaque buildup and rupture, and a blood thinner. I take 100 milligrams one to two times a day.

For brain support: phosphatidylserine, acetyl-l-carnitine, creatine, and ginkgo biloba.

SS: And finally, how important is detoxification for antiaging?

CP: We have to get rid of toxins faster than they come into the body, because this may be one of the most important factors we experience in age acceleration. This garbage accumulation can mess up every aspect of our bodies' functions; it can impair the brain, the hormones, the energy production, and the immune system.

Imagine a house where you constantly have more trash coming in and accumulating inside than you are taking out on a daily basis. How can you function if the garbage piles up?

First, let's not bring trash into the house to begin with. By this I mean toxins from food and the environment. There will always be some trash that accumulates as a result of normal metabolism. So take plenty of fiber through food and/or supplements all throughout the day, drink water, and sweat with every opportunity.

A liver-support detox formula may be very useful as a supplement on an ongoing basis. This may contain: NAC, glycine, taurine, and methionine. Designs for Health offers these in the Amino-D-Tox formula, and for additional protection, you can also take DETOX-ANTIOX, which has additional antioxidants (like green tea, grape seed), anti-inflammatories (like turmeric), and toxic metal chelating agents (like lipoic acid, selenium).

In addition, a periodical detox diet program (like spring cleaning) may be very beneficial. There are many programs out there, but I trust only the ones based on science, and they must include protein.

Everyone knows they should have annual physicals and regular blood work, but what about having periodical nutritional status checkups? It's a new concept, and most people have not even heard that nutritionists and some doctors are doing this routinely. The information found through lab work helps find the best approach to treating disease or just optimizes your health.

I am grateful that there is so much available today in the realm of tests and supplements to give us effective tools and means to support our efforts to optimize health. Supplementation is essential and necessary in order to survive in today's environment, which presents toxic challenges with nonoptimal soil and food supplies. Supplements are a gift—a way of putting back into our bodies what food once was able to do for us—and compensate to a certain extent for some age-related physiological changes we experience.

Instead of allowing nutritional deficiencies to undermine our performance and health, we can be proactive by giving our body what it wants and needs.

SS: Well said. Thank you for all this wonderful information.

CRISTIANA PAUL'S
BREAKTHROUGH BREAKOUTS

- For optimum health, multivitamins should not be "one-a-day," and multiminerals should be taken in chelated forms.

- After three months of taking quality multivitamins and multiminerals and trying to eat healthy, take nutritional tests to find out what deficiencies you may need to counteract with supplementation. Continue regular nutritional checkups.

- Taking omega-3 fish oil supplements helps alleviate depression and inflammation of the joints. Plus it builds healthy cell membranes.

- The fatty acid GLA (gamma-linolenic acid) is essential for reducing inflammation and to ensure optimal immune function and skin health, to name a few.

- R-lipoic acid, carnosine, and benfotiamine help process sugar in a way that reduces the typical damage that occurs after eating starchy or sugary foods. Taking fiber before a nonoptimal meal with refined sugar and flour slows down the sugar absorption by mixing it with fiber in the stomach. Fiber is also important in reducing the risk of constipation and helping the body get rid of the toxins that the liver pulls out of the blood.

- Herbal compounds such as grapefruit seed extract, bearberry, caprylic acid, and black walnut can kill and reduce the numbers of problematic microbes in the colon.

- Supplementing with resveratrol essentially fools the body into thinking it needs to do everything available to preserve function, rev up defenses, and keep us in top shape.

- Other powerful supplements include vitamin D, vitamin K, Co-Q$_{10}$, curcumin, phosphatidylserine, acetyl-l-carnitine, creatine, and ginkgo biloba.

29

STEP 7: EXERCISE REGULARLY

My grandmother started walking five miles a day when she
was sixty. She's ninety-three today and we don't know where
the hell she is!

    —Ellen DeGeneres

EXERCISE IS ANY TYPE OF ACTIVITY that you enjoy doing. It doesn't have to
be regimented, you don't have to go to a gym. In fact, I have never been
to a gym in my life. Instead I have always chosen to get my exercise
through things I love doing: hiking, walking, strolling, taking the stairs instead of elevators, taking the stairs in my home two at a time, gardening,
dancing . . . ah dancing, that's fun. I danced for many years. All the years
I was headlining in Las Vegas I loved it, pushing my body to its outer lim-
its, forcing injuries because I knew my young body could take it. I danced
for twenty-five years.

I also have enjoyed easy exercise devices like the ThighMaster and my
new E-Z Gym. They travel well and are simple to pick up and use in short
spurts with great results.

But my most important form of exercise for the last four years has been
yoga. Three to four times a week I faithfully practice, and I mean practice—
because yoga is a practice (for you are always progressing), but it happens
slowly and it is noncompetitive. You don't even compete with yourself.
There are some mornings my body doesn't want to be pushed. I listen to
that, I never force anything anymore. Yoga has taught me respect for my
body. There are days I am amazed at what I can do: twisting my body into
some form of pretzel or standing on my forearms with my head off the
ground in a handstand, at sixty-one! Yoga burns fat; it gets rid of those fat

deposits that come with age like no other form of exercise I have ever done.

I love yoga. I love when my teacher, Julie Carmen, arrives at the house to give so generously of her time—she and I work together for an hour. I am always lost in my practice; I am always amazed when the hour is up.

Yoga calms me, yoga strengthens me, yoga improves my breathing, improves my cardiovascular system, increases my energy, and keeps me limber. Being limber is a blessing. I am like a cat that stretches every morning and again several times during the day. Yoga is something I honestly believe I will do for life, until the day I die.

Innately I have always understood that a body needs to be worked, exercised. I have worked with a trainer but I always dreaded all the counting and monotony of repetitive movements.

Yoga is what *I* found. You will find what is right for you. There is no way you can be healthy or well without daily movement, without exercise. There is no way to avoid or skip this step. Nothing else you do for your health will be as effective unless you also add exercise to the template. You can take advantage of some of the many breakthrough advances in medicine that I mention in this book, but if you don't exercise, your body will not work at its optimum. That's why getting proper exercise is part of the 8 Steps to Wellness

Find what you love and then commit to it. So, go take a walk or a hike through the woods, breathe, think good thoughts, think about who and what you love, and discard all negative thoughts. Manifest your dream, see it before you, and then make it happen.

30

STEP 8: GET PROPER SLEEP

EVERY TIME I LECTURE to groups of women, I ask the same question: "How many of you sleep five hours or less each night?" Inevitably every hand in the room is raised. This is a typical reaction and a real disaster for women and all people who are unable to sleep. It seems like no one is sleeping well these days, and pharmaceutical companies are booming, coming up with sleeping pills that they say will take care of this problem.

It is essential to understand that sleep is as important for health as replacing low, missing, or declining hormones. Sleep is as important as supplementation, detoxification, good nutrition, and exercise. That's why I have made sleep the final part of the 8 Steps to Wellness—you cannot avoid it if you want to achieve optimal health. With a better understanding of how our hormones work and the advances that breakthrough medicine has to offer, it is possible to sleep well without having to resort to pharmaceuticals.

There are so many products these days pushed by drug companies to help people sleep, including "sedative hypnotics" like Ambien and Lunesta. These drugs are now coming with strong warnings from the Food and Drug Administration because of incidences of people crashing their cars, trying to cook, eating inedible foods, and doing other things while in a sleeping-pill–induced haze. Not everyone is affected that way, but why risk adverse side effects from pharmaceuticals when there are natural ways to get a good night's sleep? Besides, as I have said in my other books, sleep by Ambien or any other sleeping pill is not sleep! It is a suspended state, but none of the healing work of your bodily functions (namely hormones) can take place in this suspended state. It's a form of rest, but it's not restorative.

Sleep is impossible if your hormones are imbalanced. If one hormone is "off," then the entire cascade is off. For instance, if your major hormone, insulin, is high or even out of the normal bounds, then all the rest of the hormones slide downward and are put in a state of imbalance.

Imagine a teeter-totter: At one end are the minor hormones—estrogen, progesterone, and testosterone—and at the other end are the major hormones—adrenals, insulin, thyroid, and cortisol. Imagine that teeter-totter tipping to the ground on the estrogen, progesterone, and testosterone side; your major hormones on the other end of the teeter-totter have no option but to go up.

Low estrogen, progesterone, or testosterone (your minor hormones) create the imbalance that raises your insulin, thyroid, adrenals, and cortisol (your major hormones).

High adrenals and cortisol are why you are not sleeping, high insulin is why you are gaining weight even though you are eating less and exercising, and that hypothyroid is why you are getting belly fat, depressed, and gaining weight.

Hormones are a language and they all speak to one another. If the minors are low then the majors go high, and this is an unhealthy scenario for your body; you feel uncomfortable, you put on weight, you can get depressed, and you lose your ability to sleep (which can put your heart in jeopardy). When there is imbalance the "language" gets interrupted. It's as though you have a recipe but are missing an ingredient.

Imagine you were making a cake and you didn't have any eggs. You could make that cake, but it probably wouldn't taste as good, look as good, or bake as well as if you had included *all* the ingredients. That is how our hormonal system works. A number of things can throw you out of whack and leave you with that incomplete cake. If you have a stressful morning, or things are rough at work, or you have a fight with your spouse, or you are dealing with a sick child, your hormones become imbalanced because stress blunts hormone production. When that happens the entire system gets out of tune.

Cortisol is a major hormone, and if it is high, sleep is impossible. Cortisol is our stress hormone; it is meant to be used when we are in acute danger; it would have been released in our ancestors if they were being chased by a saber-toothed tiger—you would have needed superhuman strength to run from such a fast and ferocious animal.

But in today's world, instead of saber-toothed tigers, we have job pressure, financial pressure, and multitasking lifestyles, all of which trigger the stress hormone, cortisol, all the time. All of us (women and men) are constantly fighting high cortisol, and only real hormone replacement in the correct individualized ratios can keep your cortisol under control. Also it is important to note that chronic high cortisol leads to heart attack, and the leading killer of women is heart disease. That is why those women "toughing it out" and choosing to ride out their menopause without replacement are doing themselves a disservice. The hormones you have lost are not going to come back, and this constant imbalance will lead to chronic insomnia, plus all the other symptoms of hormonal imbalance. It does not get better. As women we adjust to the suffering and start to take sleeplessness as normal, but taking the steps to correct the imbalance and restore the missing hormones gives you quality of life and that includes sleeping.

Cortisol is sensitive to light. It is the hormone that wakes us up in the morning and then, in turn, makes us sleepy at the end of the day when the light starts to dim. That low light signals to the adrenals to turn down the cortisol production, that it can take it easy for the rest of the night and has no other chores until sunrise tomorrow morning (that is, if all the other hormones are in balance).

But if you are experiencing hormonal decline, the dip in those hormones throws off your cortisol and triggers it to stay "on," as if it needs to remain elevated in order to deal with the stress of the imbalance in your body. Cortisol now has a job to do and can't take it easy, which unfortunately means it won't let you sleep.

Now that you see the role hormones can play in preventing a good night's sleep, how do we fix it? It is essential to go to bed two to three hours before midnight so there is time for the "nature" in you to do its healing work. This is how our bodies have been set up. It takes at least three and a half hours of melatonin secretion before prolactin is released. Prolactin is a pituitary hormone that induces lactation and prevents ovulation. Prolactin is the domain of nursing mothers. A mother with a new infant needs to be awakened many times during the night to feed her baby . . . thus the high prolactin.

The National Institutes of Health concludes that six hours of prolactin production in the dark is the minimum necessary to maintain immune function like T-cell and beneficial killer-cell production. But you can't get six hours of prolactin secretion on six hours of sleep a night because three and a half hours of melatonin secretion are necessary before you even see prolactin.

So, if you go to bed after midnight, there just isn't enough time for it all to happen. If you can't sleep for whatever reason, including low estrogen (remember, when your estrogen is down, your cortisol can be high), then all the healing work your body needs and wants cannot happen and you are the loser. Chronic poor sleep can leave you fatigued, depressed, overweight (high cortisol can lead to high insulin and weight gain), and suffering from hypothyroidism and depleted adrenals. Eventually this scenario can leave your body in such a weakened and imbalanced state that disease and heart problems follow.

Besides going to bed three hours before midnight, you must sleep in complete darkness. Even the smallest light can raise your cortisol levels (cortisol reads light)—this extra little light could be the thing that is interfering with your ability to sleep. A recent study put subjects in a completely dark room and then put penlights on the backs of their knees. As a result of this teeny light, all the subjects showed raised cortisol levels.

There are ways to retrain your body to sleep. The most important thing is to have your hormones balanced. As with every one of the 8 Steps to Wellness, if you don't have balanced hormones, you are not going to enjoy the full benefits of good health. Everything recommended here will work so much better if your hormones are balanced.

Taking melatonin supplementation can be helpful (I discuss this in depth in chapter 31). You can also wear a nondrug sleep patch created with nanotechnology (see Nanotechnology in chapter 31). Using the supplement and the patch every night helps guarantee that I'll get eight to nine hours of sleep.

You need to set up your bedroom so that you will be able to sleep. As mentioned earlier, you need a totally dark environment. Put black tape over your TV lights, telephone lights, and computer lights. From sunset on, dim the lights in your house or light candles. This step lowers your cortisol. Remember, cortisol regards light as meaning that it is still time to be active. By turning down the lights, cortisol naturally begins to lower.

About an hour before you go to bed, take a hot bath, then get in bed at 9:00 or 9:30 P.M., put on your nanotechnology sleep patch (go to www .suzannesomers.com and there will be a direct link to LifeWave). Take your melatonin nightly, put your TV on a timer for one hour and watch something that is calm and peaceful, as opposed to news coverage. If you do this nightly, eventually you will start sleeping. In more ways than you can imagine, your restful nights will keep you healthy and happy—and even save your life.

No pessimist ever discovered the secrets of the stars, or sailed to an uncharted land, or opened a new heaven to the human spirit.

–Helen Keller

PART III

The Future of Medicine

In the next twenty years, 80% of everything you know will be new.

–Eighty-year-old Canadian futurist Frank Ogden,
The Last Book You'll Ever Read

31

THE FUTURE IS NOW

AS I SAID in the beginning of this book, breakthrough medicine is a fast-moving train. There are so many different ways we can build up the body to fight disease, through better nutrition, hormone replacement, exercise, and supplementation. Following the 8 Steps to Wellness will put you on the path toward living the breakthrough life. There are other advances in anti-aging medicine that make it even more possible to live a vital, healthy, long life, free of disease. While everyone can understand the importance of a good night's sleep or a healthy diet in staying well, there are some amazing cutting-edge things being done that will be just as important in maintaining our health and that will have a dramatic impact on how we treat disease in the future. This is not science fiction; these advances are happening now and are already helping people. I will tell you about two of the most remarkable developments in breakthrough medicine: stem cell transplants and nanotechnology. Sounds scary, I know, but what you'll learn is anything but scary. Dr. Robin Smith is in the forefront of stem cell technology, and David Schmidt is the founder of LifeWave nanotechnology patches. Their interviews really open your eyes to the potential that exists for these therapies. I have taken advantage of both of these therapies myself. I banked my stem cells and I regularly use the nanotechnology patches for detoxification, sleep, pain, and energy. I can't live without them. I haven't taken a painkiller in quite some time, and have an aversion to taking over-the-counter products when nondrug patches do the job better.

Medical science and better food and hygiene have given us more years to our lives; cell therapy is concerned with giving more life to those years.

–Dr. Peter Stephan

STEM CELLS

Stem cells are one of the most exciting new therapies on the horizon. Stem cells have the capacity to repair any tissue damage in the body, which is why cutting-edge doctors and professionals are excited about their potential. They will extend life span and retain the healthy nature of organs in the body. There is also the possibility that stem cells will help regenerate tissue, too—someday we will be able to regrow body parts from our own stem cells. It is this possibility that makes banking your stem cells now a "bio-insurance" against future problems.

What is a stem cell? A stem cell is a very early cell in our immune system—it can turn into any stage organ cell, which means it could become part of our heart or our skin or our hair or our cartilage or much more. When we are stressed, our bodies release stem cells, which can go on to rejuvenate tissue. If you are sick, your body's ability to release healthy stem cells is compromised. That is why doctors treat patients with an infusion of stem cells when they are sick—healthy stem cells will help the body fight disease.

There are three types of stem cells: fetal, umbilical, and adult. It has become routine for parents to request that umbilical stem cells are retrieved from the delivery room and banked for future use for the baby if he or she falls ill and needs them. Unfortunately, those stem cells will not work indefinitely. According to Dr. Robin Smith, the cells collected from the umbilical cord will only last that child until he or she is about seven years old—then body weight outgrows the stem cell quantities from birth. So it is a good idea to bank these stem cells as an adult; if you need stem cells when you grow older, it is better to have banked some taken from your own body as an adult.

FETAL stem cells are twenty-seven times more potent than adult stem cells and nine times more potent than umbilical cells for tissue repair. Umbilical and adult stem cells, unless they are from your own body, do have the capacity to be problematic because they could develop self-antigens, possibly resulting in immune system rejection issues when used therapeutically.

But overall, stem cells harvested from a particular individual and then frozen until later use have shown extremely promising results. There are serious moral debates about the use of fetal stem cells in treatments. However, banking your own stem cells, taken from you when you are a young and healthy adult, means that you are putting back into your body cells that were already in your body—Dr. Smith explains this in her interview. Your body will recognize these cells as your own and shouldn't reject them. You are simply reinjecting cells, originally taken from your own body, into the part of your body that needs repair.

No doubt about it, stem cells will play an important role in the future of health. These cells are manipulated to develop into specialized cells and offer the possibility to continually repair damaged tissues and prolong the life span of important organ systems, like the brain and immune system, by supplying a renewable source of new cells. Stem cell therapy can contribute greatly to the servicing of the body because of its ability to work in accordance with the body's natural system. Stem cells make things happen naturally, rather than forcing the body to accept something that is inherently unnatural, such as an organ in an organ transplant. It is obviously better to repair worn-out or damaged tissues in the body than to replace them.

The future of stem cells is actually here. You can now treat heart disease by rebuilding damaged heart muscle and blood vessels. In one study, injected stem cells from bone marrow migrated to the damaged areas of the patient and transformed into heart muscle cells. After nine days, new heart muscle cells covered 68 percent of the damaged area of the heart, and they also stimulated the formation of new blood vessels. These are the types of dramatic results we see with new medicine, and it will only get better in the future.

I have avidly embraced the idea of stem cell therapy, and recently I had my own stem cells banked by the NeoStem Company. They sit you in a chair and hook up needles in both arms: over a two- to three-hour period they extract stem cells and then at the end, they replace your blood with your own new blood. It is a fairly easy procedure and is not uncomfortable. Your body will replace those missing stem cells over the next few hours, and there are no ill effects. The frozen cells will last for your lifetime. Dr. Robin Smith talks more about the process in her interview. How great to know that if I ever get sick, I will have my own stem cells on hand to help me get better.

NANOTECHNOLOGY

What if there were ways to increase your body's antioxidant levels without having to swallow pills or juice?

What if you could experience rapid, drug-free pain relief?

What if you could control your appetite while still eating normal meals, and reduce the cravings that cause you to overeat and gain weight?

What if you could sleep all night, in a deep, satisfying way, without pills or drugs of any kind?

What if you could realize maximum energy levels every day without the benefit of drugs?

What if you could improve the look and texture of your skin, not only on your face but all over your body without expensive creams or drugs?

ALL of these advances are now available through nanotechnology. Nanotechnology is like software for the body. The future really is now!

I first became interested in nanotechnology two years ago when I met with David Schmidt, CEO/inventor of LifeWave, and Dr. Steven Haltiwanger or, as he is called, "Dr. Steve." These two men have developed a system of nanotechnology patches that help you sleep, give you energy, improve your skin, manage your pain—and help you lose weight! All of these patches work without drugs, and they are not transdermal, meaning nothing goes into your skin.

Nanotechnology operates by stimulating acupuncture points and allows you to obtain a new level of benefit that has never before been available. People (myself included) have been able to utilize these patches and have achieved remarkable results. The patches will open up an entirely new world of possibilities in medicine that once only drugs could address, but by using no chemicals and with no side effects.

The time has come for something new. People are ready for an alternative to drugs and pills, and nanotechnology will give renewed energy, pain relief, and drug-free sleep. This way of relief is a gift. You can read more about these patches in my interview with David Schmidt—I'll tell you, too, how you can order them (see page 423) if you get as excited about them as I am.

A number of years ago I was plagued with allergies . . . not just the usual "spring fever," but all year long. Certain office buildings would initiate the sneezing, parts of my home would make my eyes run, walking outside would give me a headache . . . in other words, I was miserable.

I heard about an acupuncturist who worked with allergies, and when I met with him he cautioned that "this wasn't Western medicine, as in taking an antibiotic with immediate results." After several months of weekly appointments, my allergies were gone and have been ever since. Now I think about all the over-the-counter allergy medicines and remedies I took for so many years and all the resultant toxins I put in my body. This was one of my first introductions to nondrug true healing therapies. I am no longer allergic. I watch people sneeze and cough and realize that there is a way to get on top of allergies and get off of antihistamines and allergy medications that cause dependence. Another drug gone!

Then I met with the LifeWave people and they were jumping out of their chairs with excitement about their futuristic nondrug patches for pain, energy, skin, antioxidants, and weight loss. Dr. Steve had just lost forty pounds by wearing the weight-loss patches. They diminish your appetite by working on . . . bingo . . . acupuncture points. Now, of course, there will never be a magic bullet, and naturally you have to watch your diet and follow something sensible like my Somersize eating plan, but the results of these weight-loss patches are amazing.

Recently, my thyroid suddenly became low—I think because of stress—and as a result I put on an extra five pounds. First, I increased my thyroid medication and I thought, okay, this is an opportunity to see if these weight-loss patches really work. I ate, as always, a nutritious diet and wore the patches for a couple of weeks. The five pounds just melted away.

It makes sense; acupuncture, like LifeWave patches, works on meridians. Meridians are a network of energy pathways. These energy pathways oscillate with life force. Huh, you say? Think of this force as a "life wave" that travels along, say, the string of a violin in response to a light stroke with the bow. Depending on which strings and notes are played, information is conveyed in the form of music to the listener. What actually happens is that the stimulation of the string causes the atoms to vibrate and generate a sound wave. Just as music can affect our emotional states, promoting excitement, courage, peacefulness, melancholy, and even sleep, stimulating the "notes," or acupoints, along a physical meridian string will send vibrational information to the organs, energy centers, and brain. This is what nanotechnology patches do for the human body.

The pathways, or meridians, in our bodies get blocked from stress, sickness, toxicity, and poor diet. This clogs the energy and the body gets sluggish (it's much more complex than this and involves telomeres and cell division, but I will let Mr. Schmidt explain that one!). Toxins get trapped and the lymph system can't move the fluids, hormones, or debris out of the designated channels; we get digestive problems, headaches, joint pain, and swelling ankles. Normally we run to the local drugstore and get pain medication for the headache and joint pain, diuretics for the swelling, antacids for stomach acid, plus additional medication for other digestive problems. Think about all the drugs/toxins we ingest to get rid of the toxins and sickness we already have! Pharmaceutical or over-the-counter drugs will never heal these conditions—they only mask them and so the need for more drugs increases and so on. It makes for a toxic, sluggish, overweight body.

But imagine, instead of drugs and medication to take the symptoms away, you put on these patches. Imagine, instead of having acupuncture needles inserted in your skin for forty minutes to slowly unblock and release your sluggishness, you put on the patches? A nanotechnology patch adheres to the same meridians as in acupuncture, and the energy begins to flow freely again. The results are fast and healthy and no drug has entered the body.

We are only as alive as the level of energy and information that travels as a life wave along these meridians which allows our internal machinery to work. Consider this: When a lightbulb dims, it's an indication that not enough electricity is flowing along the wires. Once the electrical flow is restored, the light brightens. It's the same way with vibrantly alive and healthy people. There is a glow to their faces, a sparkle to their eyes, and a luster to their hair because the life wave is moving along the meridians, recharging and revitalizing all the glands and organs of their physical bodies. The quantity and quality of your life is in direct proportion to the vibrations of the life wave.

The beauty of stimulating the acupoints with nanotechnology patches is that you can actually send specific information to your physical body. In essence you can place noninvasive, nontransdermal, molecular antennae on specific acupoints to instruct your body to do everything from burning fat for energy to reducing inflammation, while allowing drug-free deep sleep to increase the antioxidants to fight off the aging effects of free radicals in your body. Sounds too good to be true . . . but it's not.

According to David Schmidt: "For the disbelievers, consider this: A mere sixty-six years ago, we went from believing it was impossible for a heavier-than-air machine to fly to walking on the moon. One hundred years ago, two out of every ten adults could not read or write and only 6 percent had high school diplomas. One hundred years ago, mail was still delivered on horseback; there were only 8,000 cars and only 144 miles of paved road in the entire nation. You couldn't pick up the phone and call across the country; only 8 percent of the homes had a phone. Today you can send an e-mail instantly to the other side of the globe, and almost everyone has a cell phone in their pocket. The rate at which knowledge is expanding is mind-boggling. Our understanding of aging as a disease is approaching breakthrough proportions. Knowledge in antiaging medicine and fields such as nanotechnology is doubling every three and a half years. This is history in the making. The old secrets of ancient Chinese medicine and the new science are revolutionizing our lives."

32

DR. ROBIN SMITH

TO SAY THAT ROBIN SMITH, M.D., M.B.A., is an accomplished woman is a mild understatement. She received her medical degree from Yale and her M.B.A. from the Wharton School of Business. She has also won many awards in her field, and with NeoStem, continues to be on the cutting-edge of modern medical technology. Having spent time socializing with Robin, I discovered a woman who is passionate about her work and her promise for the future of mankind. My interview with Dr. Smith will give you a clear understanding that the future of medicine is right now.

SS: Thank you for spending this time with me. I know my readers will be intrigued to learn about stem cells. I believe if people are reading this book, it's because they want to live longer and healthier.

To begin with, I am very excited to have had my own stem cells collected by your company, NeoStem. In order to understand the process I wanted to have firsthand experience with collection, and I must say it gives me great peace of mind that in the event of need, or, God forbid, catastrophe, I have a resource for healing that will not be rejected. The reason is because, of course, these stem cells are *mine*.

Perhaps through my experience and your enthusiasm and expertise, you can make the argument to all those who are open to the idea if it could be explained properly.

We've all heard about stem cells, but we really don't know how they work or why we would want to consider having them collected and stored. So tell me, from your perspective, why are stem cells so important?

RS: Stem cells have the properties to repair and regenerate your tissues. Anytime your body is stressed or injured, you release stem cells that are found in all parts of your body; it's your body's way of responding to this type of biological event. This includes whether you are sick or experiencing emotional stress, or even environmental stress.

However, if you have a real serious medical event, there often aren't enough stem cells available, or your stem cells may not be effective in making a major lifesaving clinical impact.

SS: Then, how do you get enough stem cells in quantity in a particular area to make an impact?

RS: To get enough stem cells, NeoStem uses a method of stem cell mobilization in which the body is coaxed into producing a huge number of stem cells that enter the circulating or peripheral bloodstream. We are able to collect these cells and have them available for use in fighting certain diseases.

There are many different ways researchers have been looking to increase the number of stem cells and how best to deliver them to a particular site. New methods of introducing stem cells to tissues and organs are being developed and researched every day. Some methods include direct injection of the stem cells into the area that needs them, catherization techniques to guide the stem cell delivery to the appropriate area, and intravenous drip of stem cells directly into the bloodstream.

A common use of a stem cell transplant, for instance, is if you have leukemia and your chemotherapy treatment has stripped your immune system and you will most likely need a bone marrow transplant. Just to be clear—a bone marrow transplant is really another way of describing a stem cell transplant. In some cases, you might be able to get the bone marrow from another person, but 70 percent of people die waiting for a transplant from another donor. Those who do find an adequate match for a bone marrow transplant have a good possibility they will reject those cells because they are not from their own body. Now, if you happen to have an identical twin, you might have a chance of using their cells and not rejecting them.

SS: What about collecting stem cells from the umbilical cord at birth? I hear that's being done routinely in many of our hospitals.

RS: Yes, that's true, and it is a good idea. You can collect stem cells from the umbilical cord at birth. However, there are usually only enough stem cells for most therapies collected from cord blood to last that child until he or she is about seven years old. As a child's body weight increases, the stem cell quantities needed to treat most blood cancers, for instance, will be insufficient and potentially another donor would need to be found.

The only other way to ensure that you have stem cells for your personal use is to bank them today, while you are healthy, and have them available in clinically significant quantities for later use. The younger you are, the healthier you are, the greater the quantity you will have and the greater the chance that the existing stem cells will not be damaged.

So, the younger you are, the better.

Recently there was a segment on a popular morning TV show about a child with cerebral palsy who used stem cells from his own umbilical cord collected at his birth to treat his disease; the "befores" and "afters" were very dramatic.

The problem with a disease like that is that it's progressive and therefore there usually aren't enough stem cells from the initial umbilical collection beyond seven years; multiple treatments may be required and they would be used up. Now we have a new collection mechanism allowing people to bank significant quantities of cells produced by their own bodies and frozen in multiple bags for multiple uses in the future.

SS: Is there any other way to get stem cells if you haven't banked your own?

RS: There are public donor banks and the National Marrow Donor Program where adults and children can look for donors who may match their blood type and other important biological markers. However, there is a high probability of rejection and possible serious medical side effects and problems that are usually associated with transplants of cells that are not your own. Unfortunately, your parents are not often a good match (because each carries his or her own distinct genetic cell makeup that is only partially yours) and even a sibling may not qualify as a donor for a transplant.

SS: But what about the environment? I mean, even if we are young, in today's world our bodies and our health are being degraded by toxins and chemicals.

RS: Yes, the environment will affect the quality of all your cells, including your stem cells. That is why it is important to have your stem cells collected and stored sooner rather than later. The less exposure those cells have, the better it is for you and your medical future.

Pesticides, toxins, smoking, and environmental hazards all affect your stem cells. Polymers, which are a part of the DNA, get shorter and shorter as we age and they are often affected by our environment. So, it's clear that collecting and storing stem cells earlier and while you are healthy gives you a better chance of harvesting better quality and larger quantities of stem cells.

SS: Please explain how you collect stem cells from your clients.

RS: The technology we use today is a very safe and easy way to collect stem cells—similar to giving blood or donating platelets. An intravenous line is set in each arm, and you get to relax and watch a movie while your stem cells are slowly collected from your circulating blood (it's quite comfortable). As this process continues, your blood is returned to you and the stem cells are saved in an IV bag. Once enough cells are collected, you are finished and your body replenishes its cell population rather quickly, so there is no interruption of most normal activities. Certainly you can go back to work the next day.

SS: How many stem cells do you collect and how do you measure the amount?

RS: It varies by age and by sex. As we get older our stem cell population slowly decreases and is not as effective as when we are younger. Our collection protocols allow for the release of many stem cells into the circulating blood to enable us to collect clinically significant quantities. Generally, after a four-hour collection, we collect enough cells to be used for a repopulation of your immune system (if you need one for a blood malignancy therapy) and additional cells for regenerative therapies. Stem cells are used in treatments for heart disease, hair regrowth, or orthopedic uses in the joints, which would help to avoid knee replacement or hip replacement. Recent technology shows that stem cell therapy will affect how we treat many diseases such as neurological disease, orthopedic disease, cardiac disease, and cancer, just to name a few.

We measure the quantity of stem cells by a laboratory analysis method, which identifies particular biomarkers on the stem cells and allows us to perform an accurate cell count.

SS: It makes sense. Now, once you collect these stem cells, what do you do with them?

RS: They are delivered to one of our laboratories where they are processed and cryopreserved. Your cells are separated into two equal amounts of cells. Assuming enough cells are collected, half is stored in a sterile plastic bag (similar to an IV bag) for potential use for immune reconstitution (commonly referred to as a "bone marrow transplant") for the treatment of blood malignancies. The other half is stored in approximately twenty different vials so that you have multiple uses for cellular regenerative therapies or applications that are in use today or are being developed for future use.

Our unique process enables transplant clinicians to use only the precise amount needed for a particular therapy, while allowing for the remaining cells to be kept frozen for any future therapies, should the medical need arise. Once cells are defrosted, they cannot be refrozen and must be used or discarded. One of the main advantages of our storage technique is to have many storage containers so that only the amount used for a therapy is defrosted before transplant, thus ensuring the integrity of the remaining frozen cells.

The ability to have additional cells available for treatment is key in such diseases like lupus or multiple sclerosis. People may go into remission, but because stem cell replacement treats the *symptoms* of the disease but not the *cause* of the disease, there is the likelihood that they will eventually need more treatments. Therefore, having the cells stored in multiple packages enables future use ten, thirty, or even fifty years from now.

SS: Are there studies that show that these banked cells will be okay and available when we need them twenty or thirty years from now? I mean, this is such new technology; you are asking us to take a big leap of faith.

RS: Well, one only needs to look at bone marrow transplantation; it's been in existence for many, many years. There are some universities that have cells that have been stored frozen in their storage tanks since the eighties, and they are still viable.

Based on laboratory data, stem cells go through a degradation process at a rate of less than 5 percent over thirty years, so your stored stem cells will probably remain viable for the rest of your life.

At NeoStem we have a quality control program where we measure the viability of our frozen cells annually to ensure their integrity.

SS: What's an adult stem cell?

RS: An adult stem cell is a cell that can transform into many different types of cells, such as blood cells, nerve cells, heart cells, lung cells, or pancreatic cells. Adult stem cells are not the same as embryonic stem cells. There are no ethical or moral issues involved in using one's own stem cells, and there are no concerns about rejection of the cells, since they come from your own body.

This means that stem cells can become tissue or differentiate into beta-islet cells of the pancreas that secrete insulin for diabetes; they could become cardiac myocyte cells of the cardiac muscle; they could become chondrocyte cells, which can become precursor cells that produce the cartilage we have in our knees and our joints; or they could even differentiate into early precursor cells for hair growth.

SS: How about skin? We're all doing things to keep our skin young, to counteract the damage of the sun—would stem cells grow new young skin?

RS: There is no reason why stem cells cannot be the "secret sauce" in producing skin cells that are new, young, and pliable.

SS: That's a good reason for banking right there. What is the difference between using your own stem cells or fetal stem cells?

RS: Although they show up prior to birth, adult stem cells are developmentally older, specialized cells that exist in many places in the body, biding their time before they replace old and damaged cells and the diseased tissue in which they reside. The principal difference between adult and embryonic stem cells lies in their potential to become different types of cells and tissues. Embryonic stem cells have potential in that they can theoretically become any cell or ORGAN in the body. With early fetal stem cells there is a point where the egg and the sperm come together called the blastocyst phase where those cells ultimately evolve into a person. Those cells become *you*! Adult stem cells, by contrast, are restricted in what they can become.

The primary benefit of using your own adult stem cells versus anyone else's cells, whether they're fetal, embryonic, umbilical cord, or cells donated from another individual, is that your body will not reject your own cells and they will engraft faster and work more efficiently at repairing damaged tissue.

SS: What is the cost?

RS: We've tried to make it affordable for most people. The cost is $7,500. But NeoStem can implement a very affordable monthly financing plan through GE's division called Care Credit. Monthly payments can be as low as $200, and you can select a plan that spans three, four, or even five years. Whatever works best for you.

SS: That is reasonable!

RS: Yes, and this is true insurance—*bioinsurance*—for *you*. It allows you to be prepared for your own future and, more important, you are the beneficiary of the medical benefits—while you are alive—unlike traditional life insurance, which is designed to benefit others.

SS: Where are your collection centers and how many do you have at present?

RS: At present, NeoStem has adult stem cell collection centers in Coral Gables/Miami; New York City; Long Island, New York; Santa Monica, Sherman Oaks, Encinitas (all in California); and in Louisville, Kentucky. We will soon be opening others throughout the country and expect to open collection centers in other countries. NeoStem has one processing and storage facility in the Los Angeles area and one outside of Boston.

At present there are 106 companies working on stem cell therapy and there are more than 2 million treatments done a year.

Stem cells will absolutely impact how we treat disease in the future and they will keep people healthier, on fewer drugs, and definitely be the path to longevity.

SS: Dr. Ron Rothenberg, who has a NeoStem collection center at his office, mentioned to me that they have discovered embryonic-like stem cells in the adult body. Are you part of this discovery?

RS: Yes. NeoStem, with the work of some very fine researchers, has discovered very small embryonic-like stem cells called "VSELs" in adults. These cells live within all of us and exhibit embryonic-like characteristics. These small cells have particular biomarkers on them, which are exactly the biomarkers found on embryonic stem cells. We believe that after fertilization, and then cellular division, some of these embryonic cells that go on to become a person lay dormant in your organ tissues (like your skin, your lungs, and your bone marrow). These cells can be collected from your body and someday, hopefully, be used for tissue and organ repair.

Since some groups perceive a moral issue with fetal or embryonic cells that may even be derived from a petri dish, the discovery of the VSEL theoretically makes it possible to locate and grow true embryonic cells from your own body, with all its natural medical benefits.

Discovering these cells within our own body may be like finding the Holy Grail of cellular therapy. The potential exists to have these cells, *your own cells*, be used in therapeutic applications that only embryonic stem cells can perform. NeoStem is working hard in the laboratory to be able to isolate and increase the number of these VSELs with the hope of one day using them for therapeutic purposes.

SS: This is not about making new human beings, this is about life extension and complete body repair in ways that are so far beyond today's surgery and patch jobs that we presently refer to as "Western medicine." We are just at the tip of the iceberg relative to the usage of stem cells, right?

RS: There will be so many uses. The future of medicine is turning to cellular therapy as a means to provide true *cure-directed treatments*. For instance, many women have suffered the loss of one or both breasts due to breast cancer and surgery. We see in the future where it would be possible to regrow breast tissue (perhaps the entire breast itself) or any body part for that matter. That's where this is going.

In addition, stem cell use is not only for disease or accident victims, but also can be considered for cosmetic use. You can enhance areas where you desire improvement, using your own cells and without causing scar tissue, to produce healthy, vibrant results.

SS: One of the results of my radiation treatments was tremendous damage to the skin on my chest. I use creams and my LED light machine, and got it looking pretty good, but are you saying stem cells injected into, in my case, the chest area could grow new perfect skin?

RS: It's very promising in that regard. We are quite excited about the possibilities for skin rejuvenation, for hair regrowth, for teeth, for the jaw, and most oral surgeries. Stem cells are going to change the way we treat people once it becomes more mainstream in use and "standard of care." This field of medicine is providing such breakthroughs, we just have to work on educating and making people aware of the progress so far and to make this accessible for everyone.

SS: It makes me think about the hormonal system; as people age, we have trouble with all of our declining hormones: adrenals, thyroid, parathyroid; we have trouble with cortisol production. Could stem cells be injected into these glands or organs to rev them up again?

RS: We are starting to look at that. For instance, physicians, in treating diabetes, have been able to inject stem cells directly into the pancreas and have seen those cells differentiate into beta-islet cells, which go on to produce insulin. There are many other endocrinological diseases we could impact with stem cells. So, yes, hormones are part of the regenerative benefits of stem cell therapy.

SS: Having banked my stem cells already with your company, NeoStem, what can I expect relative to my health in the future?

RS: Well, you have taken the right steps in having your stem cells collected and stored. Remember, these are your cells for your use! Should you require them, your physician would request those cells so they can be used to treat you at the time of illness. Your stem cells represent insurance against disease and other medical maladies.

Unfortunately, stem cell treatment centers in the United States are slow to open and, at present, many people are going outside the country to get treated for Parkinson's and spinal cord injuries. Other countries seem to be more progressive in their use of stem cells than we are in America today.

SS: This is disheartening. We are usually at the forefront of new technology, especially when it comes to medical breakthroughs. Do we even *have* doctors in this country who understand what to do with stem cells?

RS: Absolutely! There are over 2,000 clinical trials using adult stem cells as treatments, with 450 clinical trials focused on cardiac therapies alone. Most of these studies are NIH (National Institutes of Health) funded, and there are many clinical trials that are going on at major universities actually treating diseases with stem cells successfully.

These studies are also discovering the best mechanisms for usage— How do you inject them? Where do you inject them? In what quantities?—and then looking at optimizing the possibilities. Every day we are learning new ways to maximize the potential of stem cell therapy.

SS: Then, what is legal in the United States relative to stem cell use? What are we allowed to use them for at present?

RS: The beauty of this is that NeoStem collects *your* stem cells for *your* use. We are not manipulating them or making them into a drug; stem cells are found in your body. We are simply returning the cells back to your body, as young, healthy, and not diseased cells, and allowing them to do the medicinal work for which they were designed to do. This idea is not very controversial nor does it represent many legal or medical concerns.

The treatment of blood cancers using bone marrow transplantation (stem cell transplants) is performed under hospital investigational review boards (IRB approval), and has been an accepted and legal treatment for over twenty years.

In the field of orthopedics, they are beginning to use stem cell therapy for joint repair, joint replacements, and the treatment of arthritis. I mean, isn't that a better modality than putting a foreign object into your body, which has a big possibility of being rejected?

Others have suggested that stem cell therapy could almost be considered a wellness infusion: to inject your cells, routinely and proactively, as you age in an attempt to keep you young.

SS: I hadn't thought of that, but I guess it's a big improvement over Botox.

RS: Yes, it is. Botox is a foreign substance with potential harmful side effects, and there is a lot of negative information coming out about it.

There are so many therapies that will be affected by stem cells, especially in the neurosciences and spinal cord injuries in particular.

In the United States, there are guidelines (often gray) with which we comply. Unfortunately, there are other countries that are more proactive in treating people with end-stage disease using stem cells. That is why U.S. citizens are flying to China and other countries to get help. They feel desperate and are willing to give it a try in foreign countries. It is important for those seeking treatment to thoroughly research those centers that are offering therapies. As in every area of medicine, there are the good and the bad.

SS: What is the objection to stem cells? It appears to be what we have been looking for; it seems more progressive than surgery (cutting and pasting) as we know it presently.

RS: People have been conditioned by the discussions offered by others, and when they hear the words "stem cells" they immediately think of embryonic cells derived from fetal cells or abortive tissue. But it's just not that way. In fact, almost all sources of embryonic cells considered for research are harvested from cellular growth in a petri dish. However, with NeoStem and most adult stem cell therapeutic applications, your own cells are simply extracted and returned to you into the area that needs repair and growth.

SS: So what's everyone so afraid of?

RS: Most people have been fed so much information that has been twisted; I believe it's the quintessential fear of the unknown. But new ideas and modalities take time. The more people learn of the successes we're having and how it changes people's lives and saves lives, the less afraid they will be.

When people realize just how this potential newfound medical safety net can impact their lives in the future, they will be more apt to embrace this therapy.

I know if I were to be diagnosed with breast cancer, or have to experience radiation exposure, or suffer from a severe burn or wound or fracture, I will have my banked stem cells to handle the situation. I feel confident about that!

Suzanne, you already took a proactive medical step in ensuring your health. Because of your history with cancer, should there ever be a reccurrence, you already have had your stem cells frozen while you were cancer free and healthy. These cells could be used to help you and others who are at risk for cancer and other diseases, to fight the disease and potentially even eliminate the cause.

SS: That is very comforting. What are your great successes?

RS: A gentleman comes to mind, in his late forties, a strong athlete, who had a terrible heart attack with almost complete blockage of all his heart arteries. He barely could get out of bed to brush his teeth and was placed on a heart transplant list. But after a successful stem cell transplant directly into his heart, using his own stem cells, he has been able to return to normal activities and is no longer in need of a heart transplant. There are so many of these stories.

More than 15,000 people have already been treated with stem cells and that number continues to grow.

The possibilities to protect our military or our first responders, like our firemen and law enforcement heroes, by collecting and storing their stem cells before they are faced with potential harmful exposure are incredible. Being able to cure terminal disease is a gift.

SS: When you think about it, injecting your own stem cells seems a lot safer to me than a heart transplant, or a liver transplant, or a kidney transplant. I would much rather produce my own real tissue from my own stem cells that my body will accept readily and not reject.

The reason I wanted to interview you for this book is to get people thinking about it. There's a kind of "Dr. Strangelove, science fiction" notion about stem cells, but really, truly, the use of stem cells is not only the future but is here right now, and the possibilities are expanding daily.

I guess the real message here is to understand that the sooner you are able to bank your stem cells, the better; sooner because younger, healthier cells are the most desirable. You don't want to wait until you are old and sick; it's almost as if this technology is a gift to the baby boomers and younger people.

RS: I am a doctor and a scientist, and I believe in stem cells. I have seen firsthand the incredible results. They will have a dramatic impact on how we treat disease in the future, whether it's in curing the patient or in prolonging life. The prospects are thrilling for their ability to keep people active, healthy, young, and able to live. It is one of the most extraordinary advances that we have available in modern medicine.

SS: Thank you so much for this exciting information.

33

DAVID SCHMIDT

DAVID SCHMIDT IS A SCIENTIST, the inventor of the LifeWave technology and founder of LifeWave nanotechnology patches. As a result of work performed for the design of emergency oxygen systems for General Dynamics and the U.S. Navy, he was invited to participate in the navy's next-generation minisub program. He has received an honorary doctorate from the International Hall of Fame. He was formally educated in management information systems and biology at Pace University in Pleasantville, New York. He went on to specialize in energy production technologies for both military and commercial applications. He developed new methods for producing hydrogen and oxygen and constructed metal-combustion rocket engines.

In other words, this is one smart guy. In this interview David will explain in layman's terms the science behind his remarkable LifeWave nanotechnology patches. I have been using these nondrug patches for pain, sleep, energy, appetite control, and detoxification for the past two years and I can't say enough about them. After you read this interview you are going to want to run to his Web site to get some for yourself. Sometimes things are too good to be true; these patches are simply good and true.

SS: Thank you for your time. I'm sure you would rather be designing spaceships or something like that. After all, you are the man who was able to turn seawater into cement! In knowing you the last couple of years it is clear that your brain just works differently from the average person's. What prompted you to develop the nanotechnology patches?

DS: I was asked by a government contractor to find new ways we could keep crews of submarines alive longer in the event of an accident. For example, it's not unusual for a helicopter pilot to have to fly thirty hours straight. There have even been B-2 bomber missions where the pilots have to stay awake for sixty hours on missions. In order to do that they have to resort to amphetamines and caffeine to stay awake and have the energy to do so. I thought this could be an opportunity to see if we could find a way to improve the crews' energy and stamina without having to resort to drugs. This led me on a journey to what became my Life-Wave nanotechnology energy patches.

SS: These patches are in sync with new medicine in that we are all trying to diminish our dependence on pharmaceuticals. You call these patches software for the body—can you explain this?

DS: Most people are ingrained in the pharmaceutical model that some form of drug will create a response within our bodies. To understand our technology (the patches), we need to know that the body has a chemical system and also a bioelectronics system.

When we go out into the sun, we understand that a frequency of light will cause our bodies to make vitamin D. This is a perfect example of how a frequency of energy—in this case, light—can trigger a chemical change within our bodies, a very beneficial change. Another example is, as Californians we go out in the sun hoping to get a tan. This is an example of how a frequency of light is causing our bodies to make melanin, which is an antioxidant and is our bodies' response to being hit with high-energy light. Our bodies do this as a protective mechanism, but most people think along the lines of aesthetics.

In order for these mechanisms to be possible (to be able to respond to light), the cells of our bodies have what are called "photoreceptors." The pharmaceutical model works with some type of drug or nutrient to produce a chemical response, but we know that our cells have photoreceptors, meaning they can take in photons of light and produce chemical changes in the presence of different frequencies of light to be used for healing.

SS: How?

DS: Let's look at one very sophisticated piece of human technology, the man-made space shuttle, that has over five million parts. The human eye, by comparison, has over one billion parts. We all know the human eye is specifically designed to process light. The light enters our eye and travels through the optical nerve around the center of our brain into the pineal, where it is filtered and then travels through the rest of our bodies.

It has been proven that the DNA in our cells actually emits specific frequencies or wavelengths of light that trigger all of the reactions that occur within the cells of our bodies. If we know and understand that light is involved in cell communication, wouldn't it make sense that if you wanted to improve the way our bodies burn fat, we could use the frequency of light from our cells to trigger fat burning?

If we know the frequency of light our bodies use to repair tissue, we simply shine that frequency of light on our bodies and we accelerate tissue repair. So with our nanotechnology patches we can use light therapy in very sophisticated ways that pharmaceutical medicine cannot address today.

SS: So, is this "light" from our own body heat, and how does this information connect to the patches?

DS: Yes. We use our body heat to access the light. In the patches I was able to use organic materials (stereoisomers) to reflect specific wavelengths of light and come up with a unique combination of organic materials, specifically amino acids, sugar, water, and oxygen, and then process these materials in such a way that they reflect the wavelengths of light that will trigger different reactions in the body.

SS: And the patches do this when we place them on the body's meridians?

DS: We place them on the meridians to stimulate the acupuncture point, because science has found that the meridians in our bodies conduct light extremely efficiently. But we don't need to place the patches on an acupuncture point in order for them to function.

SS: What are meridians made of?

DS: Western science has had a problem with the whole concept of acupuncture because they can't see meridians. Meridians are not made of collagen or muscle tissue, they are actually made of water; strings of charged water droplets, actually water molecules with charged ions such as calcium and magnesium. The water molecules line up in these very fine threads, which are charged electrical particles (electrolytes), and these meridians vibrate like a string. Each meridian is connected to an organ and vibrates at its own specific frequency. Think of a musical instrument, a violin or a guitar; each string of its own length will produce its own sound and, of course, that's a different frequency. If we can understand the meridian system we could dramatically optimize and improve our health.

SS: Okay, I think I am "seeing the light." Meridians are their own system and they conduct light.

DS: Yes, and they specifically conduct infrared light. The LifeWave patches are powered by this band of energy, meaning that you place a LifeWave patch on the body (the patch is a form of infrared energy). This band of energy will actually trigger the patch to start reflecting the wavelength of light to do whatever it is meant to do.

SS: So if you have a patch that elevates *glutathione* (which I know you do), instead of going to the antiaging doctor and getting an intravenous drip of glutathione for detoxification purposes, we simply take this patch and place as instructed on our body and our body heat activates the wavelengths of light that trigger the cells in the body that make glutathione? Did I get it?

DS: Exactly. You get an "A."

SS: Well, the glutathione patch is such an interesting way to detoxify the body, in fact downright exciting. A breakthrough!

DS: Yes. Because a glutathione drip has a half-life of somewhere around seven to ten minutes, one hour after your drip, your blood glutathione is back to normal—which is worth it from the standpoint of cleaning out heavy metals. It is extremely safe and it saves people's lives. If we are interested in detoxifying the body of heavy metals, a glutathione drip is worth it; however, if we are interested in keeping our glutathione levels elevated on a regular basis as an antiaging strategy, our patch is the only way to do it. When we look at blood tests after our patches have been worn, the results are so extraordinary that most doctors and scientists have difficulty believing the results are accurate. What we are able to show is that we can elevate glutathione levels by over 300 percent on average within just twenty-four hours. We compare that to the sixty thousand to seventy thousand clinical studies that have been done worldwide on glutathione, and what we see is that with conventional use (as in a drip) we might be getting only a 15 percent increase in glutathione over thirty days. But our Lifewave patches elevate glutathione levels very, very rapidly over a short period of time and keep them elevated.

SS: What does that mean? Do we keep them elevated for the rest of our lives, and why do we want or need to do this?

DS: It depends on your goal. If your goal is to live as long and healthy as possible, then the answer is yes. One of the things that doctors have substantiated is that how long you live is directly proportional to how high you can keep your glutathione levels.

SS: That's quite a statement. I know that glutathione is a powerful master antioxidant.

DS: Yes. Antioxidants protects our intercellular fluids and our inter-cellular environment from free-radical damage. And, of course, if we want to hold off the ravages of aging, then we should all be concerned with our whole blood levels of glutathione.

SS: Is this because we are being bombarded with so many toxins in this new world?

DS: Yes. And as a result, individuals' glutathione levels are depressed compared to what they were many years ago. So with today's toxic envi-ronment we have to have new strategies implemented daily to protect us from these harmful toxins.

SS: This is more than exciting. You have recognized the existing threat of the damaging and harmful effects of toxins and chemicals on the body and this is your answer: the magic bullet.

DS: Yes. We have to do something. Pharmaceuticals are not the an-swer for everything. We are getting hundreds of environmental toxins in-troduced into our bodies from the food we eat and the air we breathe, and some of these are in the form of heavy metals, plastics, and pesticides. It is no longer good enough just to take a vitamin pill to elevate our an-tioxidants; now we have to be concerned with protecting our bodies from free-radical damage, keeping our liver clean, and keeping the heavy metals out of our bodies.

SS: And your glutathione patch can do that, keep the liver clean and kill free radicals?

DS: Yes. The liver is a big part of it, and we know that we find elevated levels of glutathione in the liver. We also know that the liver has multiple pathways for keeping the blood clean, and glutathione is one of the pre-dominant pathways. And we know that glutathione's traditional benefit has been in removing heavy metals and protecting the body from free radicals, so, yes to your questions.

SS: This seems like it would be interesting technology for our military.

DS: Yes. The military has been exceptionally interested in elevating glutathione levels in our troops for many reasons. Glutathione holds off muscle fatigue; when you give it to an individual, their ability to exercise increases substantially. This would allow our troops to perform better be-cause they will have better endurance and stronger muscles. Also the number one disability in the military is hearing loss from weapons fire, and glutathione is the principal antioxidant that protects us from hearing loss.

SS: So, if I wear these patches, I can expect a better effect on my workout, my muscles will be stronger, and my hearing will be protected, and as well I am killing off free radicals and detoxifying my body from the chemical onslaught? This sounds too good to be true; this truly is breakthrough protection and *prevention*.

DS: Yes. Glutathione has all these benefits. Of course, if someone already has hearing loss from nerve damage, then glutathione will not be of value. The Department of Defense and the Department of Homeland Security are concerned with bioterrorism—that someone could drop a dirty bomb or anthrax or smallpox—and they've discovered that if you can elevate glutathione levels quickly enough in people who have been exposed to these bioweapons, you can actually save their lives. With these chemicals what you actually die from are the free radicals, but the glutathione goes in there and does the job to protect. It won't kill the smallpox or the anthrax, but it keeps you alive until you can get antiviral or antibacterial medication.

SS: Well, I hope we never need this antidote. Shifting gears, years ago I was plagued with allergies. I was always using over-the-counter medications to control them. Then I went to an acupuncturist and he said he could get rid of my allergies if I was patient, that this wasn't Western medicine. I committed to him, and for one year I went to acupuncture once a week, and today, ten years later, I do not have allergies, regardless of the season. Knowing that you work with acupuncture points, it seems to me that glutathione would be an approach to reducing or eliminating allergies.

DS: Well, elevating glutathione levels will happen regardless of where you place the patches. What you are referring to is how we can get energy flowing through the body normally. It's important to understand that the meridian system in the body is an electrical communication system. When an electrical system breaks down, then the biochemistry of the body will not function properly. Allergies originate from the action of the kidneys and the adrenal glands being impaired. People with severe allergies always have impaired adrenal glands, so we can make ourselves resistant to allergies by putting needles in the back of the acupuncture points, called bladder 23, and that would stimulate the flow of energy through the kidneys and adrenals. Once you restore that energy flow, you are restoring the communication system; now the adrenals can produce the necessary hormones such as cortisol, which acts like a natural antihistamine, and now we are allergy-free, which is what seems to have happened for you.

SS: Let's talk about the carnosine patches.

DS: The carnosine patches are designed to reflect wavelengths of light that will elevate the body's store of carnosine.

SS: Why do we care about carnosine?

DS: There are similarities between glutathione and carnosine. Both are antioxidants and both are found inside our cells. Glutathione is made up of three amino acids and carnosine is made up of two amino acids. However, carnosine is a little different in that we find it in the skeletal muscle and also in our heart.

Glutathione is the mechanism or material that protects *our body from the effects of aging, and carnosine is the antioxidant that* repairs *the damage done through the effects of aging.*

SS: I get it. Interesting. So even though you've got damage, carnosine is restorative?

DS: Right. It's absolutely remarkable. Carnosine also has a dramatic improvement on endurance. Right now I am working with the Olympic athletes, giving them a combination of glutathione and carnosine, and I'm told some of these athletes are expected to break world records in the upcoming games in Beijing.

SS: Well, I remember Merv Griffin's horse winning the Breeders' Cup and the horse was wearing your energy patches. That was a great photo. You must have enjoyed that.

DS: I did, but it didn't surprise me. Carnosine has a remarkable effect on improving endurance because, like I said, it's the antioxidant that sits in the heart and the skeletal muscle, and from an antiaging standpoint, it is an anticarbonylation nutrient.

SS: Meaning the aging of our cells because of a lack of energy and hydration?

DS: Yes. Our cells are designed to produce energy, and as a result of producing that energy they will have waste as a by-product coming out of the center, the mitochondria. When the cell is functioning normally, there are transport mechanisms to take that waste and remove it out of the lymphatic system and also from our bodies.

But as we age, our cells start to accumulate molecules of carbon (kind of similar to what happens to our car engines: they rust and carbon builds up). Under a microscope our aging cells begin to distort and shrink up. Carnosine introduced in a cell removes all this junk, and what you see is that the older cells get to about 90 percent of looking like a new cell. So carnosine patches get our cells acting and functioning like young, healthy cells, and it gets better. From an antiaging viewpoint, carnosine will increase the life span of your cells from 300 to 400 percent.

SS: This is fountain-of-youth stuff, and all without drugs. I cannot tell you how thrilling this is; as we are speaking I am wearing a carnosine patch, and yesterday I was wearing the glutathione patch. I have been alternating with the two patches all month. And one thing I have noticed is that my skin has gotten so much softer. My wrinkling seems much less than it was last month. Am I imagining this?

DS: These are effects you can expect, besides all the other great benefits. The good news is that your skin will keep improving in tone and texture, and it will keep getting softer because you are cleaning your body from the inside out. Total detoxification.

SS: Could this be reparative for all the millions of adults in this country on statins? Because we know that statins kill the mitochondria, the energy cells in the center of each cell.

DS: Yes. When we experience mitochondrial dysfunction, there are a number of things we can do to get the mitochondria functioning normally. If we wanted to restore energy production, which is so crucial (because that's where it all starts and ends), if our cells aren't hydrated and energy production is halted, everything else collapses. If our cells are not hydrated and our energy production isn't high, how are we going to make hormones or utilize them? How are we going to make new proteins? The best way to focus on antiaging is to find the means to not only hydrate the body but to also increase mitochondrial functioning. Statins by their very nature damage the mitochondrial energy centers of cells, so they work against energy. We came up with light therapy in the form of our patches to increase energy production by elevating fat burning. Without hydration, the energy centers of your cells are being damaged by statins, so eventually you are going to be in trouble. All of the things we are now doing to increase energy and health, as in growth hormone, or vitamin supplements, or exercising, won't have the right effect if we can't keep the body hydrated. We won't be able to get any energy production.

SS: Well, let's talk about hydration. How much water should we be drinking a day?

DS: I laugh because it gets into the subject of what type of water do you drink?

SS: Oh brother, here we go.

DS: You take your body weight and divide it in half in ounces and that's how much water a day.

SS: I weigh 127 pounds, so for me this would this be 63½ ounces? That's about eight 8-ounce glasses of water a day. I can do that.

DS: Right. But if you really want to know how we hydrate the insides of our cells, you need to understand that it's not good enough just to drink water; you have to drink water that is structured.

SS: I knew it was going to be something like that. So, what, like Penta water?

DS: Penta water is a very good example. It is a water that has a low surface tension, and the lower the surface tension, the easier it is to drive the water into the cell where it's needed. Otherwise, you can drink all the water you want and you are still going to be dehydrated.

SS: Does this connect with the fact that we have fluoride in our water in most cities in America?

DS: Fluoride is highly carcinogenic, as is chlorine.

SS: Isn't that great! [*Sigh.*] Anyway, let's get back to water and hydration.

DS: We have to keep our bodies well hydrated so we can get the toxins out of our systems. We do that by eating good food, organic food, which is pesticide-free, hormone-free, and then we need to keep the energy production in our bodies cranked up and keep it free from free radicals. If we do these things, it becomes very difficult for a disease to get a hold of our system.

SS: Well, that makes the effort worth it. I had not heard about drinking the *right* water! I did not know that regular bottled water has a hard time getting into the cells. I didn't realize that water needed to get into the cells.

DS: Here's why: The younger we are, the *larger* our cells. As we get older, our cells get *smaller;* therefore, it's harder to get the energy or the oxygen into them. From the time we are born up to about age eighteen our cells start to shrink progressively, and this is extremely damaging from two points of view. One, as the cells get smaller, it makes it more difficult to get nutrients and water into the cell, and it also makes it difficult to get waste out of the cell. Water has a positive charge around hydrogen and a negative charge around oxygen.

SS: So, it's like a magnet that pulls the negative and positive together?

DS: Yes. Almost like a magnet or like the electrostatic charges you get when you walk across a carpet. When these water molecules stick together, they form large clumps that you can't see. Imagine if these clumps of water are so big that they are actually bigger than the pores on the cell membrane. So you have water in your body but not inside the cell where you need it. It's on the outside of the cell, so it won't do anywhere near as much good as if it could get inside.

SS: But Penta water comes in a plastic bottle. How good is that?

DS: The plastic bottles are very bad for us. Yes, it's a dilemma.

SS: Okay, we've got glutathione patches for detoxification; we've got carnosine patches for skeletal repair and eating up free radicals; and both of these patches beautify and remove wrinkles by cleaning the insides of your body. We need to consume the correct water with the right surface tension to hydrate our cells, and you always say what we all really die of is dehydration, so this is pretty important stuff. What else can we do?

DS: Simple things like putting a filter on your shower and bathtubs. We get more free radicals from our morning shower than anything else we do. A filter can remove the chlorine and fluoride from coming in contact with our skin. And also put a filter on your tap for cooking water.

SS: Are we talking about reverse osmosis?

DS: Yes. That would be good, and switch over to glass bottles of water. We are getting polypropylene or polyethylene bottles that Penta and every other spring water comes in, and all that plastic leaches into the water.

SS: Let's talk about your other patches—the energy patches, for instance, which I have been using for past two years. Please explain what these do and why we want them.

DS: The energy patch was my first LifeWave invention. A number of clinical studies showed that as we get older, we not only lose the function of the mitochondria because the energy output decreases, but now the cell produces less energy and less of our energy comes from fat. Fat has twice the energy as sugar, but it's also more difficult to metabolize. As a survival mechanism the little cells say, "Wait a minute, the cells are shrinking and I've got to make energy to survive; where am I going to get that energy? How about from sugar, because it is easier to process even though we get less energy from it?"

This is terrible, of course, because we've got to do something with the fat, so we store it. Then it becomes a downward spiral because now we are burning less fat and our metabolism decreases, and this has an unfortunate end.

SS: So if we wanted to improve our energy naturally, where would be the best place to get it and how could we burn off more fat?

DS: Good question. As we age, we get less of our energy from fat burning, so I figured if we had a technology that could increase the amount of energy we get from burning fat, not only would we have a way of increasing our overall energy, but we'd also have a way of staying younger.

SS: So can you do this with your energy patches?

DS: That's correct. There is a positive and a negative patch, a white one and a tan one, and it's significant as to *where* we place them on the body. By placing them on the correct places on the body, you can burn over 20 percent more fat the very first time you use it.

SS: This is provided you are eating correctly, right?

DS: Of course.

SS: The idea of wearing simple patches instead of taking some lethal terrible drug to diminish your appetite is going to be of great interest to my readers.

DS: The incidence of overweight and obesity in this country is alarming. We are living sedentary lifestyles with enormous amounts of sugar in our diets. When we take in these sugars, it decreases fat burning and triggers fat storage; then add in all the toxins and you realize why we are experiencing this epidemic of obesity.

SS: And very few people are consuming real food.

DS: Right. We recommend a person wear our glutathione patches about a month before they start a weight-loss program and we find their results are much better. Detoxification is critical for people wanting to lose weight.

We have artificial ingredients in our foods, two of which are NutraSweet and MSG—both of which will create lesions in the hypothalamus. This is why people get a headache after having Chinese food; it's very simple: The MSG is giving us brain damage!

SS: Wow.

DS: If we were to look under a microscope, we would see that the MSG is creating scarring in one of the areas of the hypothalamus that inhibits the ability of the hypothalamus to do what it is designed to do, and one of the functions is appetite control.

SS: What a statement about chemicals. Scarring, yipes!

DS: It's just the beginning. MSG is an excitotoxin for a neurotransmitter, so it is creating other damage in our bodies than just affecting our appetite. That's one of the reasons that after consuming diet food you are still hungry.

SS: So these chemicals are killing the brain.

DS: They are killing the brain. That's why the glutathione patch is so exciting. If we give up these harmful so-called foods and detox and change our diets, it's not unusual for people to lose five, ten, or fifteen pounds in the first month of using the glutathione patches.

SS: Well, I had put on about five pounds last month because my thyroid got "off," and since I wore the patches, I've lost five pounds easily, maybe more. So let's talk about your sleep patches. As a champion of women's health, I know one of the most difficult aspects of hormonal loss, aging, and menopause is the inability to sleep. I am also hearing young people (thirties, forties) saying that they don't sleep well either. I am very excited by the sleep patches and believe they are the greatest menopause product ever made. I love that they are safe and nondrug. The amino acids are not transdermal, meaning nothing goes into the skin, and they work by "reading light" in the body, as you have stated.

DS: Inability to sleep is epidemic. In fact, in Japan about 75 percent, 80 percent, or even higher numbers of the population have chronic sleep problems. If you've ever been there, you understand why; they have very high-pressure lifestyles. It is a significant problem. As a general rule, we are overstressing our adrenals—and it is also happening to the younger generation, which is why they are starting to have sleep problems. I decided to attack this from a different point of view by elevating the production of melatonin.

SS: Tell me how.

DS: When we sleep, we get an initial shot of serotonin; then our bodies produce melatonin, and before we wake up, our bodies produces DMT. However, it's the melatonin that people are often missing, because they are going to sleep too late or they are eating too late. So we designed these patches that elevate the body's melatonin levels. We did a clinical study at a sleep clinic and found consistently that people with a sleep problem produced brain waves below 85 percent. After one week of using the sleep patches, every one of our participants was sleeping better.

SS: Does it shrink the amount of time for the melatonin to kick in?

DS: Absolutely correct. Now, if people eat late, it affects their results, or if a person doesn't have any protein in their diet, it can affect results. The sleep patch is like taking the right amount of melatonin, which induces deep natural sleep.

SS: Does this patch have anything to do with calming down the adrenals?

DS: I think that it does. There is certainly enough information to show that when you elevate melatonin levels, you are reducing adrenal stress.

SS: Like I said, this is a great product for menopausal women as well as the "young burnout people," which I once was. Now, and finally, let's talk about the pain patches. These blow my mind because they work. Once again, a nondrug, nontransdermal patch to eliminate pain.

DS: These are remarkable and among my favorites because they are the easiest to demonstrate. I have applied these pain patches to myself as well as to over five thousand people, and the results never fail to amaze people. In less than one minute we can get a 50 percent or better reduction in pain by properly applying these patches.

Pain is a bioelectrical phenomenon. We've done experiments where we can see the electrical conductivity of tissue increasing in about one minute from the application of the patches. What that means is that we are restoring the natural electrical property to the body by placing a patch at the site of pain where the tissue is damaged; the inflammation diminishes and the result is that the pain drops dramatically.

SS: Do athletes use these patches?

DS: Absolutely. The first doctor to do a clinical study on the pain-relief patches was Dr. Dean Clark, in Portland, Oregon (the doctor for the U.S. Olympic team). He tested two hundred people in a double-blind placebo-controlled environment, using medical infrared imaging. He was able to show that in just five minutes of applying pain-relief patches, there were significant decreases of inflammation.

SS: Why don't these materials, the amino acids, go into the skin? And what would happen if they did?

DS: Well, first of all, the materials are all natural and cleared by the FDA as being safe, and all the materials in the patches are ingredients you would consume anyway. These amino acids have very specific properties, because in addition to reflecting light, we can also create what are called "polarization effects." When you place these patches on the body, they act like positive and negative terminals. All we are doing is generating the flow of energy into our bodies without the need for electrical equipment.

SS: This has been great. What remarkable achievements you have made in your young life, and you still have so much curiosity. It is thrilling to think of what you will come up with next.

DS: Well, Suzanne, Albert Einstein showed that everything in the world around us is made of light. In quantum physics today we are beginning to understand and appreciate this, but now we can go a step further and say everything around us is made of light and information. Many doctors and scientists now refer to this new and emerging field as informational medicine, meaning that instead of using a drug, instead of using a vitamin, we can use *information* to improve the function of our bodies. We are putting specific frequencies of light into the body, causing beneficial chemical changes. In all the double-blind placebo-controlled studies we have proved that indeed this method works.

SS: Your patches are a breakthrough. They are advancing the health of people rather than degrading it, as with (in most cases) the present allopathic approach. I love the concept, I understand it, I use it, and I take my hat off to you for using your considerable talents and brainpower to create something so positive.

DS: Thank you. This is true antiaging and more. This gives quality of life.

DAVID SCHMIDT'S
BREAKTHROUGH BREAKOUTS

- Our cells have photoreceptors that take in different frequencies of light and trigger chemical changes, such as the production of melatonin and vitamin D, that can encourage healing.

- Antioxidants like glutathione protect our intercellular fluids and our intercellular environment from free-radical damage and hold off the ravages of aging.

- Carnosine is an antioxidant like glutathione that helps cells rid themselves of waste; glutathione is the mechanism that protects our bodies from the effects of aging, while carnosine is the antioxidant that repairs the damage done through the effects of aging.

- By staying well hydrated, eating good organic foods, and increasing the energy production in our bodies to keep it free from free radicals, we are able to prevent disease.

- Installing water filters on taps and showerheads and switching to water in glass bottles can help us avoid ingesting potentially carcinogenic chemicals.

- Nanotechnology patches induce sleep, repair, protect, provide energy, and assist in weight loss.

34

THE WRAP-UP

It's the passion; antiaging doctors are excited and passionate. My patients are intrigued by this new approach to medicine. When you get someone balanced and they feel better than they did when they were younger, they will stick with the programs. When, as a doctor, you can really, truly help someone, it's very rewarding.

—Dr. Andy Jurow, Burlingame, California

I HOPE YOU'VE ENJOYED this journey with me. The interesting part of writing this book was having the 8 Steps to Wellness emerge organically as a recurring theme. Each doctor at some point rattled off all of the steps to wellness unbeknownst to one another. At one point in writing, it became very clear. This is the message: Make these simple changes and open yourself up to the possibilities of this new breakthrough medicine while taking advantage of all that good health provides. The gift to yourself is your long, healthy life.

We can all do this: Replace missing hormones with real ones, avoid chemicals and detoxify all the chemicals in your body, avoid taking unnecessary pharmaceuticals, create a healthy GI tract, take nutrition seriously, supplement what we no longer get from our food supply, exercise regularly, and sleep. Even as you reread these steps, you can feel in your gut that they make sense.

In an unhealthy world, good health is the treasure. We are in a new millennium, and the medicine we have been practicing up until now is obsolete. Change is essential for survival. New technologies are exciting—nanotechnology, stem cells, energy medicine—all of these things are new ways of dealing with conditions that once required pharmaceuticals.

Imagine a world that is not dependent on drugs, where people have energy, vitality, and good working brains. Where sickness is not the norm, where aging is not commensurate with sickness, where health is normal, energy is normal, sexuality is normal. This is breakthrough medicine.

The opportunity of spending this kind of time with the top doctors of the world has made me to realize the marvel called our human body. This "house" we all live in will endure self-imposed and environmental destruction to a point, but it responds so quickly to good treatment, like a happy, trusting puppy. . . . quick to forgive and receive love.

When you feed it properly, rest it, take care of it, treasure it, love it, the body will give back again and again and again.

Breakthrough medicine is the new choice; the choice to start in a new direction that doesn't require drugs to keep ourselves together.

Breakthrough medicine is about prevention and restoration; we can now prevent it from happening in the first place and restore what has begun to decline by using natural treatments.

Vitality and energy have no bounds in the practice of this medicine. The new expected life span is 90 to 120 years. I look forward to all those years because I am taking the steps I have learned through the writing of this book, which I know will enable me to have that luxury.

I hope you see the possibilities for yourself and that this book has turned you on to the notion that you really don't have to age or be sick if you are willing to start a new course of health for yourself right now.

If so, I accomplished what I set out to do: to change the face of medicine by giving the best and the brightest doctors on the planet the opportunity to teach all of us about the breakthroughs that will improve our lives.

INFORMATION IS POWER.

Thank you.

NOTE: If you have found the information in *Breakthrough* helpful and wish to receive regular updates on new medical developments, procedures, supplementation, progressive doctors, and cutting-edge research, please register at www.suzannesomers.com. Click on BREAKTHROUGH and then on HEALTH UPDATE REGISTRY and provide your contact information. Our privacy policies apply.

RESOURCES

This Web site will help you find a
  doctor in your area:
www.lef.org/docs

ALABAMA

Dr. Marla Wohlman
3351 Main St.
Millbrook, AL 36054
866-780-7808

ARIZONA

Dr. Shaida Sina
851 S. Main St., Suite E
Cottonwood, AZ 86326
928-649-0269

Dr. Shawn Tassone
LaDea Ob-Gyn
1845 W. Orange Grove Rd.,
  Suite 109
Tucson, AZ 85704
520-544-0906
520-544-5690 (fax)

BAHAMAS

Dr. Norman R. Gay
Bahamas Anti-Aging Medical
  Institute
P. O. Box N3222, W. Bay St.
Nassau, Bahamas
242-328-4100
242-328-4104
E-mail: drnormangay@yahoo.com

CALIFORNIA

Dr. David Allen
2211 Corinth Ave., Suite 204
Santa Monica, CA 90064
310-966-9194

Dr. Daniel Amen (Integrative
  psychiatry)
4019 Westerly Place, Suite 100
Newport Beach, CA 92660
949-266-3700
949-266-3750 (fax)
www.amenclinics.com

American College for the
  Advancement of Medicine (ACAM)
23121 Verdugo Dr., Suite 204
Laguna Hills, CA 92653
800-532-3688

American Health Institute
Dr. Michael Galitzer
12381 Wilshire Blvd.
Los Angeles, CA 90025
800-392-2623
www.ahealth.com

Dr. Catherine Arvantely
4121 Westerly Place, Suite 102
Newport Beach, CA 92660
949-660-1399
949-660-1333 (fax)
www.drarvantely.com

Dr. Dan Asimus (Integrative
  psychiatry)
200 E. Del Mar Blvd., Suite 208
Pasadena, CA
626-578-7111
E-mail: lifefitness@earthlink.net

Dr. Harvey S. Bartnof
Founder–Medical Director
California Longevity & Vitality
  Medical Institute
450 Sutter St., Suite 2433
San Francisco, CA 94108
415-986-1300
Email: DrBartnof@DrBartnof.com
www.longevitymd.net

Dr. Arash Bereliani (Integrative
  medicine, cardiology)
125 N. Robertson Blvd.
Beverly Hills, CA 90211
310-550-8000
www.optimalvitalemd.com

Dr. Jennifer Berman
444 N. Camden Dr.
Beverly Hills, CA 90210
888-849-9933
www.bermansexualhealth.com

Dr. Hyla Cass (Integrative psychiatry)
1608 Michael Lane
Pacific Palisades, CA 90272
310-459-9866
310-459-9466
www.drcass.com

The Center for Antiaging Medicine
1270 Coast Village Circle, Suite 2
Montecito, CA 93108
800-392-2623

Dr. Yun-Ching Chen (Internal
  medicine)
720-A Capitola Ave.
Capitola, CA 95010
831-462-6013
www.ching@emotrics.com

Dr. Marc Darrow
Sports Medicine Center
11645 Wilshire Blvd., Suite 120
Los Angeles, CA 90025
310-231-7000

Dr. Joe Filbeck
8929 University Center Lane, Suite
  202
San Diego, CA 92122
858-457-5700
www.palmlajolla.com

Dr. Drew Francis, Lac, OMD
  (Integrative medicine)
2019 Sawtelle Blvd.
West Los Angeles, CA 90025
310-575-5611
310-575-9885 (fax)
www.goldencabinet.com

Dr. Michael Galitzer (my personal
  physician)
12381 Wilshire Blvd., Suite 102
Los Angeles, CA 90025
800-392-2623
www.ahealth.com

Dr. Allen Green (Integrative
  medicine)
2211 Corinth Ave., Suite 204
Los Angeles, CA 90064
310-907-6126
E-mail: admin@allengreenmd.com
www.allengreenmd.com

Dr. David L. Greene
459 W. Line St.
Bishop, CA 93514
760-873-8982

Dr. Robert Greene
1255 East St., Suite 201
Redding, CA 96001
530-244-9052
www.specialtycare4women.com
www.robertgreenemd.com

Dr. Hans Gruenn
Longevity Medical Center
2211 Corinth Ave., Suite 204
Los Angeles, CA 90064
310-966-9194
E-mail: ceo@drgruenn.com
www.drgruenn.com
www.i4sh.com

Dr. Prudence Hall
The Hall Center
1148 4th St.
Santa Monica, CA 90403
866-933-HALL (4255)
310-458-0179 (fax)
E-mail: info@thehallcenter.com
www.thehallcenter.com

Dr. Lisa Hirsch (Integrative medicine,
  gynecology)
360 San Miguel, Suite 308
Newport Beach, CA 92660
949-720-0511
949-720-9404 (fax)
www.newportwomenshealthandwell
  ness.com

Dr. Andrew H. Jurow
Board-Certified Anti-Aging Medicine
1828 El Camino Real, Suite 804
Burlingame, CA 94010
650-552-0395
650-552-0382 (fax)
www.physiciansyouthfulresolutions
  .com

Dr. Candice Lane
1250 La Venta Dr., Suite 206
Westlake Village, CA 91361
805-496-7869
877-496-4289
805-496-7879 (fax)

Dr. Howard Liebowitz
The Hall Center
1148 4th St.
Santa Monica, CA 90403
866-933-HALL (4255)
310-458-0179 (fax)
E-mail: info@thehallcenter.com
www.thehallcenter.com

Dr. Cathie Lippman
The Lippman Center for Optimal
  Wellness ·
291 S. La Cienega Blvd., Suite 409
Beverly Hills, CA 90211
310-289-8430
310-289-8165 (fax)
www.cathielippmanmd.com

Dr. Gary London (Ob-gyn)
9201 Sunset Blvd., Suite 401
Beverly Hills, CA 90069
310-207-4500
www.garylondonmd.com

Dr. Hilda Maldonado
Functional & Anti-Aging Medicine
1240 Westlake Blvd., Suite 133
Westlake Village, CA 91361
805-496-6698
805-557-0223 (fax)
www.drhildamaldonado.com

Dr. Alex Martin (Integrative
  medicine)
Ergonique
359 San Miguel Dr., Suite 110
Newport Beach, CA 92660
949-721-8304
949-721-9194
www.ergonique.com

Dr. Robert Mathis
9 E. Mission St.
Santa Barbara, CA 93101
805-569-7100
www.baselinehealth.net

Dr. Philip Lee Miller
Los Gatos Longevity Institute
15215 National Ave., Suite 103
Los Gatos, CA 95032
408-358-8855
www.antiaging.com

Dr. Steven Nelson
74-133 El Paseo, Suite 5
Palm Desert, CA 92260
760-776-5001
760-776-5005 (fax)
www.wholehealthamerica.com/
  drstevenelson
www.drstevenelson.com

Dr. Christine Paoletti (Integrative
  medicine, gynecology)
1304 15th St., Suite 405
Santa Monica, CA 90404
310-319-1819
310-319-1335 (fax)
www.drpaoletti.com

Cristiana Paul, MS (Nutrition)
Los Angeles, CA
E-mail: cristiana@cristianapaul.com
www.cristianapaul.com

Dr. Allen Peters (Integrative
  medicine)
3655 Lomita Blvd., Suite 307
Torrance, CA 90505
310-373-7830
www.nourishingwellness.com

Dr. Bijan Pourat (Integrative
  medicine, cardiology)
125 N. Robertson Blvd.
Beverly Hills, CA 90211
310-550-8000
E-mail: antiagingbybijan@hotmail.com

Dr. Wendy Miller Rashidi
Women's View Medical Group
299 W. Foothill Blvd.
Upland, CA 91786
909-982-4000
www.womensviewmedical.com

Dr. Uzzi Reiss
414 N. Camden Dr., Suite 750
Beverly Hills, CA 90210
www.uzzireissmd.com

Dr. Christian Renna (Integrative
  medicine)
2811 Wilshire Blvd., Suite 610
Santa Monica, CA 90403
310-453-2335
310-453-2337 (fax)
www.lifespanmedicine.com

Dr. Ron Rothenberg, FACEP
Founder, California HealthSpan
  Institute
320 Santa Fe Dr., Suite 301
Encinitas, CA 92024
(Located on the campus of Scripps
  Memorial Hospital, Encinitas, CA)
760-635-1996
800-943-3331
www.ehealthspan.com

Dr. Neal Rouzier
Preventive Medicine Clinics
  of the Desert
2825 Tahquitz Canyon Way, Suite
  200
Palm Springs, CA 92262
760-320-4292
www.hormonedoctor.com

Dr. Gary Ruelas
Integrative Medical Institute of
  Orange County
707 E. Chapman Ave.
Orange, CA 92866
714-771-2880
www.integrative-med.org

Dr. Joseph Sciabbarrasi
2001 S. Barrington Ave., Suite 208
Los Angeles, CA 90025
310-268-8466
310-268-8122 (fax)
www.drjosephmd.com

Dr. Allan Sosin (Integrative medicine)
Institute for Progressive Medicine
4 Hughes, Suite 175
Irvine, CA 92618
949-600-5100
949-600-5101 (fax)
www.iprogressivemed.com

Dr. Svetlana R. Stivi
New Health Institute
180 Newport Center Dr., Suite 120
Newport Beach, CA 92660
949-644-6969
949-644-6959
www.newhealthinstitute.com

Dr. Jennifer Sudarsky (Integrative
medicine)
3201 Wilshire Blvd., Suite 211
Santa Monica, CA 90403
310-315-9101
E-mail: jsudarsky@mednet.ucla.edu

Dr. Julie Taguchi
317 W. Pueblo St.
Santa Barbara, CA 93105
805-681-7500
Email: drtaguchi@thewileyprotocol
.com

Dr. Cheryl Thomas (Integrative
medicine)
Total Wellness Medical Corp.
195 S. C St., Suite 100
Tustin, CA 92780
714-669-4700
www.TMWC.meta-ehealth.com

Dr. Duncan Turner (Ob-gyn)
219 Nogales Ave., Suite A
Santa Barbara, CA 93105
805-682-6340
www.duncanturner.com

Dr. Karlis Ullis (Integrative medicine)
1807 Wilshire Blvd., Suite 205
Santa Monica, CA 90403
310-829-1990
310-829-5134 (fax)
www.agingprevent.com

Dr. Cynthia Watson
Watson Wellness
3201 Wilshire Blvd., Suite 211
Santa Monica, CA 90403
310-315-9101
310-829-9860
www.watsonwellness.org

Dr. Ronald Wempen
Health and Energy Medical Clinic,
Inc.
14795 Jeffrey Rd., Suite 101
Irvine, CA 92618
949-551-8751
949-551-1272 (fax)
E-mail: lifenergy@cox.net

COLORADO

Dr. David Leonardi
8400 W. Prentice Ave., Suite 700
Greenwood Village, CO 80111
303-462-5344

Dr. Ron Rosedale (Integrative
medicine)
Advanced Metabolic Laboratories
LLC
Bioscience Park Center
12635 Montview Blvd., Suite 100
Aurora, CO 80045
720-859-4132
www.rosedalescience.com

CONNECTICUT

Dr. Peggy Fishman
Institute of Integrative and
Age-Management Medicine
267 Westport Rd.
Wilton, CT 06897
203-834-7747
www.iaamed.com

Dr. Henry Sobo
111 High Ridge Rd.
Stamford, CT 06905
203-348-8805

FLORIDA

Jean Allen, DO
1502 S. MacDill Ave.
Tampa, FL 33629
813-253-3223

Dr. Robert G. Carlson
1901 Floyd St., Suite 302
Sarasota, FL 34239
941-955-1815
866-955-1815
www.andlos.com

James Cennamo, DO
2708 E. Oakland Park Blvd.
Fort Lauderdale, FL 33306
954-318-0873

Dr. Peter Holyk
600 Schumann Dr.
Sebastian, FL 32958
772-388-5554

Herbert Pardell, DO
4330 Sheridan St.
Hollywood, FL 33021
954-987-4455

Dr. Juan Remos
The Miami Institute for Age
  Management & Intervention
1441 Brickell Ave., 3rd Floor–Sky
  Lobby
Miami, FL 33131
305-624-0009

Dr. Herbert Slavin
7200 W. Commercial Blvd., Suite 210
Lauderhill, FL 33319
954-748-4991
www.drslavin.com

Dr. Paul Wand
Neurological Pain Management, Inc.
2885 N. University Dr.
Suite 210
Coral Springs, FL 33065
954-344-9772
954-344-9760 (fax)
www.integrativeneurology.com

GEORGIA

Dr. Donovan Christie
227 Idlewood Rd.
Tucker, GA 30084
678-205-2039
678-205-2039 (fax)
www.anwanwellness.com

Dr. Michelle Fischer
Anti-Aging & Vitality Center of
  Atlanta
325 Hammond Dr., Suite 204
Sandy Springs, GA 30328
404-255-5583

Dr. Milton Fried
4426 Tilly Mill Rd.
Atlanta, GA 30360
770-451-1928

Dr. Linda Kelly
Cobb Longevity & Wellness
4343 Shallowford Rd., Bldg. B,
  Suite 4
Marietta, GA 30062
770-649-0094

Dr. Ralph Lee
110 Lewis Dr. NE, Suite B
Marietta, GA 30060
770-423-0064

Metametrix Clinical Laboratories
4855 Peachtree Industrial Blvd.
Norcross, GA 30092
770-446-5483

Dr. Daniella Paunesky
11300 Atlantis Place, Suite A
Alpharetta, GA 30002
770-777-7707

Elizabeth L. Schultz, DO
1351 Stonebridge Pkwy., Suite 106
Watkinsville, GA 30677
706-769-0720

HAWAII

Dr. Alan D. Thal
55-3327 Akoni Pule Hwy.
Hawi, HI 96719
808-889-5556
808-889-5411 (fax)
www.drthal.com

IDAHO

Dr. Paul Brillhart
1110 E. Polston Ave.
Post Falls, ID 83854
208-773-1311
www.drpaulbrillhart.com

ILLINOIS

American Academy of Anti-Aging
  Medicine
1510 W. Montana St.
Chicago, IL 60614
773-528-4333
www.worldhealth.net

Laura Berman, Ph.D.
Berman Center
211 E. Ontario St.
Chicago, IL 60611
800-709-4709
www.bermancenter.com

Dr. William Epperly
245 S. Gary Ave., Suite 105
Bloomingdale, IL 60108
630-893-9661

Dr. Paul Savage, FACEP
Chief Medical Officer, BodyLogicMD
4753 N. Broadway Ave., Suite 101
Chicago, IL 60640
866-535-BLMD (2563)
866-344-BLMD (2563) (fax)
www.bodylogicmd.com
Other locations may be found on
  their Web site, including Chicago,
  IL; Hartford, CT; Ft. Lauderdale, FL;
  Naples, FL; Jacksonville, FL

INDIANA

Dr. Tammy Born
Crossroads Healing Arts
21764 Omega Court
Goshen, IN 46528
574-875-4227
www.bornclinic.com

Linda J. Spencer, MSN, CPNP, FNP
Complementary Family Medical Care
  of Indiana
3850 Shore Dr., Suite 205
Indianapolis, IN 46254
317-298-3850
www.complementaryfamilymedicare
  .com

Dr. Charles Turner
3554 Promenade Parkway, Suite H
Lafayette, IN 47909
765-471-1100
www.charlesturnermd.com

Dr. George Wolverton
647 Eastern Blvd.
Clarksville, IN 47129
812-282-4309

KENTUCKY

Dr. Peggy Fishman
Institute of Integrative and
  Age-Management Medicine
2932 Breckenridge Lane
Louisville, KY 40220
502-451-7720
502-451-7737 (fax)
www.iaamed.com

Dr. Paul Hester
812 E. High St.
Lexington, KY 40502
859-266-5483

Dr. Stephen Kiteck
600 Bogle St.
Somerset, KY 42503
606-677-0459

MASSACHUSETTS

Dr. Alan Altman
Assistant Professor, Obstetrics,
  Gynecology and Reproductive
  Biology
Harvard Medical School
55 Pond Ave.
Brookline, MA 02445
617-232-0202

Dr. Barry Elson
Dr. Darren Lynch
Dr. Liz O'Dair
Northampton Wellness Associates
395 Pleasant St.
Northampton, MA 01060
413-584-7787

MICHIGAN

Dr. Tammy Born
3700 52nd St. SE
Grand Rapids, MI 49512
616-656-3700
www.bornclinic.com

Dr. David Brownstein
Center for Holistic Medicine
5821 W. Maple Rd., Suite 192
West Bloomfield, MI 48322
248-851-1600
www.drbrownstein.com

Robert DeJonge, DO
350 Northland Dr. NE
Rockford, MI 49341
616-866-4474

Dr. Steven Margolis
43956 Mound Rd.
Sterling Heights, MI 48314
586-323-1122

David Nebbeling, DO
3918 W. Saint Joseph Hwy.
Lansing, MI 48917
517-323-1833

MINNESOTA

Dr. Khalid Mahmud
4005 W. 65th St., Suite 212
Edina, MN 55435
952-922-2345
www.idinhealth.com

NEVADA

De. James W. Forsythe
ReVage Medical Spa
1225 S. Fort Apache Rd., Suite 145
Las Vegas, NV 89117
702-989-2410
www.revagemedicalspa.com

Dr. James W. Forsythe
Century Wellness Clinic
521 Hammill Lane
Reno, NV 89511
775-827-0707
www.drforsythe.com

NEW JERSEY

Dr. Vladimir Berkovich
1707 Atlantic Ave., Bldg. B
Manasquan, NJ 08736
732-292-2101

Gary Klingsberg, DO
66 N. Van Brundt St.
Englewood, NJ 07631
201-503-0007

Dr. Allan Magaziner, DO
Magaziner Center for Wellness and
  Anti-Aging Medicine
1907 Greentree Rd.
Cherry Hill, NJ 08003
856-424-8222
www.drmagaziner.com

Dr. Neil Rosen
555 Shrewsbury Ave.
Shrewsbury, NJ
732-219-0895

Dr. Judith Volpe
107 Monmouth Rd.
West Long Branch, NJ 07764
732-542-2638

NEW YORK

Dr. Kenneth Bock
Dr. Steven Bock
Dr. Michael Compain
The Rhinebeck Health Center
108 Montgomery St.
Rhinebeck, NY 12572
845-876-7082
www.rhinebeckhealth.com

Dr. Kenneth Bock
Dr. Steven Bock
The Center for Progressive Medicine
Pinnacle Place
10 McKown Rd., Suite 224
Albany, NY 12203
518-435-0082
www.rhinebeckhealth.com

Dr. Eric Braverman, Clinical Assistant
  Professor, New York Weill Cornell
PATH Medical
304 Park Ave. S., 6th Floor
New York, NY 10010
212-213-6155
212-889-5204 (fax)
E-mail: pathmedical@aol.com
www.pathmed.com

Dr. Rashmi Gulati
31 E. 28th St., 6th floor
New York, NY 10021
212-794-4466
E-mail: info@patientsmedical.com
www.patientsmedical.com

Dr. Ronald Hoffman
The Hoffman Center
40 E. 30th St.
New York, NY 10016
212-779-1744
www.drhoffman.com

Dr. Alexander N. Kulick
625 Madison Ave.
New York, NY 10022
212-838-8265
www.ostrow.medem.com

Dr. Richard Linchitz
Linchitz Medical Wellness
70 Glen St., Suite 240
Glen Cove, NY 11542
516-759-4200
www.linchitzwellness.com

Dr. Ron Livesey
30 Central Park South
New York, NY 10003
877-888-7074

Dr. Jeffrey A. Morrison, CNS
103 Fifth Ave., 6th Floor
New York, NY 10003
212-989-9828
212-989-9827 (fax)
Email: drmorrison@themorrison
  center.com
www.themorrisoncenter.com

Dr. John Salerno
14 W. 49th St., Suite 1401
New York, NY 10020
212-582-1700
www.salernocenter.com

NORTH CAROLINA

Dr. R. Ernest Cohn
Dr. Robert G. Apgar
Holistic Medical Clinic of the
  Carolinas
308 E. Main St.
Wilkesboro, NC 28697
336-667-6464
336-667-4488 (fax)
E-mail: info@holisticmedclinic.com
www.holisticmedclinic.com

Dr. Larry Webster
3605 Peters Court
High Point, NC 27265
336-841-1850
866-266-8869
336-841-1855 (fax)
www.lwebster.org
Also does compounding

OHIO

Dr. Josephine Aronica
1867 W. Market St.
Akron, OH 44313
330-494-8641

Dr. James Frackelton
24700 Center Ridge Rd.
Westlake, OH 44145
440-835-0104

Dr. Felicitas Juguilon
Anti-Aging & Vitality Center of
  Cleveland
6000 Lombardo Center Dr., Suite
  150
Seven Hills, OH 44131
216-573-5600

OREGON

Dr. Daniel Laury
786 State St.
Medford, OR 97504
541-773-5500

PENNSYLVANIA

Dr. Adrian J. Hohenwarter
Family Practice & Alternative
  Medicine
745 S. Grant St.
Palmyra, PA 17078
717-832-5993
Also compounds hormones

Ruth Jones, DO
342 S. Richard
Bedford, PA 15522
814-623-8414

Conrad Maulfair, DO
403 N. Main St.
Topton, PA 19562
610-682-2104

TENNESSEE

Dr. Marc Houston (Integrative
  medicine)
Hypertension Institute
4230 Harding Rd., Suite 400
Nashville, TN 37205
615-297-2700
615-467-0365

Dr. L. Morgan Williams
321 Billingsly Court, Suite 20
Franklin, TN 37067
615-771-8832

TEXAS

Dr. Sakina Davis
Woodlands Wellness & Cosmetic
  Center
9595 Six Pines Dr., Suite 6250
The Woodlands, TX 77380
281-362-0014
281-466-8044 (fax)
www.woodlandswellness.com

Dr. Linda Ho
Anti-Aging & Vitality Center of Dallas
6101 Chapel Hill Blvd.
Plano, TX 75093
972-312-8881

Dr. Steven Hotze
20214 Braidview Dr., Suite 215
Katy, TX 77450
281-698-8698
877-698-8698
www.hotzehwc.com
www.drhotze.com

Alice Pangle, DO
3303 University Ave.
Lubbock, TX 79410
806-795-6466
800-772-6466

Dr. Christian Renna (Integrative
  medicine)
Dr. Courtney Ridley (Ob-gyn)
2706 Fairmount St.
Dallas, TX 75201
214-303-1888
214-303-1550 (fax)
www.lifespanmedicine.com

John Sessions, DO
1609 S. Margaret
Kirbyville, TX 75956
409-423-2166

UTAH

Rachel Burnett, ND
Utah Natural Medicine
242 S. 400 East, Suite A
Salt Lake City, UT 84111
801-363-8824

Dr. Paul Navar
166 N. 300 West, Suite 3
St. George, UT 84790
435-619-1577

Dr. Gordon Reynolds
Green Valley Spa
1871 W. Canyon View
St. George, UT 84770
435-628-8060

VIRGINIA

Dr. George Guess
2776 Hydraulic Rd., Suite 5
Charlottesville, VA 22901
434-295-0362

WASHINGTON

Dr. Jonathan V. Wright
Tahoma Clinic
801 S.W. 16th St., Suite 121
Renton, WA 98057
www.tahomaclinic.com

WISCONSIN

Dr. Steven Meress
180 Knights Way
Fond du Lac, WI 54935
920-922-5433

CANADA AND EUROPE

This Web site will help you find a
doctor in your area: www.lef.org/docs

OTTAWA

Metalife BioMedical Clinic
The International Center for
  MetabolicTesting (ICMT)
NutriChem
1303 Richmond Rd.
Ottawa, Ontario, Canada K2B 7Y4
613-820-4200
613-829-2226 (fax)
www.nutrichem.com

TORONTO

Dr. Alvin Pettle
The Ruth Pettle Wellness Center
3910 Bathurst St., Suite 207
Toronto, Ontario, Canada M3H 3N8
416-633-4101
416-633-3400 (fax)
www.drpettle.com

Dr. Maria Schleifer
H.O.P.E. Clinic of Integrative
  Medicine
4195 Dundas St. West
Toronto, Ontario, Canada M8X 1Y4
416-236-8788

VANCOUVER

Ronald Conn
Ubiquity Wellness Centre
4255 Arbutus St., Suite 260
Vancouver, BC, Canada V6J 4R1
604-228-1183
866-329-1183
604-228-1184 (fax)
www.ubiquitywellness.ca

Dr. Nishi Dhawan
Dr. Bal Pawa
Dr. Karla Dionne
Westcoast Women's Clinic
1003 W. King Edward Ave.
Vancouver, BC, Canada V6H 1Z3
604-738-9601
604-738-9605 (fax)
www.westcoastwomensclinic.com

Dr. Karla Dionne
Dr. Brian Martin, BSc, ND
EnerChanges Clinic—Canada's First
  Medically Supervised Anti-Aging
  and Weightloss Clinic
M11-601 W. Broadway
Vancouver, BC, Canada V5Z 4C2
604-681-8380
604-681-7003 (fax)
www.enerchanges.com

BRUSSELS, BELGIUM

Dr. Thierry Hertoghe
7 Avenue Van Bever
B-1180 Brussels
+3227366868
+3227325743 (fax)
E-mail: secretariathertoghe@hotmail
  .com (only for appointments)
www.hertoghe.eu

THE WILEY PROTOCOL—RHYTHMIC CYCLING

Dr. Yun-Ching Chen (Internal
  medicine)
720-A Capitola Ave.
Capitola, CA 95010
831-462-6013
www.ching@emotrics.com

Dr. Karla Dionne
EnerChanges Clinic—Canada's First
  Medically Supervised Anti-Aging
  and Weightloss Clinic
M11-601 W. Broadway
Vancouver, BC, Canada V5Z 4C2
604-681-8380
604-681-7003 (fax)
www.enerchanges.com

Dr. Allan Magaziner
Medical Director and Founder
Magaziner Center for Wellness and
  Anti-Aging Medicine
1907 Greentree Rd.
Cherry Hill, NJ 08003
856-424-8222
www.drmagaziner.com

Dr. Robert Mathis
9 E. Mission St.
Santa Barbara, CA 93101
805-569-7100
www.baselinehealth.net

Dr. Courtney Ridley (Ob-gyn)
2706 Fairmount St.
Dallas, TX 75201
214-303-1888
www.lifespanmedicine.com

Dr. Julie Taguchi
317 W. Pueblo St.
Santa Barbara, CA 93105
805-681-7500
E-mail: drtaguchi@thewileyprotocol
.com

Dr. Duncan Turner (Ob-gyn)
219 Nogales Ave., Suite A
Santa Barbara, CA 93105
805-682-6340
www.duncanturner.com

NEW TECHNOLOGIES

All three of these companies can be contacted by direct links on my Web site:

LifeWave
David Schmidt
1020 Prospect St., Suite 200
La Jolla, CA 92037
858-459-9876
866-420-6288
www.suzannesomers.com (click on LIFEWAVE)

NeoStem Company
Dr. Robin Smith
420 Lexington Ave., Suite 450
New York, NY 10170
212-584-4180
646-514-7787 (fax)
www.suzannesomers.com (click on NEOSTEM)

Ondamed
www.suzannesomers.com (click on ONDAMED)

MASTER HERBALIST

Paul Schulick
New Chapter
99 Main St.
Brattleboro, VT 05301
802-257-9345
www.newchapter.info

OTHER HELPFUL WEB SITES

Dr. Russell L. Blaylock
Advanced Nutritional Concepts, LLC
www.russellblaylockmd.com

Julie Carmen (Yoga)
juliecarmen@charter.net
www.intlhormonesociety.org

Suzanne Somers
www.suzannesomers.com

Don Tolman
www.dontolmaninternational.com

TESTING HORMONE LEVELS

Aeron LifeCycles
1933 Davis St., Suite 310
San Leandro, CA 94577
800-631-7900
www.aeron.com

Sabre Sciences, Inc.
2233 Faraday Ave., Suite K
Carlsbad, CA 92008
www.sabresciences.com

Life Extension Foundation
Fort Lauderdale, FL
888-884-3666
www.lef.org/goodhealth

TESTING FOR NUTRITIONAL DEFICIENCIES

Cristiana Paul, MS (Nutritionist)
Los Angeles, CA
E-mail: cristiana@cristianapaul.com
www.cristianapaul.com

NONSURGICAL FACIAL REJUVENATION

Dr. Peter Hanson
Cherry Creek Center for Healing
3300 E. First Ave., Suite 600
Denver, CO 80206
303-733-2521
www.peterhansonmd.com

COMPOUNDING PHARMACIES

These Web sites list compounding
pharmacies by state:

www.angelfire.com/fl/endohystnhrt/
   pharmacy.html

Professional Compounding Center of
   America (PCCA), www.pccarx.com

ARIZONA

Women's International Pharmacy
12012 N. 111th Ave.
Youngtown, AZ 85363
800-279-5708
www.womensinternational.com

CALIFORNIA

Compounding Pharmacy of Beverly
  Hills
9629 W. Olympic Blvd.
Beverly Hills, CA 90212
310-284-8675
888-799-0212
www.compounding-expert.com

Dr. Eleanor Kong, PharmD
Wellness Clinician/Educator of BHRT
3435 Ocean Park Blvd., Suite 105B
Santa Monica, CA 90403
310-393-2755
E-mail: Eleanor155@aol.com

Medical Center Pharmacy
Sue Decker
Pharmacist: Nilesh Bhakta
Redondo Beach, CA
310-540-3312

San Diego Compounding Pharmacy
Jerry Greene, RPh, FACA
5395 Ruffin Rd., Suite 104
San Diego, CA 92123
858-277-8884
866-413-2673
858-277-8889 (fax)
E-mail: sdcprx@gmail.com

Steven's Pharmacy
1525 Mesa Verde Dr. E.
Costa Mesa, CA 92626
800-352-3784
www.stevensrx.com

Town Center Drugs and
  Compounding Pharmacy
72624-A El Paseo
Palm Desert, CA 92260
760-341-3984
877-340-5922

COLORADO

College Pharmacy
3505 Austin Bluffs Pkwy., Suite 101
Colorado Springs, CO 80918
719-262-0022
719-262-0035 (fax)
800-888-9358
800-556-5893 (fax)

FLORIDA

The Compounding Shop
4000 Park St. N.
St. Petersburg, FL 33709
727-381-9799
866-792-6731
727-347-2050 (fax)
www.gotocompoundingshop.com

MARYLAND

Village Green Apothecary
Paul Garcia
Marketing Director
5415 W. Cedar Lane
Bethesda, MD 20814
301-530-0800
240-644-1362 (fax)
www.myvillagegreen.com

NEVADA

Kronos Pharmacy (formerly Medical
  Center Pharmacy)
3675 South Rainbow Blvd.
Las Vegas, NV 89103
800-723-7455

OHIO

The Medicine Shoppe Pharmacy
649 W. High St.
Piqua, OH 45356
937-773-1778
888-723-5344
www.hormoneconnection.biz

PENNSYLVANIA

Hazle Compounding
7 N. Wyoming St.
Hazleton, PA 18201
570-454-2958
800-213-0592
800-400-8764 (fax)
E-mail: info@hazlecompounding.com
www.hazlecompounding.com

TENNESSEE

Solutions Pharmacy
4632 Highway 58 N.
Chattanooga, TN 37416
423-894-3222
800-523-1486
www.solutions-pharmacy.com

TEXAS

ApotheCure, Inc.
4001 McEwen Rd., Suite 100
Dallas, TX 75244
972-960-6601
800-969-6601
www.apothecure.com

International Academy of
  Compounding Pharmacists
P.O. Box 1365
Sugar Land, TX 77478
800-927-4227
www.iacprx.org
You may call them or go to their Web
  site and enter your zip code for a
  referral to the closest compounding
  pharmacy in your area.

VERMONT

Custom Prescription Shoppe
Scott W. Brown, PD
42 Timber Lane
South Burlington, VT 05403
802-864-0812
800-928-1488
scott@customrxshop.com

VIRGINIA

Blue Ridge Apothecary
Graham Stephens, RPh, PharmD
621-F Townside Rd.
Roanoke, VA 24014
540-345-6480
540-345-6844 (fax)

Leesburg Pharmacy
Jay Gill, PharmD
36 C Catoctin Circle
Leesburg, VA 20175
703-737-3305

WISCONSIN

Health Pharmacies
2809 Fish Hatchery Rd., Suite 103
Madison, WI 53713
800-373-6704

CANADA

NutriChem Pharmacy
1303 Richmond Rd.
Ottawa, Ontario, Canada K2B 7Y4
613-820-4200
613-829-2226 (fax)
www.nutrichem.com

York Downs Pharmacy
3910 Bathurst St.
Toronto, Ontario, Canada M3H 5Z3
416-633-2244
800-564-5020
416-633-3400 (fax)
www.yorkdownsrx.com

Sexual Aids

www.goodvibes.com www.grandopening.com

Natural Beauty Products

www.SUZANNE.com
All active ingredients used in my Beauty Care Line are "naturally derived" (plants, minerals, herbs, flowers, wheat, fruits and vegetables, sea algae, etc.). We use high-quality, effective ingredients, organic ingredients when possible, and a paraben-free preservative system. All facial skin care products are synthetic free and fragrance free and contain essential oils and plant infusions.

Spa Masks
Botanical Spa—Apple Pectin Mask
Botanical Spa—Cleansing Clay
  Herbal Mask

Basic Skin Care
Hydrating Therapy—Gentle
  Exfoliating Cleanser
Hydrating Therapy—Soothing Aloe
  Vera Toner
Hydrating Therapy—Daily
  Moisturizer SPF 30
Balancing Therapy—Clarifying
  Cleanser
Balancing Therapy—Healing Enzyme
  Toner
Balancing Therapy—Daily
  Moisturizer

Antiaging Therapy—Night Repair
  Cream
Antiaging Therapy—Intensive Eye
  Cream
Antiaging Therapy—Hydra Lift
  Serum AM Treatment
Antiaging Therapy—Hydra Lift
  Serum PM Treatment
Antiaging Therapy—Hydra Lift
  Finishing Gel
Fresh Face Gentle Cleansing Gel
Hydra Lift & Soft As Silk Firming Set

Body Care
Energizing Body Scrub & Cool Sorbet
  Body Moisturizer
Fit to Be Tight Firming Body
  Treatment—AM with Natural Tint
  and PM

Cosmetics (also available at
  www.SuzanneSomers.com)
Spray On Makeup—Professional
  Foundation
Spray On Primer—Perfecting Base

FaceMaster
800-770-2521
www.facemaster.com

Exercise Products

ThighMaster
www.thighmaster.com

EZ Gym
www.ezgym.com

THE LIFE EXTENSION FOUNDATION

FOUNDED IN 1980, the Life Extension Foundation is a nonprofit organization dedicated to discovering innovative approaches to prevent aging and treat degenerative disease.

Since its inception, Life Extension has introduced evidence-based approaches to enhance human longevity that are often five to ten years ahead of conventional medicine. These scientific advances are chronicled each month in *Life Extension* magazine, read by over 300,000 people worldwide.

Consumers and medical professionals alike join the Life Extension Foundation to obtain the latest information about achieving optimal health and long life while protecting against common age-related disorders.

In addition to authoritative medical updates, Life Extension members gain access to unique low-cost blood tests that provide critical data about their state of health. The results from these blood tests enable Life Extension to design customized antiaging programs for each member.

Perhaps the greatest benefit of Life Extension membership is free phone access (seven days a week) to a team of knowledgeable health advisers who provide personalized guidance based on one's individual profile. Foundation members also enjoy substantial discounts on a wide array of health products.

To join the Life Extension Foundation or to speak to a health adviser, call 1-888-884-3666 or go to www.lef.org/goodhealth for a free copy. New members receive a 1,500-page reference book called *Disease Prevention and Treatment*, which provides invaluable health information published by the foundation over the past three decades.

Supplements

Here is a list of supplements available through Life Extension. They are listed by category and will be helpful to you in deciding which supplements will give you the best support.

To order, call 800-544-4440 or visit www.lifeextension.com.

AMINO ACIDS

Acetyl-L-Carnitine
Acetyl-L-Carnitine-Arginate
Arginine Capsules
Arginine/L-Ornithine HCL Complex
Arginine/L-Ornithine HCL Powder
Branched Chain Amino Acids
D, L-Phenylalanine Capsules
GABA Powder
Glycine Capsules
Glycine Powder
L-Arginine Free Base Powder
L-Carnitine Capsules
L-Carnitine Powder
L-Cysteine Capsules
L-Glutamine Capsules
L-Glutamine Powder
L-Glutathione, L-Cysteine & C
L-Lysine Capsules
L-Lysine Powder
L-Methionine Powder
L-Tyrosine Powder
L-Tyrosine Tablets
Mega L-Glutathione Capsules
N-Acetyl-Cysteine Capsules
Optimized Carnitine w/ GlycoCarn™
PharmaGABA
Super Carnosine Capsules
Taurine Capsules
Tryptopure™ Tryptophan
(Optimized) Tryptopure™ Plus

BONE AND JOINT HEALTH

ArthroMax™ w/ FruiteXB
Bone Restore
Bone-Up™
Chondroitin Sulfate
Chondrox
Fast Acting Joint Formula
Glucosamine Chondroitin Capsules

BRAIN HEALTH

Acetyl-L-Carnitine
Acetyl-L-Carnitine-Arginate
CDP Choline Capsules
Cognitex w/ NeuroProtection Complex
Cognitex w/ Pregnenolone & NeuroProtection Complex
DMAE
DMAE-Ginkgo
DMAE Powder (37% DMAE)
Ginkgo Biloba Certified Extract™
Huperzine A
Lecithin w/ B_5 and BHA
Lecithin Granules
Methylcobalamin Lozenges

Optimized Ashwagandha Extract
Phosphatidylserine Capsules
Rhodiola Extract
Super Ginkgo Extract
Vinpocetine

DIGESTIVE

Bromelain Powder
Carnosoothe w/ PicoProtect
Digest RC™
Enhanced Super Digestive Enzymes
Florastor
Life Flora™
Natural EsophaGuard
NutraFlora (FOS) Powder
N-Zimes™
Pancreatin
Papain Powder
Regimint™

DURK AND SANDY PRODUCTS

Blast™
Choline Cooler™
Dual-C
Fast Blast™
Power Maker II
Power Maker II Sugar Free
Rise & Shine™
Root Food

EYE CARE

Bilberry Extract
Brite Eyes III
Lutein Plus Powder
Overxcast Polarized Sunglasses
Solarshield Sunglasses
Super Zeaxanthin w/ Lutein & Meso-Zeaxanthin
Viva Drops

FIBER

Apple Pectin Powder
Chitosan
Enhanced Fiber Food
Hi-Lignan® Nutri-Flax®
SlimStyles™ PGX
WellBetX PGX™ Soluble Fiber Blend

HAIR CARE

Dr. Proctor's Advanced Hair Formula
Dr. Proctor's Shampoo
Life Extension Conditioner
Life Extension Shampoo

HEART HEALTH

D-Ribose Capsules
D-Ribose Powder
Endothelial Defense
Enhanced Co-Q_{10} w/ Brewer's Yeast
Fibrinogen Resist
Forskolin
Herbal Cardiovascular Formula
Homocysteine Resist
Low Dose Aspirin (enteric coated)
Maitake SX-Fraction™
Natural BP Management
Peak ATP™ w/ GlycoCarn™
Policosanol
Super Absorbable Co-Q_{10}™ w/ d-Limonene
Super Omega-3 EPA/DHA w/ Sesame
Lignans & Olive Fruit Extract
Super Ubiquinol Co-Q_{10}
Sytrinol™
TMG Powder
TMG Tablets

HERBAL/PHYTO PRODUCTS

Artichoke Leaf Extract

Astaxanthin

Blueberry Extract

Blueberry Extract w/ Pomegranate and Cocoa Gold

Butterbur Extract w/ Standardized Rosmarinic Acid

Calcium D-Glucarate

Chloroplex

Cilantro Herbal Extract

Citrus Bioflavonoid

Cocoa Gold™

Dual-Action Cruciferous Vegetable Extract w/ Cat's Claw

Dual-Action Cruciferous Vegetable Extract w/ Resveratrol/Cat's Claw

Grapeseed Extract w/ Resveratrol

Green Tea Leaves

Hesperidin Complex Powder

Huperzine A w/ Natural Vitamin E

Kyolic® Garlic Formula 105

Kyolic® Reserve

Long Life Organic Green Tea Bags

Mega Green Tea Extract (98%)

Mega Green Tea Extract (98% decaffeinated)

Mega Lycopene

Mega Silymarin w/ Isosilybin B

Optimized Ashwagandha Extract

Phyto-Food

Pomegranate Extract

Pomegranate Extract w/ Cocoa Gold

Pomegranate Juice Concentrate

Pure-Gar™

Pure-Gar™ w/ EDTA

Resveratrol

Rhodiola Extract

Rosmarinic Acid Extract

Rutin Powder

Silibinin Plus

Silymarin

SODzyme™ w/ GliSODin®

Stevia Extract

Super Bio-Curcumin

Super Ginkgo Extract

Super Curcumin w/ Bioperine®

Super Polyphenol Extracts w/ Cocoa Gold

Venotone

Whole Grape Extract

HORMONES

DHEA

DHEA Complete

Melatonin

Melatonin Timed Release

Natural Estrogen w/ Pomegranate Extract

Pregnenolone

ProFem Cream

7-Keto® DHEA

Super Miraforte w/ Maximum Strength Chrysin

IMMUNE ENHANCEMENT

AHCC® (Active Hexose Correlated Compound)

Buffered Vitamin C Powder

Echinacea

Enhanced Life Extension Whey Protein

Immune Protect w/ Paractin®

Lactoferrin

Maitake SX-Fraction

Norwegian Shark Liver Oil

Primal Defense™

ProBoost™ Thymic Protein A

Pure-Gar™

Sambu® Guard

Thymic Immune Factors

Vitamin C w/ Dihydroquercetin

Zinc Lozenges w/ Vitamin C

INFLAMMATORY REACTIONS

ArthroMax™ w/ FruiteX B

Barlean's Kids DHA

Boswella

Boswella™ Topical Cream

Bromelain (specially coated)

Coromega Kids Brain and Body (DHA)

DHA 240

Emulsified Norwegian Cod Liver Oil

Fast Acting Joint Formula

Korean Angelica

5-Loxin

Mega EPA/DHA

Mega GLA w/ Sesame Lignans

MSM

Natural Relief 1222™ Cream

Perilla Oil

Serraflazyme

Shark Cartilage

SODzyme™ w/ GliSODin and Wolfberry

Super GLA/DHA

Super MaxEPA

Super Omega-3 EPA/DHA with Sesame Lignans & Olive Fruit Extract

Udo's Choice Oil

LIVER HEALTH

Branch Chain Amino Acids

HepatoPro

Mega Silymarin w/ Isosilybin B

N-Acetyl Cysteine

SAMe

Silibinin Plus

Silymarin

MINERALS

BioSil™

Bone Restore

Bone-Up™

Boron Capsules

Calcium Citrate w/ D_3

Chromium Ultra

Copper

Iron Protein Plus

Magnesium

Magnesium Citrate

Mineral Formula for Men

Mineral Formula for Women

Only Trace Minerals

OptiZinc

Selenium

Se-Methylselenocysteine

Vanadyl Sulfate

Zinc w/ Lozenges Vitamin C

MISCELLANEOUS

Blood Pressure Monitor Arm Cuff Medium

The Capsule Filler Machine

Cell Sensor Gauss Meter™

Empty Gelatin Capsules

The Pill Cutter and Grinder

MITOCHONDRIAL SUPPORT

Acetyl-L-Carnitine

Acetyl-L-Carnitine-Arginate

ChronoForte w/ Luteolin

Mitochondrial Energy Optimizer w/ SODzyme

Optimized Carnitine w/ GlycoCarn™

R-Dihydro-Lipoic Acid

Super Absorbable Co-Q$_{10}$™ w/ d-Limonene

Super Alpha Lipoic Acid w/ Biotin

Super Ubiquinol Co-Q10

MOOD RELIEF
Adapton
L-Theanine
Natural Stress Relief
SAMe
St. John's Wort Extract
Tryptopure L-Tryptophan

MOUTH CARE
Dr. Tung's Tongue Cleaner
Life Extension Toothpaste
MistOral III™ w/ Co-Q$_{10}$

MULTIVITAMIN
Children's Formula Life Extension Mix
Comprehensive Nutrient Pack
Life Extension Booster
Life Extension Herbal Mix w/ Stevia
Life Extension Mix Capsules
Life Extension Mix Powder
Life Extension Mix Tablets
Life Extension Mix w/o Copper Capsules
Life Extension Mix w/o Copper Powder
Life Extension Mix w/o Copper Tablets
Life Extension Mix w/ Extra Niacin
Life Extension Mix w/ Extra Niacin w/o Copper
Life Extension Mix w/ Stevia Powder
Life Extension Mix w/ Stevia w/o Copper Powder
Life Extension One-Per-Day
Life Extension Two-Per-Day
Super Booster Softgels w/ Advanced K$_2$ Complex

PET CARE
Life Extension Cat Mix w/ Resveratrol
Life Extension Dog Mix

PROSTATE AND URINARY HEALTH
BetterWOMAN®
Cran-Max
5-Loxin
Super Saw Palmetto with Beta-Sitosterol
Super Saw Palmetto/Nettle Root Formula w/ Beta-Sitosterol
Ultra Natural Prostate Formula

SKIN CARE
Anti-Aging Mask
Antioxidant Rejuvenating Foot Cream
Antioxidant Rejuvenating Foot Scrub
Antioxidant Rejuvenating Hand Cream
Antioxidant Rejuvenating Hand Scrub
Anti-Redness & Blemish Lotion
Corrective Clearing Mask
Dual-Action MicroDerm Abrasion
Essential Plant Lipids Reparative Serum
Face Rejuvenating Antioxidant Cream
Fine Line-Less
Healing Mask
Hyaluronic Facial Moisturizer
Hydroderm®
Lavilin Underarm Deodorant
Life Extension Sun Protection Spray
Lifting & Tightening Complex
Living Skin
Mild Facial Cleanser
NaPCA w/ Aloe Vera
Neck Rejuvenating Antioxidant Cream
New Feeling
Peel Off Cleansing Mask

Pigment Correcting Cream

Rejuvenex®

Rejuvenex® Body Lotion

RejuveneX Factor

RejuvenEyes®

Rejuvenating Serum

Skin Lightening Serum

Total Sun Protection Cream

Ultra Lip Plumper

Ultra Rejuvenex

Ultra RejuveNight® w/ Progesterone

Ultra RejuveNight® w/o Progesterone

Ultra Wrinkle Relaxer

Under Eye Refining Serum

Under Eye Rescue Cream

Vitamin C Serum

Vitamin K Healing Cream

SOY

EcoGen® Super Soy Extract

Natural Estrogen w/ Pomegranate

Soy Power Powder

Soy Protein Concentrate

Super Absorbable Soy Isoflavones

Ultra Soy Extract

SPECIAL PURPOSE FORMULA

Anti-Alcohol Antioxidants w/ HepatoProtection Complex

Benfotiamine w/ Thiamine

Breast Health Formula

Butterbur Extract w/ Standardized Rosmarinic Acid

Chlorella

Chlorophyllin w/ Zinc

Cocoa Gold w/ Beta Glucan

Enhanced Cinnulin PF® w/ Glucose Management Proprietary Blend

Fem Dophilus

Feverfew

GlucoFit™

Hemorcream

Migra-eeze™

Pecta-Sol®

Pork Pancreas Enzymes

Potassium Iodide

Rosmarinic Acid Extract

SPORTS PERFORMANCE

Creatine Whey Glutamine

DMG (N, N-dimethylglycine)

Enhanced Life Extension Protein

Inosine

L-Glutamine Capsules

L-Glutamine Powder

Micronized Creatine Capsules

Micronized Creatine Powder

Octacosanol

VITAMINS

Ascorbic Acid Powder

Ascorbyl Palmitate Capsules

Ascorbyl Palmitate Powder

B_1

B_2

B_{12}

Beta-Carotene

Biotin Capsules

Biotin Powder

Buffered Vitamin C Powder

Calcium Ascorbate Powder

Complete B Complex

Folic Acid + B_{12}

Folic Acid Powder

Gamma E Tocopherol w/ Sesame Lignans

Gamma E Tocopherol/Tocotrienols

Inositol Capsules

Inositol Powder

Liquid Emulsified Vitamin A

Mega Lycopene Extract
Methylcobalamin
MK-7
No-Flush Niacin
PABA Capsules
PABA Powder
Super Ascorbate C Capsules
Super Ascorbate C Powder
Super K w/ Advanced K_2 Complex
Tocotrienols w/ Sesame Lignans
Vitamin B_1 Powder
Vitamin B_2 Powder
Vitamin B_3 (Niacin) Capsules
Vitamin B_5 Powder
Vitamin B_6
Vitamin B_{12} Powder
Vitamin C
Vitamin D
Vitamin D_3
Vitamin E Succinate
Vitamin K_1

WEIGHT MANAGEMENT

Chitosan
CitriChrome
DHEA Complete
Enhanced Fiber Food
Fucoxanthin Slim
HCA
Life Mix
Natural Appetite Control
Natural Weight Control
7-Keto DHEA
SlimStyles™ PGX
Stevia Liquid Extract
Super CLA Blend w/ Guarana and Sesame Lignans
Super CLA Blend w/ Sesame Lignans
Udo's Choice Wholesome Fast Food Blend
WellBetX PGX™ Soluble Fiber Blend

RECOMMENDED READING

I HAVE READ all these books—and authored a few of them—and used them for research, and I highly recommend them.

Begley, Ed. *Living Like Ed: A Guide to the Eco-Friendly Life.*

Blaylock, Russell L., M.D. *Excitotoxins: The Taste That Kills.*

———. *Health and Nutrition Secrets That Can Save Your Life*, revised edition.

———. *Natural Strategies for Cancer Patients.*

———. *Nuclear Sunrise* (e-booklet).

Braverman, Eric R., M.D. *The Edge Effect: Achieve Total Health and Longevity with the Balanced Brain Advantage.*

———. *Younger You: Unlock the Hidden Power of Your Brain to Look and Feel 15 Years Younger.*

Brownlee, Shannon. *Overtreated: Why Too Much Medicine Is Making Us Sicker and Poorer.*

The Burton Goldberg Group. *Alternative Medicine: The Definitive Guide.*

Canton, James M., Ph.D. *The Extreme Future: The Top Trends That Will Shape the World for the Next 5, 10, and 20 Years.*

Graveline, Duane, M.D.. *Lipitor, Thief of Memory.*

Greene, Robert A., M.D., and Leah Feldon. *Perfect Balance: Dr. Robert Greene's Breakthrough Program for Finding the Lifelong Hormonal Health You Deserve.*

Hertoghe, Thierry, M.D. *The Hormone Solution.*

Kurzweil, Ray, and Terry Grossman, M.D. *Fantastic Voyage.*

Life Extension Foundation. *Disease Prevention and Treatment,* expanded
    fourth edition.

Mahmud, Khalid, M.D. *Keeping aBreast: Ways to Stop Breast Cancer.*

Mercola, Joseph. *Take Control of Your Health.*

Miller, Philip Lee, M.D., and the Life Extension Foundation. *Life Extension
    Revolution: The New Science of Growing Older Without Aging.*

Murphy, Christine (editor). *Iscador, Mistletoe and Cancer Therapy.*

Niehans, Paul. *Cell Therapy* (usedbooksearch.co.uk).

Ragnar, Peter. *The LifeWave Experience to a New You: The Official Handbook.*

Rogers, Sherry A., M.D. *Detoxify or Die.*

Rothenberg, Ron, Kathleen Becker, and Kris Hart. *Forever Ageless.*

Schwarzbein, Diana, M.D. *The Program: Losing Weight the Healthy Way.*

Small, Gary, M.D. *The Longevity Bible.*

Somers, Suzanne. *Ageless.*

———. *Slim and Sexy Forever.*

———. *The Sexy Years.*

Starr, Mark, M.D. *Hypothyroidism Type 2.*

Thomas, John. *Young Again: How to Reverse the Aging Process.*

Van Zyl, Bernard. *Stem Cells Saved My Life: How to Be Next.*

Watson, Brenda. *The H.O.P.E. Formula.*

Watson, Brenda, M.D., and Leonard Smith, M.D. *Gut Prescriptions: Natural
    Solutions to Your Digestive Problems.*

Wiley, T. S. *Sex, Lies, and Menopause.*

Wright, Jonathan V., M.D. *D-Mannose and Bladder Infection.*

———. *Dr. Wright's Book of Nutritional Therapy: Real-Life Lessons in
    Medicine Without Drugs.*

———. *Maximize Your Vitality and Potency.*

———. *Natural Hormone Replacement for Women over 45.*

———. *Natural Medicine, Optimal Wellness* (formerly *Patient's Book of
    Natural Healing*).

———. *The Natural Pharmacy.*

———. *Thriving Through Dialysis.*

———. *Why Stomach Acid Is Good for You.*

———. *Xylitol—Dental & Upper Respiratory Health.*

Young, Simon. *Designer Evolution: A Transhumanist Manifesto.*

SELECTED STUDIES

Alexander, GM, RS Swerdloff, C Wang, et al. Androgen-behavior correlations in hypogonadal men and eugonadel men. II. Cognitive abilities. *Hormones and Behavior* 33, no. 2 (1998): 85–94.

Alpert, C, et al. Blood levels of long-chain n-3 fatty acids and the risk of sudden death. *New England Journal of Medicine* 346, no. 15 (April 11, 2002).

Barrett-Connor, E, et al. Endogenous sex hormones and cognitive function in older men. *Journal of Clinical Endocrinology and Metabolism* 84, no. 10: 3681–85.

Braunstein, GD. Safety of testosterone treatment in postmenopausal women. *Fertility and Sterility* 88, no. 1 (July 2007): 1–17.

Campagnoli, C, et al. Pregnancy progesterone and progestins in relation to breast cancer risk. *Journal of Steroid Biochemistry and Molecular Biology* 97 (2005): 441–50.

de Lignieres, B. Effects of progestogens on the menopausal breast. *Climacteric* 5, no. 3 (September 2002): 229–35.

de Lignieres, B, et al. Combined hormone replacement therapy and risk of breast cancer in a French cohort study of 3,175 women. *Climacteric* 5, no. 4 (December 2002): 332–40.

Dimitrakakis, C. Breast cancer incidence in postmenopausal women using testosterone in addition to usual hormone therapy. *Menopause* 11, no. 5 (September–October 2004): 531–35.

Endogenous Hormones and Prostate Cancer Collaborative Group. Endogenous sex hormones and prostate cancer: A collaborative analysis of 18 prospective studies. *Journal of the National Cancer Institute* 100 (2008): 170–83.

English, KM, et al. Low-dose transdermal testosterone therapy improves angina threshold in men with chronic stable angina: A randomized, double-blind, placebo-controlled study. *Circulation* 102, no. 16 (October 17, 2000): 1906–11.

Feneley, MR, et al. PSA monitoring during testosterone replacement therapy: Low long-term risk of prostate cancer with improved opportunity for cure. *Andrologia* 36 (2004): 212.

Fourniet, A., et al. Unequal risks for breast cancer associated with different hormone replacement therapies: Results from the E3N cohort study. *Breast Cancer Research and Treatment* 107, no. 1 (January 2008): 103–11.

Grodstein, F, JE Manson, and MJ Stampfer. Hormone therapy and coronary heart disease: The role of time since menopause and age at hormone initiation. *Journal of Women's Health* (Larchmont) 15, no. 1 (January–February 2006).

Grodstein, F, et al. Postmenopausal hormone therapy and mortality. *New England Journal of Medicine* 336, no. 25 (June 19, 1997): 1769–75.

Gunawardena, L, A Campbell, and A Meikle. Antiandrogen-like actions of an antioxidant on survivin, Bcl-2 and PSA in human prostate cancer cells. *Cancer Detection and Prevention* 29 (4):389–95K.

Khaw, KT, et al. Endogenous testosterone and mortality due to all causes, cardiovascular disease, and cancer in men. *Circulation* 116 (2007): 2694–2701.

Lappe, JM, et al. Vitamin D and calcium supplementation reduces cancer risk: Results of a randomized trial. *American Journal of Clinical Nutrition* 85, no. 6 (June 2007): 1586–91.

Laughlin, GA, et al. Low-serum testosterone and mortality in older men. *Journal of Clinical Endocrinology and Metabolism* 93(1):68–75.

Marchioli, R, et al. Early protection against sudden death by n-3 polyunsaturated fatty acids after myocardial infarction: Time-course analysis of the results of the Gruppo Italiano per lo Studio della Sopravvivenza nell'infarto Miocardico (GISSI)–Prevensione. *Circulation* 105, no. 16 (April 23, 2002): 1897–1903.

Morgentaler, A. Guideline for male testosterone therapy: A clinicians perspective. *Journal of Clinical Endocrinology and Metabolism* 92, no. 2 (2007): 416–17.

Morgentaler, A. Testosterone and prostate cancer: An historical perspective on a modern myth. *European Urology*, July 26, 2006.

Pantuck, AJ, et al. Phase II study of pomegranate juice for men with rising prostate-specific antigen following surgery or radiation for prostate cancer. *Clinical Cancer Research* 12 , no. 13 (July 2006): 4018–26.

Rhoden, EL, and A Morgentaler. Risks of testosterone-replacement therapy and recommendations for monitoring. *New England Journal of Medicine* 350 (January 2004): 482–92.

Saiko, P, et al. Resveratrol and its analogs: Defense against cancer, coronary disease and neurodegenerative maladies or just a fad? *Mutation Research* 658, no. 1–2 (January–February 2008):68–94.

Shores, MN, et al. Low-serum testosterone and mortality in male veterans. *Archives of Internal Medicine* 166, no. 15 (August 14, 2006): 1660–65.

Travison, TG, et al. A population-level decline in serum testosterone levels in American men. *Journal of Clinical Endocrinology and Metabolism* 92, no. 1 (October 24, 2006): 196–202.

INDEX

Acetyl-CoA, 289
Acetyl-l-carnitine, 364
Acetylcholine, 216–218, 220–222, 325
ACTH (adrenocorticotropic hormone), 132
Acupuncture, 260, 320, 378–380, 395, 398
Adderall, 224
Adrenal glands, 27, 34–35, 37, 114, 126, 132, 156, 162, 163, 228, 253–255, 258–259, 272, 369–371, 405
  nature/function of, 122–123
Ageless (Somers), 105, 107, 108, 153, 161, 169, 198, 296, 350, 354
AgePrint, 140, 211, 215, 220
AIDS (acquired immune deficiency syndrome), 19, 56, 116
Albumin, 51
Alcohol consumption, 138, 258–259, 280–281, 309
Alcoholism, lithium and, 32–33
Aldosterone, 114, 122, 132
  hearing loss and, 27–28
Alpha-linolenic acid, 202–203
Alpha-tocopherol vitamin E, 86
ALS (amyotropic lateral sclerosis), 33
Alternative Medicine (Chaitow), 179
Aluminum, 31, 203–204, 205, 234, 324–325
Alzheimer's disease, 19, 30, 102, 103
  glutamate and, 195
  heavy metals and, 325
  hormones and, 191–192
  lithium and, 33
  melatonin and, 279
  testosterone and, 155
Ambien, 152, 255, 285, 310, 368
American Academy for the Advancement of Medicine (ACAM), 249

American Academy of Anti-Aging Medicine, 129, 175
American College of Allergy and Immunology, 42
American Dental Association (ADA), 204, 205
American Heart Association (AHA), 50
American Medical Association (AMA), 297
Anabolic steroids, 24, 114
Anarazmia, 164
Anderson, Dr. Robert, 40–41
Anderson, Joyce, 296
Androgens, 132
Andropause, 49, 156–159
Androstenedione, 115
Antibiotics, 86, 361
  bladder infections and, 22, 23
  secondary infections and, 18, 24
  side effects of, 24
  Dr. Wright's views on, 23–24
  yeast infections and, 342
Antidepressants, 153, 224, 285, 341–342
Antioxidants, 20, 54, 87, 116, 174, 186, 200–201, 203, 261, 277, 304, 317
Anus, 246
Apoptosis, 53
Applied kinesiology, 321
Arachidonic acid, 75–76, 362
Aristotle, 21
Armour dessicated thyroid, 122, 134, 340
Arteriosclerosis, 202, 288
Aspartame, 192, 197, 208
Aspartate, 189
Asyra scan, 230
Atherosclerosis, 288, 327
  DHEA and, 115
  factors in, 83–84, 203
  pomegranate juice and, 84